AAOS

ALS Skills Review

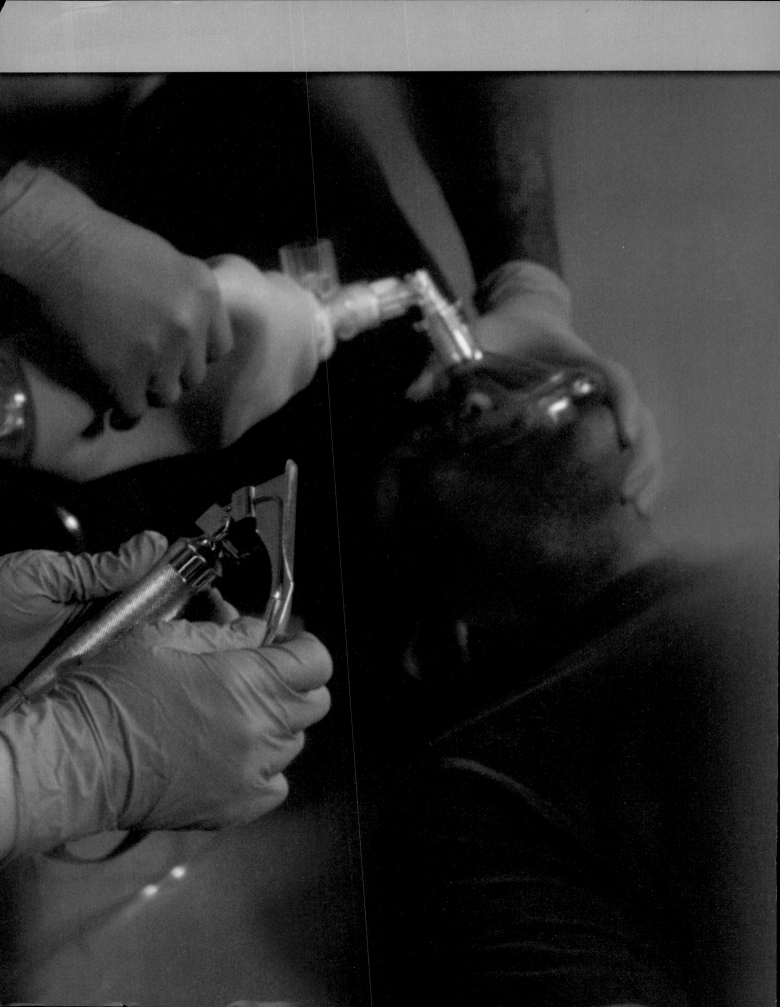

ALS Skills Review

AAOS
AMERICAN ACADEMY OF ORTHOPAEDIC SURGEONS

Jeff McDonald, NREMT-P
Author
Tarrant County College
Fort Worth, Texas

Joseph A. Ciotola, MD, FAAOS
Medical Editor
Department of Emergency Services
Queen Anne's County, Maryland

JONES AND BARTLETT PUBLISHERS
Sudbury, Massachusetts
BOSTON   TORONTO   LONDON   SINGAPORE

World Headquarters
Jones and Bartlett Publishers
40 Tall Pine Drive
Sudbury, MA 01776
978-443-5000
info@jbpub.com
www.jbpub.com

Jones and Bartlett Publishers Canada
6339 Ormindale Way
Mississauga, Ontario L5V 1J2
Canada

Jones and Bartlett Publishers International
Barb House, Barb Mews
London W6 7PA
United Kingdom

Jones and Bartlett's books and products are available through most bookstores and online booksellers. To contact Jones and Bartlett Publishers directly, call 800-832-0034, fax 978-443-8000, or visit our website, www.jbpub.com.

Substantial discounts on bulk quantities of Jones and Bartlett's publications are available to corporations, professional associations, and other qualified organizations. For details and specific discount information, contact the special sales department at Jones and Bartlett via the above contact information or send an email to specialsales@jbpub.com.

AAOS
AMERICAN ACADEMY OF ORTHOPAEDIC SURGEONS

Editorial Credits
Chief Education Officer: Mark W. Wieting
Director, Department of Publications: Marilyn L. Fox, PhD
Managing Editor: Barbara A. Scotese
Associate Senior Editor: Gayle Murray

Production Credits
Chief Executive Officer: Clayton Jones
Chief Operating Officer: Don W. Jones, Jr.
President, Higher Education and Professional Publishing:
    Robert W. Holland, Jr.
V.P., Sales: William J. Kane
V.P., Design and Production: Anne Spencer
Publisher: Kimberly Brophy
Acquisitions Editor—EMS: Christine Emerton
Associate Managing Editor: Amanda J. Green
Senior Production Editor: Susan Schultz

Director of Marketing: Alisha Weisman
Associate Marketing Manager: Meagan Norland
V.P., Manufacturing and Inventory Control: Therese Connell
Composition: Appingo
Text Design: Anne Spencer
Cover Design: Kristin E. Parker
Photo Research Manager and Photographer: Kimberly Potvin
Assistant Photo Researcher: Jessica Elias
Cover Image: © Jones and Bartlett Publishers. Courtesy of MIEMSS
Printing and Binding: Courier Companies
Cover Printing: Courier Companies

The procedures and protocols in this book are based on the most current recommendations of responsible medical sources. The American Academy of Orthopaedic Surgeons, the author, and the publisher, however, make no guarantee as to, and assume no responsibility for, the correctness, sufficiency, or completeness of such information or recommendations. Other or additional safety measures may be required under particular circumstances.

This textbook is intended solely as a guide to the appropriate procedures to be employed when rendering emergency care to the sick and injured. It is not intended as a statement of the standards of care required in any particular situation, because circumstances and the patient's physical condition can vary widely from one emergency to another. Nor is it intended that this textbook shall in any way advise emergency personnel concerning legal authority to perform the activities or procedures discussed. Such local determination should be made only with the aid of legal counsel.

Library of Congress Cataloging-in-Publication Data
McDonald, Jeff, 1960-
  ALS skills review / Jeff McDonald, author.
    p. ; cm.
  ISBN 978-0-7637-5121-0 (pbk.)
  1. Emergency medicine. 2. Emergency medical technicians. I. Title. II. Title: Advanced life support skills review.
  [DNLM: 1. Emergency Treatment—methods—Outlines. WB 18.2 M478a 2009]
  RC86.7.M287 2009
  616.02'5—dc22
                            2008047110

6048
Printed in the United States of America
12 11 10 09 08   10 9 8 7 6 5 4 3 2 1

Contents

Acknowledgments

We would like to thank the following people for their review of the *ALS Skills Review* manuscript:

Vicki Bacidore, RN, MSN, ACNP
Loyola University Medical Center
Maywood, Illinois

Leaugeay Barnes, BS, CC/NREMT-P
Oklahoma City Community College
Oklahoma City, Oklahoma

**Cindy Branscum, BS, MICT Instructor/
   Coordinator**
Cowley County Community College
Winfield, Kansas

Katrina L. Bryant, BS, NREMT-P
East Central Community College
Decatur, Mississippi

Brandon Burgess, BAS, NREMT-P
Phoenix College
Phoenix, Arizona

Bruce Butterfras, MEd, LP
The University of Texas Health Science Center
   at San Antonio
San Antonio, Texas

Wesley Carter, NREMT-P
Lenoir County EMS
Lenoir Community College
Kinston, North Carolina

Anthony Cuda, NREMT-P
Community College of Allegheny County
Public Safety Institute
Pittsburgh, Pennsylvania

Peter Cunnius, MS, NREMT-P
Montgomery County EMS Training Institute
Boyertown, Pennsylvania

Joseph A. DeAngelis, NREMT-P, CCEMT-P
Community College of Rhode Island
Providence, Rhode Island

Brian R. Dose, BS, FF/EMT-P
Ottawa Fire Department
Ottawa, Illinois
Illinois Valley Community College
Oglesby, Illinois

Mike Dymes, NREMT-P
Durham Technical Community College
Durham, North Carolina

Steven D. Glow, FNP, RN, MSN, CEN, EMT-P
Montana State University
Missoula, Montana

Eryq Hastings, NREMT-P
Southwest Ambulance
Tucson, Arizona

Lindi Holt, PhD, NREMT-P
Clarian Health/Methodist Hospital
Indianapolis, Indiana

C. H. Johnson, DVM, EMT-P
Colorado Mountain College
Carbondale, Colorado

Edward J. Kalinowski, MEd, DrPH
Kapiolani Community College
Honolulu, Hawaii

Timothy M. Kimble, NREMT-P
Culpeper County Office of Emergency Services
Culpeper, Virginia
BOD, Rappahannock EMS Council
Fredericksburg, Virginia

Patricia Maher, MPA, EMT-P
Daytona Beach Community College
Daytona Beach, Florida

Kyle Pierce, BA, LP
Austin Community College
Austin, Texas

Ryan Sittig, BA, NREMT-P
Avera McKennan School of EMS
Sioux Falls, South Dakota

Laura L. Walker, MSED, NREMT-P
Kent J. Weber Simulation Center
Norfolk, Virginia

Student Resources

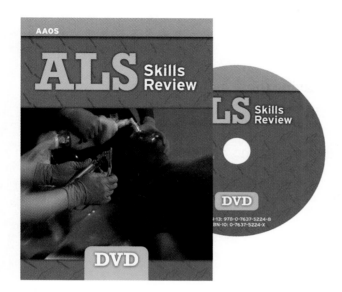

ALS SKILLS REVIEW DVD
ISBN 13: 978-0-7637-5224-8

Designed for individual student use, this action-packed DVD demonstrates the proper techniques for each skill presented in the manual. Capturing real-life scenes, each skill is clearly broken down, demonstrated, and applied in a variety of drills. This DVD is an invaluable resource for every ALS provider and gives students a chance to witness providers in action and in "real" time.

Note to Reader:

The skills depicted in this book reflect a training situation. Other or additional safety precautions may be required in an actual emergency.

The measure of our greatness is not in saving those lives that everyone else can save, for that is the standard of care.

Our greatness is measured by saving those that no one else can save.

—Roy K. Yamada, MD

Personal Safety

Personal Protective Equipment

Introduction

Personal Protective Equipment (PPE) is used to provide a barrier between the EMS responder and infectious agents that may be found in blood, body fluids, and exhaled air. It is the responsibility of the employer to provide EMS personnel with personal protective equipment (gloves, eye protection, masks, and gowns) sufficient to provide reasonable protection. It is the responsibility of EMS personnel to wear the personal protective equipment at the appropriate times and in the appropriate manner.

It is important for EMS personnel to understand that we work in an uncontrolled environment. To provide the best protection for unseen dangers, EMS personnel should enter every call with the assumption that the patient has an infectious disease and have appropriate PPE in place at the time of patient contact.

Procedures

 Step 1 ▶ **Prepare for patient contact.**

Prior to making patient contact, don protective gloves and eye protection. This should be performed on every patient regardless of risk of infectious disease.

Because of the prevalence of latex allergies, it is best to always use nonlatex gloves. This will prevent the development of latex allergies in the wearer and the stimulation of a reaction in latex-sensitive patients.

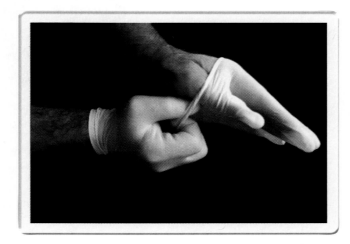

Getting into the habit of always wearing eye protection is a must. This will protect your eyes from unforeseen infectious exposures.

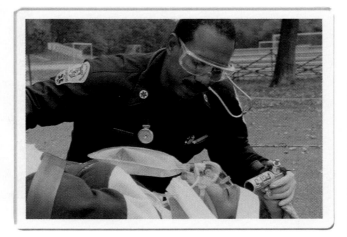

Safety Tips

Handwashing and Gloves

Studies have shown that gloves provide a barrier, but that neither vinyl nor latex procedure gloves are completely impermeable. It is important that you wash your hands every time you remove a pair of gloves.

Step **2** **Add personal protective equipment as needed.**

Upon initial contact, assess the need for additional body substance isolation. Don as appropriate the following pieces of equipment:

- **Masks or barrier devices** should be used for any invasive procedure requiring close facial contact. For instance, a pocket mask should be used to provide artificial ventilations.

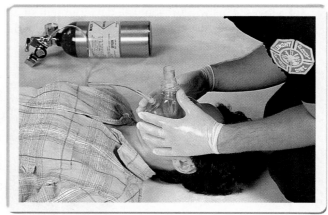

- **HEPA filter masks** should be worn any time your patient has or is suspected to have tuberculosis.

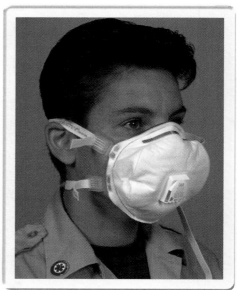

- **Gowns** should be worn to protect duty uniforms from becoming contaminated by blood or body fluids.

Body Substance Isolation

Body Substance Isolation (BSI) is the process of containing blood and other body fluids that may harbor infectious agents. The process starts by wearing personal protective equipment, but also includes procedures for containment, cleanup, and disposal of contaminated supplies and other objects.

Procedures

Step  1 ▶ **Remove contaminated clothing.**

Gowns and other protective devices prevent the contamination of clothing. However, in cases where clothing does become contaminated it is important to remove the clothing carefully. Shirts should never be removed over the head. Pullover shirts may need to be cut off and destroyed.

Once contaminated clothing is removed it should be bagged as a contaminated material. The clothing must be properly laundered and decontaminated by the EMS employer and not by the employee's home laundry.

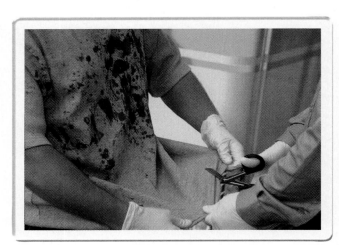

▼

Step   2 ▶ **Clean spilled blood and body fluids.**

Spilled blood and body fluids must be cleaned and the area disinfected before the equipment is returned to service. Depending on the size of the spill, it may be as simple as applying a bleach solution and a paper towel or as complicated as applying gallons of absorbent gels. In either case, it is important to place all materials used in the cleanup in biohazard bags for proper disposal.

While cleaning up body fluid spills, it is important to wear gloves and eye protection. Standard EMS gloves are sufficient for light spills with simple disinfectants. Larger spills where strong disinfectants are used may require thicker gloves intended for use with harsh chemicals.

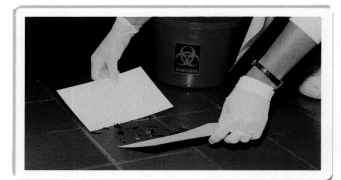

Handwashing

Handwashing is needed as a component in the preparation for, or the cleanup following patient contact.

Procedures

Step **Grasp towel.**

Remove towel from towel dispenser.

Step **Turn on water, discard towel.**

Use towel to turn water on. Discard towel into waste bin.

Step  **Apply soap and scrub vigorously.**

Apply soap to both hands and bring to lather. This may be done before or after wetting the hands depending on the type of soap used. Scrub vigorously for at least 15 seconds. When preparing for sterile procedures or preparing for delivery the hands should be scrubbed for at least 2 minutes, aided by brush or sponge.

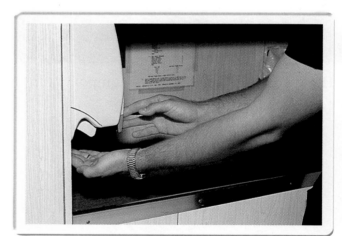

Step  **Rinse thoroughly.**

Rinse hands well.

Step  **Grasp towel and dry.**

Remove clean towel from towel dispenser. Dry your hands well. Several towels may be needed.

6 ▶ **Dispose of towel.**

Discard towel into waste bin.

▼

 7 ▶ **Grasp towel and turn off water.**

Remove clean towel from towel dispenser and turn water off. Discard towel into waste bin.

▼

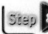 **8** ▶ **Grasp towel and open door.**

Remove clean towel from towel dispenser and open the door.

▼

 9 ▶ **Dispose of towel.**

Discard towel into waste bin.

In the Field

Waterless Cleansers
It is often difficult to find water in the prehospital environment. In these cases the use of waterless, alcohol-based cleansers can be very beneficial. They should be used routinely when the driver of the ambulance removes his or her gloves and enters the cab of the ambulance.

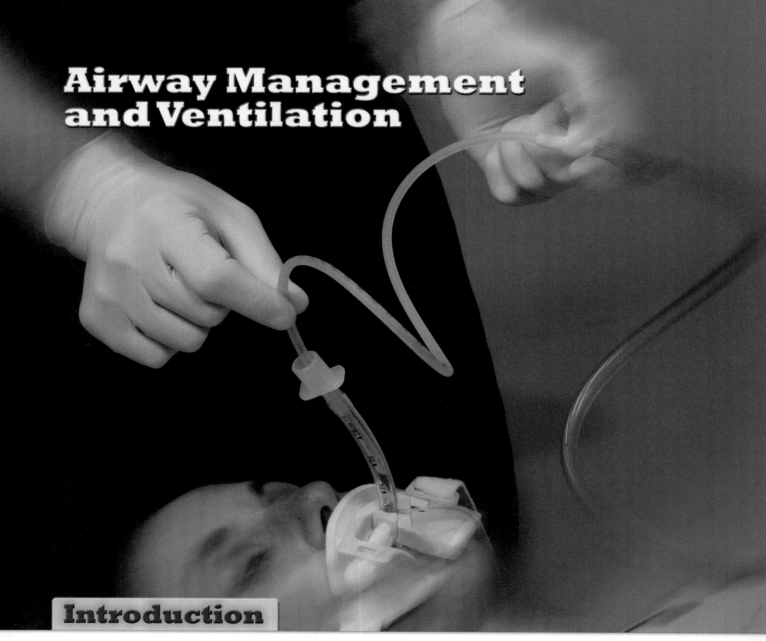

Airway Management and Ventilation

Introduction

Airway management means employing airway and ventilation skills appropriate to the needs of the patient, often in conjunction with other skills. In trauma management, we have seen a shift from thinking that cervical spine immobilization precedes airway management. In reality, it is important to use these skills together—managing the airway with concern for the cervical spine.

Airway management accomplishes nothing if oxygenation and ventilation are not included. Oxygenation and ventilation must be performed at the proper rates and adjusted to meet the needs of the individual patient.

Advanced airway management takes the process to a higher level. Properly placed, an advanced airway helps to ensure the appropriate ventilatory status of the patient. Improperly placed, the advanced airway can lead to fatal consequences for the patient. Thus, it is important to remember that advanced airways are simply adjuncts to secure and maintain the patient's airway. They assist in the delivery of oxygenation and ventilation by ensuring a direct route through the larynx and into the lungs.

The skills in this section will guide the responder through the process of securing and maintaining the airway and in performing airway management skills appropriately, and in a timely manner.

SKILL 1

Jaw-Thrust Maneuver

Performance Objective

Given an adult patient, the candidate shall demonstrate the use of the jaw-thrust maneuver using the criteria herein prescribed, in 1 minute or less.

Equipment

The following equipment is required to perform this skill:
- Appropriate body substance isolation/personal protective equipment

Equipment that may be helpful:
- Oropharyngeal airways (various sizes)
- Nasopharyngeal airways (various sizes)
- Bag-mask device
- Oxygen cylinder, regulator, and key

Indications

- Immediate opening of the airway in unresponsive patients prior to determining cause of unconsciousness and with potential for spine injury
- Maintenance of the airway in nonbreathing trauma patients

Contraindications

- Difficulty achieving an open airway using the procedure. The International Liason Committee on Resuscitation (ILCOR) recommends that if you cannot achieve an open airway with the jaw-thrust maneuver, you should abandon the procedure and use the head tilt–chin lift maneuver (see Skill 3).

Complications

- None if properly performed and maintained

Procedures

 Ensure body substance isolation before beginning procedures.

Prior to beginning patient care, appropriate body substance isolation procedures should be employed.

▼

Step 2 **Assume proper position.**

Position yourself at the patient's head, facing the long axis of the body.

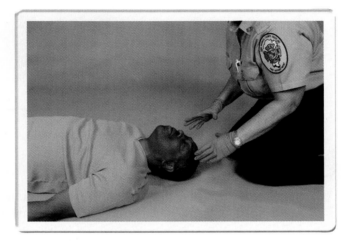

▼

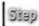 **Position hands on face.**

Using both hands, place your thumbs on the cheek bones with the base of the thumb just below the patient's eyes. Reach forward with your index fingers and place them behind the lower jaw just below the ear.

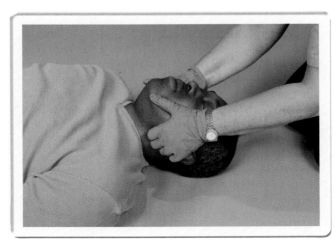

▼

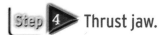 **Thrust jaw.**

Without moving the patient's neck, push the lower jaw forward (anteriorly) to lift the tongue off the posterior pharynx. It is important to maintain this position until airway adjuncts can maintain the airway.

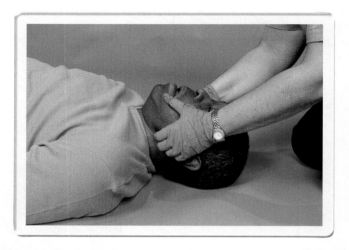

Step 5   Assess breathing.

Once the airway is open, assess the patient's ability to breathe spontaneously. If the patient is breathing on his or her own, maintain the open airway until artificial adjuncts can be inserted. If the patient is not breathing, begin artificial ventilation using either mouth-to-mask or bag-mask ventilation.

Tongue–Jaw Lift Maneuver

Performance Objective

Given an adult patient, the candidate shall demonstrate the use of the tongue–jaw lift maneuver using the criteria herein prescribed, in 1 minute or less.

Equipment

The following equipment is required to perform this skill:

- Appropriate body substance isolation/personal protective equipment

Equipment that may be helpful:

- Oropharyngeal airways (various sizes)
- Nasopharyngeal airways (various sizes)
- Bag-mask device
- Oxygen cylinder, regulator, and key

Indications

- Immediate opening of the airway in unresponsive patients prior to determining cause of unconsciousness
- Airway obstruction caused by the tongue in supine, unresponsive patients

Contraindications

- Nonbreathing patients

Complications

- None if properly performed and maintained

Procedures

 Step **1** **Ensure body substance isolation before beginning procedures.**

Prior to beginning patient care, appropriate body substance isolation procedures should be employed.

▼

 Step **2** **Assume proper position.**

Position yourself at the patient's head and shoulder, facing across the body.

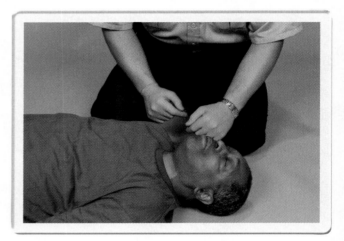

To ensure that the cervical spine does not move, place the hand closest to the patient's head on the patient's forehead. Confirm that the patient is unresponsive before beginning the next step of the procedure.

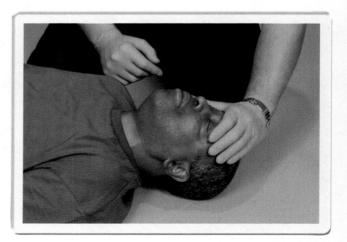

▼

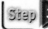 **Step 3 Grasp tongue and jaw.**

With the hand closest to the patient's feet, insert your thumb into the patient's mouth.

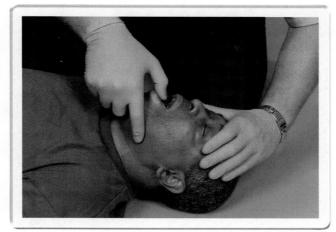

Grasp the tongue under the thumb and keep the index finger tight against the underside of the lower jaw.

 Step 4 Lift tongue and jaw.

Gently lift the tongue and jaw to pull the tongue straight up from the posterior wall of the pharynx.

 Step 5 Assess breathing.

Once the airway is open, assess the patient's ability to breathe spontaneously. If the patient is breathing, use the jaw-thrust maneuver to maintain the airway until artificial adjuncts can maintain the airway. If the patient is not breathing, switch to the jaw-thrust maneuver and begin artificial ventilation using mouth-to-mask or bag-mask ventilation (see Skill 6).

 Safety Tips

Grasping and Lifting the Tongue and Jaw
Injury may occur to the rescuer's thumb or finger if the patient begins biting motions or has seizure activity. Use extreme caution when using this procedure.

SKILL 3 — Head Tilt–Chin Lift Maneuver

Performance Objective

Given an adult patient, the candidate shall demonstrate the use of the head tilt-chin lift maneuver using the criteria herein prescribed, in 1 minute or less.

Equipment

The following equipment is required to perform this skill:
- Appropriate body substance isolation/personal protective equipment

Equipment that may be helpful:
- Oropharyngeal airways (various sizes)
- Nasopharyngeal airways (various sizes)
- Bag-mask device
- Oxygen cylinder, regulator, and key

Indications

- Immediate opening of the airway in unresponsive patients with no potential for cervical spine injury

Contraindications

- Patients with a potential or known cervical spine injury

Complications

- None if properly performed and maintained

Procedures

 **Step 1** ▶ **Ensure body substance isolation before beginning procedures.**

Prior to beginning patient care, appropriate body substance isolation procedures should be employed.

▼

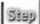 **Step 2** ▶ **Assume proper position.**

Position yourself at the patient's head and shoulder, facing across the body.

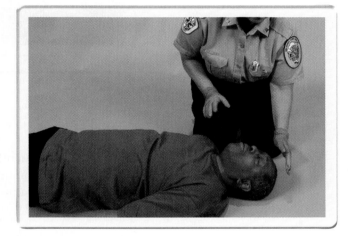

Place the hand closest to the patient's head on the patient's forehead.

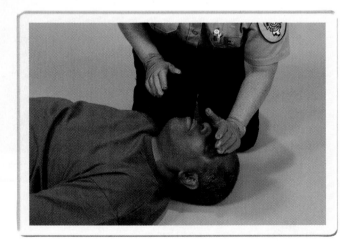

Step **2** continued

Place the hand closest to the patient's feet on the underside of the mandible just below the chin.

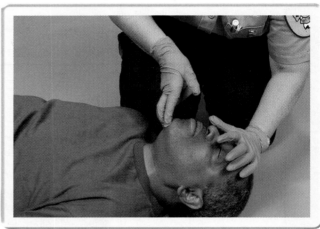

Step **3** Hyperextend the neck.

Maintaining hand position, pull up on the patient's chin while pushing down on the patient's forehead. Hyperextend the neck until the face is at least 45° to the floor. It is important to maintain this position until airway adjuncts maintain the airway.

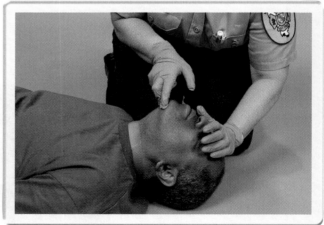

Step **4** Assess breathing.

Once the airway is open, assess the patient's ability to breathe spontaneously. If the patient is breathing, maintain the airway until artificial adjuncts can maintain the airway. If the patient is not breathing, begin artificial ventilation using mouth-to-mask or bag-mask ventilation.

Oxygen Administration

Performance Objective

Given an adult patient and appropriate oxygen delivery devices, the candidate shall demonstrate proper attachment of the regulator, ability to read the pressure gauge accurately, and ability to deliver oxygen using the criteria herein prescribed, in 5 minutes or less.

Equipment

The following equipment is required to perform this skill:
- Appropriate body substance isolation/personal protective equipment
- Oxygen cylinder, regulator, and key
- Oxygen delivery device (appropriate to patient)
  - Nasal cannula
  - Simple face mask
  - Nonrebreathing mask
  - Bag-mask device

Equipment that may be helpful:
- Pulse oximeter
- End-tidal carbon dioxide meter

Indications

- Oxygen supplement for patients in:
  - Respiratory distress
  - Respiratory failure
  - Respiratory arrest
  - General hypoxia
  - Shock
  - Myocardial infarction
  - Stroke

Contraindications

- Paraquat poisoning

Complications

- Rate dependant. High-flow oxygen levels can cause constriction of cerebral and coronary vessels. It is important to base oxygen administration on assessment of oxygen saturation as measured by pulse oximetry(S_pO_2) and end-tidal carbon dioxide concentration.

Procedures

 Step 1 Ensure body substance isolation before beginning procedures.

Prior to beginning patient care, appropriate body substance isolation procedures should be employed.

 Step 2 Assemble regulator to tank.

It is important to be able to recognize the cylinder as an oxygen cylinder by color (green, white, or chrome) and pin index (2:5), and to ensure that the cylinder is labeled as medical oxygen (Oxygen USP).

Point the oxygen port away from self, patient, and bystanders so no debris gets blown at a person. Open and close the valve quickly to blow out debris.

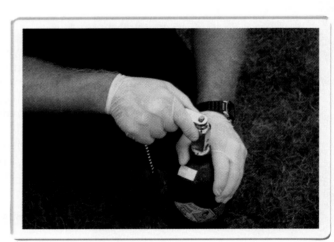

Confirm the presence of an O-ring at the oxygen port.

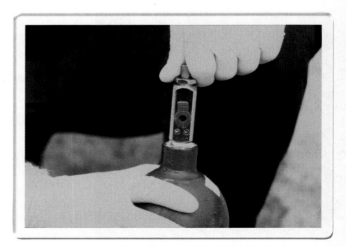

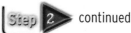 continued

Carefully attach the regulator and secure tightly by hand.

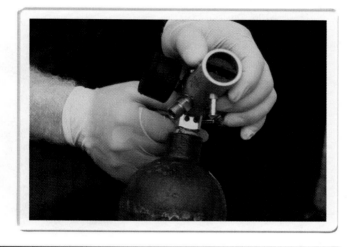

 Open tank.

With the face of the gauges pointing away from you and bystanders, open the cylinder.

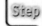 **Check for leaks.**

Check for and correct any leaks that occur.

Safety Tips

Oxygen Safety
Although oxygen is not combustible and will not explode, it does support combustion. Be extremely cautious using oxygen near open flames, and never allow patients to smoke while oxygen is being administered.

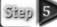 **Check tank pressure.**

Oxygen regulators have one or two gauges. The first gauge, closest to the valve stem, measures the pressure inside the cylinder. The pressure is used to identify the volume of oxygen available to the patient, and is measured in *pounds per square inch* (psi). It is important to read the pressure accurately to within 100 psi. The safe residual, the minimal amount of usable oxygen, is considered 200 psi.

The second gauge identifies the amount of oxygen delivered from the cylinder. The amount of oxygen is measured in *liters per minute* (L/min) and is controlled by the regulator knob. Some regulators do not have a liter flow gauge. Instead, they have a knob that dials in the liter flow.

6 **Attach oxygen delivery device.**

Attach the oxygen connective tubing to the flowmeter. Ensure that oxygen is flowing through the delivery device and attach it to the patient.

Most patients do not need high-flow oxygen. Studies have shown that high levels of oxygen may actually harm the patient, or at the very least provide little benefit. Which oxygen delivery device is used will depend on the patient's physical condition. Diagnostic equipment and medical control will help determine which device is to be used. As a general rule, delivery of oxygen by nonrebreathing mask is reserved for patients experiencing severe dyspnea, patients in shock, and patients with an oxygen saturation below 94%. Patients experiencing chest pain or stroke should receive only 4 L/min by nasal cannula, unless the oxygen saturation is low.

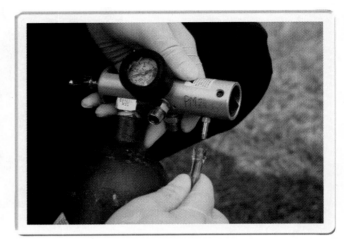

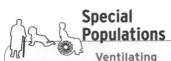
Special Populations

Ventilating Infants and Children

It may be very difficult to convince infants and small children to wear an oxygen mask or cannula. In these cases, blow-by oxygen administration may be your best option. To deliver blow-by oxygen, attach oxygen connective tubing to the cylinder and set at 4 to 6 L/min. Hold, or have the patient hold, the distal end near the patient's face to enrich the inspired air around the patient.

Oxygen Delivery Devices			
Device	Flow Rate	Use	Oxygen Delivered
Nasal Cannula	2–6 L/min	Used for basic oxygen supplementation.	Delivers an oxygen concentration between 24% and 44%.
Face Mask	6–10 L/min	Used when oxygen supplementation must be higher than can be achieved by nasal cannula.	Delivers up to 60% oxygen.
Rebreathing/ Nonrebreathing Mask	12–15 L/min	Used in treating conditions of hypoxia and shock. Always prefill the reservoir by reaching into the mask and placing a finger over the top of the reservoir bag. Hold until the bag has inflated.	Delivers an oxygen concentration between 80% and 90%.
Bag-Mask Device	15 L/min or greater	Used when the patient's ventilatory status is insufficient. Begin ventilations without supplemental oxygen if necessary, but establish oxygen flow within 1 minute.	Without oxygen: 21% oxygen Oxygen without reservoir: 60% oxygen Oxygen with reservoir tube: 90% oxygen Oxygen with reservoir bag: 100% oxygen

Step 7 ▶ Remove delivery device.

Remove the delivery device from the patient while the oxygen is still flowing. *Never* leave a dead mask on a patient.

▼

Step 8 ▶ Shut off the regulator.

Turn the oxygen flow off at the regulator.

▼

Step 9 ▶ Shut off the tank.

Close the cylinder valve.

▼

Step 10 ▶ Relieve the pressure within the regulator.

Turn the regulator valve on and allow all oxygen to bleed from the gauges. When the gauges are both at zero (0), turn the regulator valve off. Detach the regulator from the cylinder.

Calculating Usable Oxygen

To calculate how long oxygen will last in a cylinder, use the formula below with the appropriate conversion factor. Look at the oxygen bottle to determine the psi.

Oxygen Cylinders: Duration of Flow

This equation will give an estimate of how long the cylinder will last before needing to be replaced. Using this formula, a full D cylinder running 15 L/min will last for 21 minutes. This is an essential piece of information when working a cardiac arrest using a portable cylinder.

Formula:

$$\frac{(\text{Gauge pressure [psi]} - \text{safe residual pressure}) \times \text{cylinder constant}}{\text{Flow rate [L/min]}}$$

$$= \text{duration of flow in minutes}$$

Safe residual pressure = 200 psi

Cylinder constant:

D = 0.16	G = 2.41	E = 0.28
H = 3.14	M = 1.56	K = 3.14

Mouth-to-Mask Ventilation

Performance Objective

Given an adult patient, mouth-to-mask resuscitators with one-way valves, and all appropriate equipment, the candidate shall demonstrate artificial ventilation using the criteria herein prescribed, in 5 minutes or less.

Equipment

The following equipment is required to perform this skill:
- Appropriate body substance isolation/personal protective equipment
- Oxygen cylinder, regulator, and key
- Oxygen connecting tubing
- Pocket mask with
  - One-way valve
  - Oxygen connecting port

Equipment that may be helpful:
- Oropharyngeal airway
- Suction device
- Pulse oximeter
- End-tidal carbon dioxide meter

Indications

- Immediate ventilation of a nonbreathing patient
- Preferred alternative to mouth-to-mouth ventilation

Contraindications

- None if properly applied

Complications

- May cause abdominal distension and subsequent vomiting if proper airway position is not maintained

Procedures

 Ensure body substance isolation before beginning procedures.

Prior to beginning patient care, appropriate body substance isolation procedures should be employed.

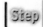 **Connect one-way valve to mask.**

Assemble the mask by forming the cup and connecting the one-way valve.

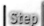 **Open patient's airway or confirm patient's airway is open (manually or with adjunct).**

Before opening the airway, consider the possibility of cervical spine injury. If spinal injury is suspected, use a jaw-thrust maneuver to open the airway (see Skill 1). If no spinal cord injury is suspected, open the patient's airway using the head tilt–chin lift maneuver (see Skill 3).

An oropharyngeal airway may be employed if available. Although not necessary initially, long-term ventilations should include its use.

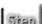 **Establish and maintain a proper mask-to-face seal.**

Position the mask with the apex over the bridge of the nose and the base between the lower lip and the prominence of the chin. Using firm pressure around the sides of the mask, form a tight seal to prevent air leakage.

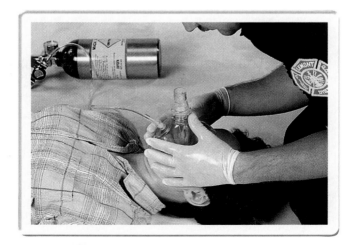

Step 5 Ventilate the patient at the proper volume and rate.

Begin ventilations as soon as the mask is sealed and assess for air leakage. Effective ventilations (ie, those breaths that cause the chest to rise adequately for the size of the patient) must be started within 30 seconds. Ventilate at a rate of 10 to 12 breaths/min.

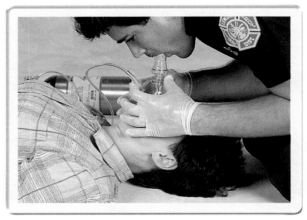

Watch for chest rise and fall during exhalation.

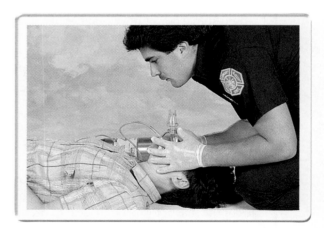

Step 6 Connect mask to high-concentration oxygen.

Attach oxygen tubing to inlet on mask and oxygen source.

Step 7 Adjust flow rate to 15 L/min.

Open the cylinder valve and adjust liter flow to 15 L/min.

Step 8 ▸ Ventilate the patient at the proper volume and rate.

Resume effective ventilations within 15 seconds of last breath. Be careful not to overventilate. Each ventilation should be delivered slowly and easily, lasting approximately 1 second. Fast and high-pressure ventilations can cause air to enter the stomach, increasing the risk of vomiting. If a second rescuer is available, the Sellick maneuver (cricoid pressure) may be applied.

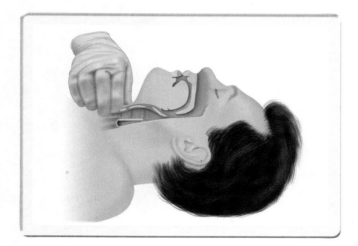

Continue the ventilations at a rate of 10 to 12 breaths/min until the patient begins spontaneous respirations, you are exhausted, you are relieved, or you are told to stop.

SKILL 6

Bag-Mask Ventilation

Performance Objective

Given an adult patient, a bag-mask device, and all appropriate equipment, the candidate shall demonstrate artificial ventilation using the criteria herein prescribed, in 5 minutes or less, with and without assistance from additional rescuers.

Equipment

The following equipment is required to perform this skill:
- Appropriate body substance isolation/personal protective equipment
- Oxygen cylinder, regulator, and key
- Oxygen connecting tubing
- Bag-mask device with appropriate-sized mask
- Oropharyngeal airway (various sizes)

Equipment that may be helpful:
- Suction device
- Pulse oximeter
- End-tidal carbon dioxide meter

Indications

- Assisting the patient with shallow or slow respirations
- Providing ventilations to the nonbreathing patient

Contraindications

- None when properly applied

Complications

- May cause abdominal distension and subsequent vomiting if proper airway position is not maintained

Procedures

 Ensure body substance isolation before beginning procedures.

Prior to beginning patient care, appropriate body substance isolation procedures should be employed.

▼

 Open the airway.

Before opening the airway, consider the possibility of cervical spine injury. If spinal injury is suspected, use a jaw-thrust maneuver to open the airway (see Skill 1).

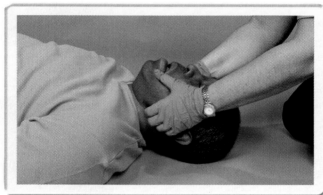

If no spinal cord injury is suspected, open the patient's airway using the head tilt–chin lift maneuver (see Skill 3).

 Insert appropriate-sized oropharyngeal airway.

Measuring from the corner of the mouth to the base of the earlobe, choose the correct-sized airway for your patient.

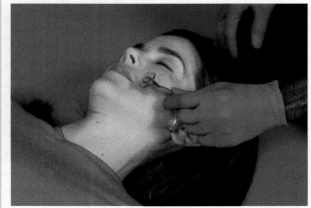

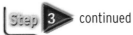

Step 3 > continued

Insert airway in front of mouth with tip pointed toward roof of mouth, or insert from side of mouth with tip toward inside of cheek.

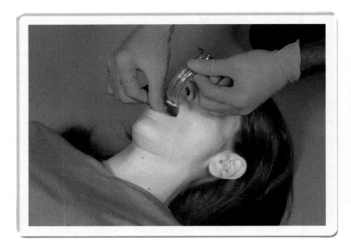

Rotate the tip of the airway toward the patient's feet as it is advanced into the oropharynx. When completely inserted, the flange of the airway should rest on the patient's lips.

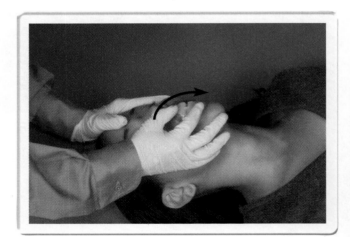

A tongue depressor can be used to hold the tongue inferior and the airway inserted tip down. If the patient starts to gag, remove the airway by pulling the flange anterior and inferior.

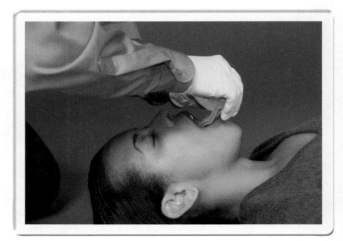

SKILL 6   Bag-Mask Ventilation

 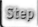

Step 4 Select appropriate-sized mask and bag.

Select the appropriate-sized bag and mask for the patient. Bag and mask sizes are normally listed as adult, pediatric, and infant. These sizes are adequate for the average-sized person meeting the age definition criteria. However, large children will require a bag that will deliver the appropriate volume. Likewise, pediatric bags may be appropriate for small adults or adults in whom overpressurization could cause pulmonary damage. Masks should be chosen to fit the patient without air leakage.

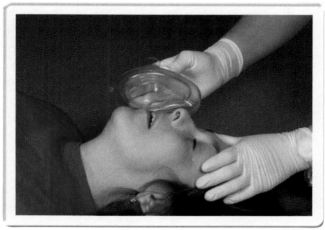

Step 5 Create a proper mask-to-face seal.

Position the mask with the apex over the bridge of the nose and the base between the lower lip and the prominence of the chin. Although this procedure can be performed by a single person, bag-mask ventilation should be performed by two people whenever possible. The first rescuer will assume the responsibilities of obtaining and maintaining the mask-to-face seal.

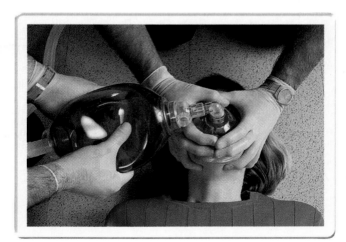

In the Field

Ventilating the Patient

Once the patient is intubated, ventilations can be performed by a single rescuer. Ensure that ventilations are slow and meticulous, adjusting the rate based on the patient's end-tidal carbon dioxide concentration if available and allowed under local protocol.

Special Populations

Ventilating the Patient With a Tracheostomy

You must make a few simple adjustments to ventilate the patient with a stoma or tracheostomy tube. For patients with a tracheostomy tube, the bag-mask device can be attached directly and ventilated as you would an endotracheal tube. Tracheostomy tubes require specialized care and can easily become clogged with mucus. If you experience difficulty ventilating the patient, you may need to suction the tracheostomy tube using a flexible suction catheter. For patients without a tracheostomy tube, place a pediatric mask over the stoma on the patient's neck. Be careful to use sufficient pressure to achieve a good seal, but not so much pressure that you occlude circulation through the carotid arteries or jugular veins.

Step 6 ▸ Ventilate patient at no less than 800 mL volume, and between 10 and 20 breaths/min.

Begin ventilations as soon as the mask is sealed and assess for air leakage. For adults, deliver ventilations at a rate of 10 to 20 breaths/min with a tidal volume of at least 800 mL. Pay close attention to ensure that each ventilation is of the appropriate volume and of a consistent rate. Allow adequate exhalation between each breath.

If a second rescuer is available, he or she should assume the responsibilities of appropriate ventilations.

Effective ventilations (ie, those breaths that cause the chest to rise adequately for the size of the patient) must be started within 30 seconds. Be careful not to overventilate. Each ventilation should be delivered slowly and easily, lasting 1 full second. Fast and high-pressure ventilations can cause air to enter the stomach, increasing the risk of vomiting.

▼

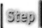

Step 7 ▸ Connect reservoir and oxygen.

Attach oxygen tubing to inlet on bag-mask device and to oxygen source.

▼

Step 8 ▸ Adjust liter flow to 15 L/min.

Open the cylinder valve and adjust liter flow to 15 L/min.

▼

Step 9 ▸ Reopen the airway.

Using the same procedure as seen in Step 2 (keeping cervical spine injury in mind if suspected), reopen the patient's airway.

▼

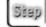

Step 10 ▸ Create a proper mask-to-face seal.

Position the mask with the apex over the bridge of the nose and the base between the lower lip and the prominence of the chin.

▼

Step 11 **Instruct assistant to begin ventilations.**

If a second rescuer is available, he or she should ventilate the patient while the first rescuer maintains the airway and mask seal (see Step 5). Two rescuers should always be used when available because this provides better control of the mask seal and of the volume delivered. Both rescuers are responsible for monitoring proper rate and depth of each ventilation. If a third rescuer is available, the Sellick maneuver (cricoid pressure) should be applied.

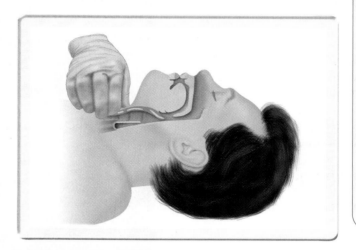

 ## Special Populations

Ventilating Geriatric Patients

When ventilating the geriatric patient with known or suspected lung disease, consider using a pediatric bag-mask device instead of the adult bag. The use of a pediatric bag will prevent the patient from receiving too deep a ventilation, which could cause injury to weakened lungs. Confirm that this will be acceptable by local protocol and that the patient's ventilations are sufficient. Monitoring of the patient's condition, arterial oxyhemoglobin saturation (S_pO_2), and end-tidal carbon dioxide concentration is important.

 ## In the Field

Determining Appropriate Tidal Volume

The best method of determining adequate ventilations is to watch for effective, not excessive, chest rise. Since most bag-mask devices have no direct means of identifying how many milliliters are being delivered, direct calculation is not possible. However, knowing how much should be delivered and estimating the size and abilities of your bag, you can better ensure that adequate volumes are being delivered. The average person uses between 7 to 10 mL/kg for every breath. Calculate the tidal volume by multiplying the patient's weight in kilograms by 7. This will provide an effective volume for most patients. If chest rise seems minimal, increase the depth slightly.

Oropharyngeal Airway

Performance Objective

Given an adult patient and appropriate equipment, the candidate shall demonstrate proper procedures for placing an oropharyngeal airway using the criteria herein prescribed, in 1 minute or less.

Equipment

The following equipment is required to perform this skill:

- Appropriate body substance isolation/personal protective equipment
- Oropharyngeal airway (various sizes)

Equipment that may be helpful:

- Tongue depressor
- Bag-mask device
- Oxygen cylinder, regulator, and key

Indications

- Basic airway adjunct used to keep the tongue from occluding the airway in unresponsive patients
- Should be used in all unresponsive patients being ventilated with a bag-mask device

Contraindications

- Patients with an intact gag reflex
- Patients with foreign body airway obstruction

Complications

- If not properly inserted, may cause the tongue to be pushed back into the hypopharynx
- Aspiration may occur if the airway is not removed before the patient regains consciousness

Procedures

 I Ensure body substance isolation before beginning procedures.

Prior to beginning patient care, appropriate body substance isolation procedures should be employed.

 2 Select appropriate-sized airway.

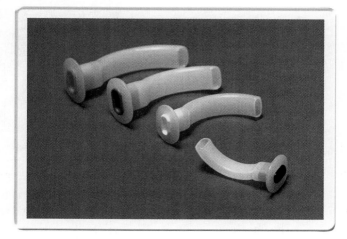

Measuring from the corner of the mouth to the base of the earlobe or angle of the jaw, choose the correct-sized airway for your patient.

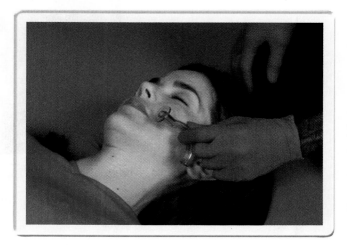

Step 3 Safely insert airway without pushing tongue posteriorly (must create patent airway).

Before opening the airway, consider the possibility of cervical spine injury. If spinal injury is suspected, use caution opening the airway and maintain in-line cervical stabilization. Open the mouth using the jaw-thrust or cross-finger technique. Insert the airway with the tip pointed toward the hard palate.

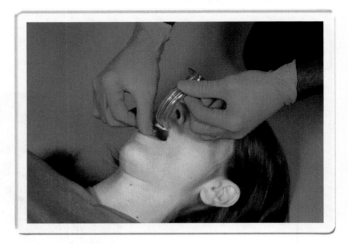

Rotate the airway 180° when no resistance is felt and the airway reaches the soft palate, or insert from the side of the mouth with the tip toward the inside of the cheek.

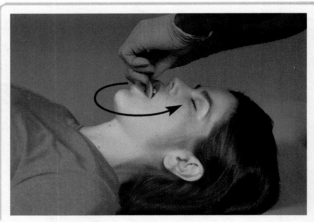

A tongue depressor can be used to hold the tongue inferior and the airway inserted tip down.

Special Populations

Infant Oropharyngeal Airways

In infants, insert the oropharyngeal airway from the side or with the aid of a tongue depressor. Rotating the airway from the top can cause trauma to an infant's palate.

Step 4 Remove oropharyngeal airway.

If the patient starts to gag, remove the airway by pulling the flange anterior and inferior.

Oral Suctioning

Performance Objective

Given an adult patient and appropriate equipment, the candidate shall demonstrate proper procedures for performing oral suctioning using the criteria herein prescribed, in 2 minutes or less.

Equipment

The following equipment is required to perform this skill:
- Appropriate body substance isolation/personal protective equipment
- Suction device and tubing
- Suction catheter
  - Rigid wand (Yankauer type)   • Flexible catheter

Equipment that may be helpful:
- Adjustable manometer
- Pulse oximeter

Indications

- Removal of blood or liquid emesis from the oropharynx
- Prevention of aspiration of secretions in patients without the ability to protect their own airway

Contraindications

- None

Complications

- Deep suctioning can stimulate the gag reflex, worsening vomiting and promoting bradycardia.
- Suctioning can cause increased intracranial pressure.
- Prolonged suctioning can promote hypoxia and anoxia.
- Incomplete suctioning can lead to forced aspiration in nonbreathing patients ventilated by bag-mask device.

Procedures

Step **Ensure body substance isolation before beginning procedures.**

Prior to beginning patient care, appropriate body substance isolation procedures should be employed.

Step  **Turn patient's head to side.**

Turn the patient's head to the side and begin manual removal of emesis. In the case of cervical spine injury the patient should be turned as a unit, secured to a backboard if possible.

Step **Turn on and prepare suction device.**

Turn on suction device and adjust manometer if available.

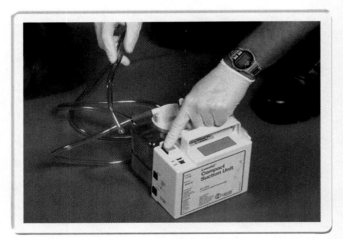

Step **Confirm presence of mechanical suction.**

Confirm that suction is working by checking suction and power.

Step 5 ▶ Insert suction tip without suction.

Measure the depth of catheter insertion from the earlobe to the corner of the mouth.

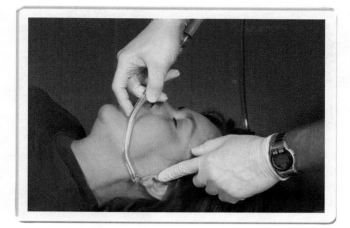

Insert the suction catheter to the proper depth with the suction turned off.

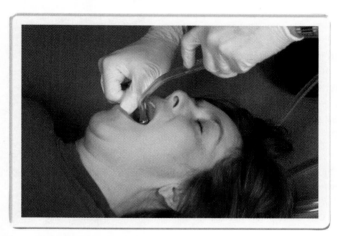

▼

Step 6 ▶ Apply suction to the oropharynx.

Apply suction to the catheter. Remove emesis by moving the catheter tip from side to side. Suction the patient for no more than 15 seconds. If the patient is not breathing or is otherwise unable to protect his or her own airway, suction until the airway is clear. Ensure no emesis remains in the nares before providing mechanical ventilation.

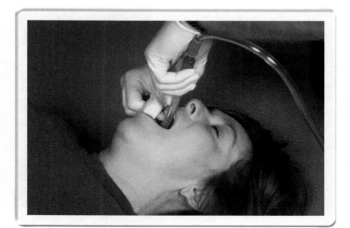

Nasopharyngeal Airway

Performance Objective

Given an adult patient and appropriate equipment, the candidate shall demonstrate proper procedures for placing a nasopharyngeal airway using the criteria herein prescribed, in 1 minute or less.

Equipment

The following equipment is required to perform this skill:
- Appropriate body substance isolation/personal protective equipment
- Nasopharyngeal airway (various sizes)
- Water-soluble lubricant

Indications

- Basic airway adjunct in patients with intact gag reflexes

Contraindications

- Facial fractures
- Anomalous facial features
- Deviated septum
- Bleeding disorders (use caution)

Complications

- Trauma to the nasal mucosa may cause bleeding and secondary aspiration of blood.
- Nasopharyngeal airways that are too long may cause esophageal intubation or laryngospasm.
- Rarely, vomiting may occur if the gag reflex is stimulated.

Procedures

 Step 1 Ensure body substance isolation before beginning procedures.

Prior to beginning patient care, appropriate body substance isolation procedures should be employed.

▼

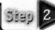 **Step 2** Select appropriate-sized airway.

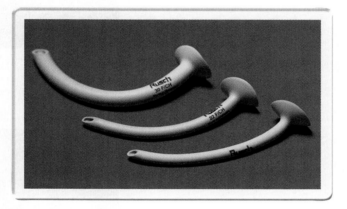

Nasopharyngeal airways are sized to fit the opening of the nose (the nares). Choose an airway that will fit the patient's nares.

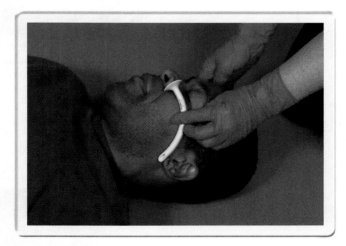

▼

 Step 3 Lubricate the nasal airway.

Lubricate the airway with a water-soluble jelly (such as K-Y jelly) or water-soluble anesthetic jelly (such as lidocaine jelly).

▼

Step **Safely insert the airway with the bevel facing toward the septum.**

Insert the nasopharyngeal airway into the chosen nostril with the bevel toward the septum.

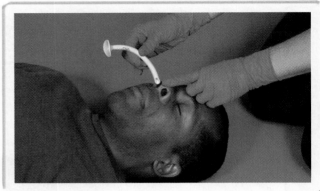

Carefully advance the airway straight down, perpendicular to the face. *Do not* push the airway upward, following the shape of the nose.

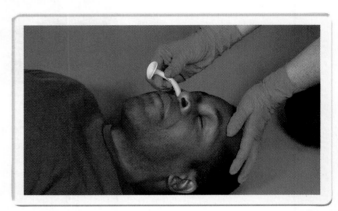

Step  **Maintain the airway.**

Frequently check the airway for proper position and to ensure it has not become occluded with mucus.

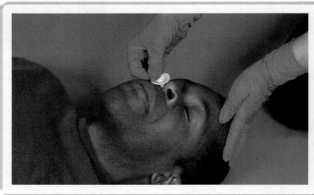

Adult Endotracheal Intubation

Performance Objective

Given an adult patient and appropriate equipment, the candidate shall insert an endotracheal tube and verify proper placement using criteria herein prescribed, in 6 minutes or less.

Equipment

The following equipment is required to perform this skill:
- Appropriate body substance isolation/personal protective equipment
- Oxygen cylinder, regulator, and key
- Oxygen delivery device (appropriate to patient)
  - Bag-mask device
- Oropharyngeal airway (adult sizes)
- Laryngoscope handle and blades (straight and curved)
- Endotracheal tubes, cuffed (6.0 to 9.0)
- Malleable intubation stylet (appropriate size for endotracheal tube)
- Water-soluble lubricant
- Towel or other padding
- Colorimetric end-tidal carbon dioxide detector
- Suction device and tubing
- Syringes (10 mL, 20 mL)
- Endotracheal tube holder or tape
- Stethoscope
- Suction catheter
  - Rigid wand (Yankauer type)
  - Flexible catheter

Equipment that may be helpful:
- Pulse oximeter
- End-tidal carbon dioxide meter
- Spare bulb, batteries

Indications

- Ensure definitive airway
- Assist with long-term ventilation

Contraindications

- None

Complications

- Unrecognized and uncorrected esophageal intubation
- Right mainstem bronchial intubation
- Laryngeal injury
- Dental injury

Procedures

 Ensure body substance isolation before beginning procedures.

Prior to beginning patient care, appropriate body substance isolation precautions should be employed.

▼

 Open the airway manually.

Before opening the airway, consider the possibility of cervical spine injury. If spinal injury is suspected, use a jaw-thrust maneuver to open the airway (see Skill 1). If no spinal cord injury is suspected, open the patient's airway by performing the head tilt–chin lift maneuver (see Skill 3).

▼

 Elevate the patient's tongue and appropriately insert simple adjunct (see Skill 7).

Measuring from the corner of the mouth to the base of the earlobe, choose the correct-sized airway for your patient.

Open the mouth using the jaw-thrust or cross-finger technique. Insert the airway in front of the mouth with its tip pointed toward the roof of the mouth, or insert it from the side of the mouth with its tip toward the inside of the cheek, rotate the airway as it is inserted until the flange rests on the patient's lips.

A tongue depressor can be used to hold the tongue inferior and the airway inserted tip down. If the patient starts to gag, remove the airway by pulling the flange anterior and inferior.

▼

Ventilate the patient immediately with bag-mask device.

Begin ventilations immediately with a bag-mask device. If the bag-mask device is not already attached to oxygen, begin ventilations with room air.

Select the appropriate-sized bag for the patient. Bag and mask sizes are normally listed as adult, child, and infant. These sizes are adequate for the average-sized person who meets the age definition criteria. However, large children require a bag that will deliver the appropriate volume. Likewise, pediatric bags may be appropriate for small adults or adults where overpressurization can cause pulmonary damage. Masks should be chosen to fit the patient without air leakage.

Position the mask with the apex over the bridge of the nose and the base between the lower lip and the prominence of the chin. Begin ventilations as soon as the mask is sealed, and assess for air leakage.

Begin ventilations at a rate of 10 to 12 breaths/min, with a tidal volume that achieves chest rise. Pay close attention to ensure that each ventilation is of the appropriate volume and of a consistent rate. Allow adequate exhalation between each breath.

Effective ventilations are those breaths that cause the chest to rise adequately for the size of the patient. In addition to assessing chest rise, consider checking breath sounds. Be cautious not to overventilate. Each ventilation should be delivered slowly and easily, lasting approximately 1 second. Fast and high-pressure ventilations can cause air to enter the stomach, increasing the risk of vomiting.

If a second rescuer is available, the Sellick maneuver (cricoid pressure) may be applied. Assisting personnel can also attach a pulse oximeter.

Although it will be necessary to stop ventilations for assessment and other procedures, you should never allow a nonbreathing patient to go without ventilations for longer than 30 seconds.

▼

 Provide supplemental oxygen.

If not previously performed, attach oxygen tubing to the inlet on the bag-mask device and to the oxygen source. Open the cylinder valve and adjust liter flow to between 12 and 15 L/min (see Skill 4).

▼

Step 6 ▶ **Ventilate the patient at a rate of 10 to 12 breaths/min with appropriate volumes.**

Continue ventilations at a rate of 10 to 12 breaths/min and ensure adequate chest rise with each.

Ventilations should be associated with capnometry. The rate of ventilation should be adjusted to achieve a capnometry reading of between 35 and 45 mm Hg. In patients with head injuries the reading should be 35 to 39 mm Hg. To drive the patient's carbon dioxide level, follow the reading. If the end-tidal carbon dioxide level is too high, ventilate faster. If the reading is too low, ventilate slower.

Consider checking breath sounds. Knowing the status of breath sounds before tube placement can be helpful when determining the correct position.

▼

 Step 7 ▶ **Direct assistant to take over ventilations.**

Direct a qualified assistant to take over ventilations at a rate of 10 to 12 breaths/min with appropriate volumes, and ensure adequate chest rise with each.

▼

Step 8 ▶ **Select, check, and prepare the equipment.**

While the patient is being hyperventilated, the person responsible for the intubation must ensure that all the necessary equipment is available and in working order. Ensure that the endotracheal tube is the proper size for the patient.

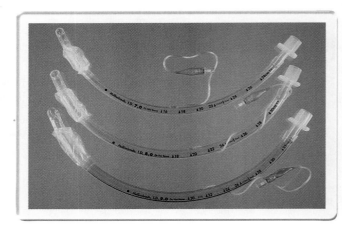

Using aseptic technique, insert an intubation stylet into the endotracheal tube and bend into a gentle curve. A properly curved stylet will allow the stylet to be removed without causing the tip of the tube to move. The stylet should be positioned so that the end of the stylet does not extend past the Murphy's eye.

Assemble the laryngoscope with the desired blade and check the brightness of the bulb. A bright white light is best for all intubations. A yellow or dull light will cause the tissues of the hypopharynx to take on similar color schemes and result in difficulties visualizing landmarks and the vocal cords. Make sure the light is turned off until the laryngoscope is placed in the patient's mouth.

 In the Field

Curved or Straight: Which Blade Is Best?

There seems to be a lot of discussion and conflict concerning which laryngoscope blade is the best blade to use. Both straight and curved blades have advantages. It is best for each person to practice with both types of blades to develop skills and abilities rather than preferences. Resist the temptation to use only one type of blade for all intubations, and don't hesitate to switch blades should the need arise.

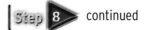

Step **8** ▶ continued

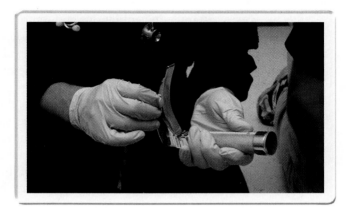

Attach a 10-mL syringe to the endotracheal tube cuff port and inflate until the balloon is tight (this will usually take less than 10 mL of air) and check for leaks. Remove the air from the cuff and remove the syringe. Place the syringe next to the patient's head. Leaving the syringe attached to the endotracheal tube can cause tearing and detachment of the balloon tubing, resulting in leaks from the cuff. There is also the possibility that the syringe may slip off and become lost. It is better to get in the habit of always removing the syringe and placing it at the patient's head.

Prepare for the intubation by placing a 1″ pad under the patient's head.

This will assist in lining up the three planes of the patient's airway. Although this step will make intubation easier, it is not required and is often difficult to accomplish in the prehospital setting. It is a good practice to learn to intubate both with and without the 1″ pad.

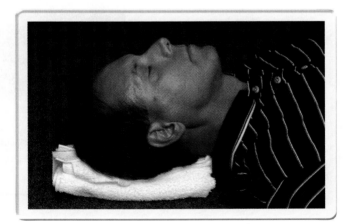

Finally, always ensure that suction is available and working before beginning intubation. Both a rigid suction tip and a flexible catheter, appropriate for the size of the endotracheal tube, should be available.

▼

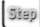

Step 9 ▶ Position patient's head properly.

Have your assistant stop ventilations and remove the mask from the bag-mask device. You will now have only 20 seconds to position the patient, place the endotracheal tube, and reestablish ventilations. Should you fail to intubate the patient, your assistant should quickly place the mask back on the bag-mask device and begin hyperventilating the patient.

Remove the oropharyngeal airway and place it next to the patient's head or in another readily available location. It will be necessary to replace this airway upon successful intubation or in the event the patient is unable to be intubated.

Gently extend the patient's neck so that the head is positioned with the chin and forehead approximately 45° from the floor. In the event the patient has had an injury to the neck or for other reasons cannot be hyperextended, refer to the procedures for in-line endotracheal intubation.

▼

Step 10 ▶ Insert blade while displacing tongue, lift mandible, and visualize larynx without using teeth as a fulcrum.

Carefully insert the blade of the laryngoscope into the patient's mouth to the depth of the uvula. Using a sweeping motion, move the patient's tongue to the left as you lift at a 45° angle along the facial plane to lift the mandible, keeping the laryngoscope off of the teeth.

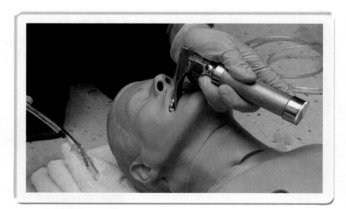

Lifting should be performed with a free hand. The habit of resting or placing the left forearm against the patient's forehead frequently causes prying and can be a dangerous practice. Placing the forearm in this position greatly limits and potentially eliminates the ability to lift the patient's lower jaw and tongue. In effect, it promotes the use of the teeth as a fulcrum as the only lifting option.

▼

11 **Introduce the endotracheal tube and advance it to the proper depth.**

Upon visualization of the vocal cords, pass the tube through the cords and into the trachea.

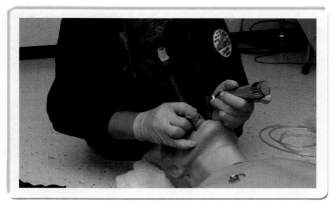

As the cuff of the tube passes the cords, stop the insertion process and maintain its position as you remove the laryngoscope. Usually this will place the tube at a depth of 22 to 24 cm at the patient's teeth. This is roughly three times the diameter of the tube. Be sure to document the position of the tube relative to the teeth.

If after two attempts you are unable to perform endotracheal intubation, strongly consider using an alternative airway device or procedure.

 12 **Remove the laryngoscope from the patient's mouth and remove the stylet from the endotracheal tube.**

Remove the laryngoscope from the patient's mouth.

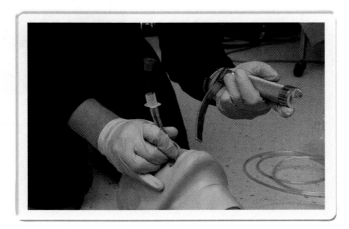

continued

Remove the stylet from the endotracheal tube.

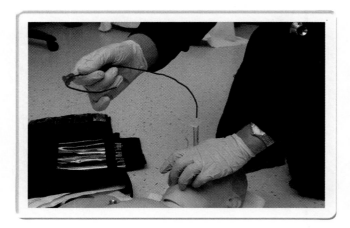

 Inflate the distal cuff to proper pressure and immediately disconnect the syringe.

Inflate the distal cuff of the endotracheal tube with 5 to 10 mL of air. Most patients will need less than the full 10 mL to fill the cuff. Remove the syringe from the inflation port.

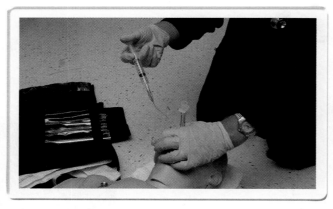

In the Field

End-Tidal Carbon Dioxide Meters

By far the most effective tool in monitoring tube placement is the use of continuous capnographic monitoring. Consistent wave forms and carbon dioxide (CO_2) readings are evidence of proper tube placement as well as the effectiveness of ventilation and oxygenation.

Measuring end-tidal carbon dioxide can be done through three simple means. The first is colorimetric, which is simply a litmus test. After applying the colorimetric device to the end of the endotracheal tube, the detection filter will change color in response to the percentage of CO_2 in the exhaled air. The colors range from purple (no CO_2) to yellow (high CO_2). Remember this: Yellow = *Yes*, Tan = *Think about it*, Purple = *Problem*.

The remaining forms of monitoring end-tidal carbon

Step 14 Attach a colorimetric end-tidal carbon dioxide detector.

Attach a colorimetric end-tidal carbon dioxide detector to the endotracheal tube.

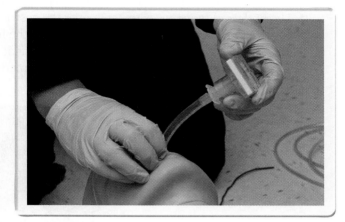

 Step 15 Direct ventilation of the patient.

While still holding the tube in place, have your partner attach the bag-mask device to the endotracheal tube and begin ventilations. Instruct your partner to deliver breaths as you move your stethoscope over the patient's abdomen and chest.

 In the Field

End-Tidal Carbon Dioxide Meters (continued)

dioxide are usually combined in the electrocardiogram monitors used in EMS. Capnometry means that a numerical value is displayed. Capnography means that a graph is formed as the patient exhales and inhales. Square wave forms, consistent with the pauses in ventilation (remember that capnography measures exhalation, not ventilation), are evidence that the endotracheal tube is in the proper position. In most cases, this will mean that the patient will have an end-tidal carbon dioxide reading of between 35 and 45 mm Hg. However, for patients in cardiac arrest, you can expect numbers to be considerably lower. An end-tidal carbon dioxide reading of 25 to 35 mm Hg may be a very good reading for a patient who is receiving cardiopulmonary resuscitation. Consistent readings below 10 mm Hg, especially if associated with asystole, are an indication that the patient has died and termination of resuscitative efforts should be considered.

Safety Tips

Checking Breath Sounds

The pattern of checking breath sounds to determine the proper placement of an endotracheal tube is different than the pattern of patient assessment. When checking tube placement, you want to determine *improper* placement in as few breaths as possible. It is best to follow these steps:

- Start by assessing the epigastric region over the stomach. If ventilatory sounds are heard here, the tube is in the esophagus. Immediately pull the tube, ventilate the patient with a bag-mask device, and consider reintubation or other airway procedures.
- Next check the breath sounds on the lower left chest, then move up to the upper left chest. If ventilatory sounds are *not* heard here, the tube has been placed in the right primary bronchus (right mainstem intubation). Carefully pull back on the endotracheal tube, 1 cm at a time, until breath sounds are heard.
- Compare the ventilations of the left chest with the right chest, upper chest to upper chest, and lower chest to lower chest. Adjust the depth as needed.

Using this process, you will determine the correct placement in just a few breaths and will determine improper placement in as little as one breath.

Step 16 ▶ **Confirm proper placement by auscultation over the epigastrium and bilaterally over each lung.**

Auscultate the abdomen and the chest to determine the correct tube placement. The preferred sequence is to listen over the gastric region first, then over the lower left, upper left, upper right, and finally the lower right chest. By using this sequence, you can determine incorrect placement with a minimal amount of unnecessary ventilations. After confirming placement, move to the next step.

If air is heard over the epigastric region, remove the tube and begin ventilating the patient with a bag-mask device. Some practitioners prefer to leave endotracheal tubes in the esophagus upon finding missed intubation, preferring instead to intubate around this first tube. Their philosophy is that this 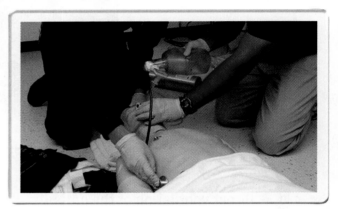 reduces the chances of missing a second time. However, this may confuse the landmarks and definitely limits the visibility in the hypopharynx. A problem of inefficient ventilations is also created.

Absent breath sounds on the left are an indication of right mainstem intubation. Deflate the cuff. Gently and carefully pull back on the endotracheal tube until breath sounds are heard over the left chest. Reinflate the cuff. Note and document the tube's position in relation to the teeth.

Step **17** ▶ **Secure the endotracheal tube.**

Maintaining a hold on the tube, attach a commercially made endotracheal tube holder.

Commercial devices are preferred over other techniques because they provide the most effective control of the airway. These devices also eliminate the need for an oral airway because they include a bite block.

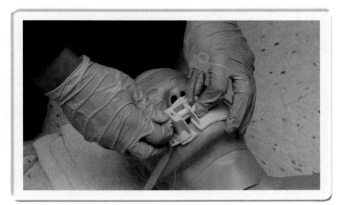

If a commercially made device is not available, secure the endotracheal tube using tape.

If you have secured the endotracheal tube using tape, place a bite block in the patient's mouth.

▼

Safety Tips

Esophageal Detectors

Esophageal detector devices (EDD) are a simple means of identifying a missed intubation. The EDD is really nothing more than a modified bulb syringe. It operates from a very simple principle. Simply squeeze the bulb and attach it to the end of the endotracheal tube. If the endotracheal tube is placed in the trachea, the bulb will reexpand because it was able to suck air from the lungs. If, however, the tube is in the esophagus, the bulb will not reexpand because it will collapse the sides of the esophagus, which prevents air from filling the bulb.

Unless specifically designed and packaged for children, EDDs should not be used on pediatric patients.

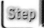 **Ensure tube placement by additional means and apply extrication collar.**

Reassess the tube placement through assessment of gastric and breath sounds. At least two additional means of ensuring tube placement should be used. These include:

- Visualization of the tube passing between the cords
- End-tidal carbon dioxide meters
- Fogging of the endotracheal tube
- Esophageal detectors
- Capnographic monitors

Finally, when placement is ensured, an appropriately sized extrication collar should be applied to maintain position of the head and neck and thus the airway.

All findings should be verbalized so that all members of the team are aware of the airway status.

It should go without saying, but, it is *essential* that the endotracheal tube be placed in the trachea for proper airway control. Missed intubations (those placed in the esophagus) must be identified and removed immediately to prevent brain damage and even death from suffocation anoxia. Failure to identify and correct an esophageal intubation constitutes gross negligence. The conscious discussion to leave an endotracheal tube placed in the esophagus under the premise that it is "the best we could get" is willful and wanton negligence, and it can result in criminal charges in many jurisdictions. Airway management carries extreme responsibility and should not be taken lightly.

Pediatric Endotracheal Intubation

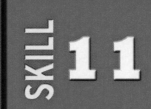

Performance Objective

Given a pediatric patient and appropriate equipment, the candidate shall insert an endotracheal tube and verify proper placement using the criteria herein prescribed, in 6 minutes or less.

Equipment

The following equipment is required to perform this skill:
- Appropriate body substance isolation/personal protection equipment
- Oxygen cylinder, regulator, and key
- Oxygen delivery device (appropriate to patient)
  - Bag-mask device
- Oropharyngeal airway (pediatric sizes)
- Laryngoscope handle and blades (straight and curved)
- Endotracheal tubes, uncuffed (2.5 to 5.5)
- Malleable intubation stylet (appropriate size for endotracheal tube)
- Water-soluble lubricant
- Towel or other padding
- Colorimetric end-tidal carbon dioxide detector (infant/child size)
- Endotracheal tube holder or tape
- Stethoscope
- Suction device and tubing
- Suction catheter
  - Rigid wand (Yankauer type)   • Flexible catheter

Equipment that may be helpful:
- Pulse oximeter   ■ End-tidal carbon dioxide meter
- Spare bulb, batteries

Indications

- Ensure definitive airway   ■ Assist with long-term ventilation

Contraindications

- None

Complications

- Unrecognized and uncorrected esophageal intubation
- Right mainstem bronchial intubation
- Laryngeal injury   ■ Dental injury

Procedures

 Ensure body substance isolation before beginning procedures.

Prior to beginning patient care, appropriate body substance isolation procedures should be employed.

 Open the airway manually.

Before opening the airway, consider the possibility of cervical spine injury. If spinal injury is suspected, use the jaw-thrust maneuver to open the airway (see Skill 1). If no spinal cord injury is suspected, open the child's airway by performing the head tilt–chin lift maneuver (see Skill 3).

 Elevate the child's tongue and appropriately insert simple adjunct.

Measuring from the corner of the mouth to the base of the earlobe, choose the correct-sized airway for your patient.

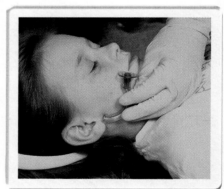

Gently open the airway and insert the oropharyngeal airway from the side of the mouth with the tip toward the inside of the cheek. A tongue depressor can be used to hold the tongue inferior and the airway inserted tip down.

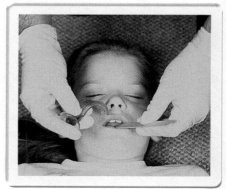

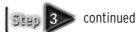

Step 3 continued

If the child starts to gag, remove the airway by pulling the flange anterior and inferior. Be aware that a gag reflex in children can lead to serious bradycardia.

▼

 ## Ventilate the child immediately with bag-mask device.

Select the appropriate-sized bag for the child. Bag and mask sizes are normally listed as adult, child, and infant. These sizes are adequate for the average size person who meets the age definition criteria. However, large children will require a bag that will deliver the appropriate volume. Likewise, pediatric bags may be appropriate for small adults or adults where overpressurization can cause pulmonary damage. Masks should be chosen to fit the child without air leakage.

Position the mask with the apex over the bridge of the nose and the base between the lower lip and the prominence of the chin. Begin ventilations as soon as the mask is sealed and assess for air leakage.

Begin ventilations at a rate of 12 to 20 breaths/min, with a tidal volume adequate to create chest rise. Pay close attention to ensure that each ventilation is of the appropriate volume and of a consistent rate. Allow adequate exhalation between each breath.

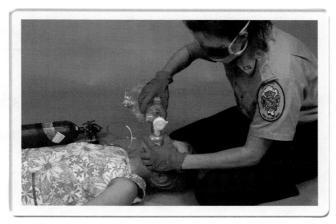

The initial ventilations of a nonbreathing patient should be performed in a controlled and accelerated manner. Deliver 6 to 10 breaths in 30 seconds. Use extreme caution not to overventilate. Each breath should be given slowly, with adequate time for exhalation in between.

Effective ventilations are those breaths that cause the chest to rise adequately for the size of the patient and must be started within 30 seconds. In addition to assessing chest rise, consider checking breath sounds. Be cautious not to overventilate. Each ventilation should be delivered slowly and easily, lasting approximately 1 second. Fast and high-pressure ventilations can cause air to enter the stomach, increasing the risk of vomiting. The Sellick maneuver should never be performed on children or infants. Although it will be necessary to stop ventilations for assessment and other procedures, you should never allow a nonbreathing patient to go without ventilations for longer than 30 seconds.

▼

 **Step 5** ▶ **Provide supplemental oxygen.**

If not previously performed, attach oxygen tubing to the inlet on the bag-mask device and to the oxygen source. Open the cylinder valve and adjust liter flow to between 12 and 15 L/min (see Skill 4).

▼

 Step 6 ▶ **Ventilate the patient at a rate of 12 to 20 breaths/min with appropriate volumes.**

Continue ventilations at a rate of 12 to 20 breaths/min, with a tidal volume adequate to achieve chest rise. Pay close attention to ensure that each ventilation is of the appropriate volume and of a consistent rate. Allow adequate exhalation between each breath.

Effective ventilations, those breaths that cause the chest to rise adequately for the size of the patient, must be started within 30 seconds. Be cautious not to overventilate. Each ventilation should be delivered slow and easy, lasting 1 second each. Fast and high-pressure ventilations can cause air to enter the stomach, increasing the risk of vomiting.

In addition to assessing chest rise, also consider checking breath sounds. Knowing the status of breath sounds before tube placement can be helpful when determining the correct position. Oxygen saturation as measured by pulse oximetry (S_pO_2) and end-tidal carbon dioxide levels should be obtained as time permits.

▼

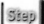 **Step 7** ▶ **Direct assistant to take over ventilations.**

Direct a qualified assistant to take over ventilations at a rate of 12 to 20 breaths/min with appropriate volumes, and ensure adequate chest rise with each breath.

▼

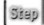 **Step 8** ▶ **Select, check, and prepare the equipment.**

While the child is being hyperventilated, the person responsible for the intubation must ensure that all the necessary equipment is available and in working order. Ensure that the endotracheal tube is the proper size for the child.

Proper sizing can be achieved by comparing the diameter of the endotracheal tube to the diameter of the child's little finger or the open-

Special Populations

Cuffed Tubes in Children

Most people would never consider placing a cuffed tube in a child or infant. However, cuffed tubes in pediatric intubation have a place. The purpose of the cuff is to seal the airway. In children, this is done anatomically by the cricoid ring, in most cases. However, there is an assumption here that the chosen tube is the correct size for the patient. In EMS and all aspects of emergency medicine, it is very likely that the tube size estimate will be small for the patient. For this reason, a cuffed tube would solve the problem. The airway would be secure, and the patient could be adequately ventilated. A small amount of air in a cuffed tube would fix a poor anatomic seal. If a cuffed tube is used, be sure to limit the amount of air in the cuff and monitor it frequently.

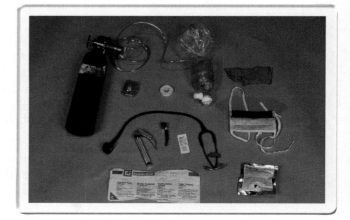

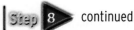

Step 8 continued

ing of the child's nares. Under most normal circumstances, an intubation stylet will not be necessary. If a stylet is used, make sure it is positioned so that the end of the stylet does not extend past the Murphy's eye.

Uncuffed endotracheal tubes are traditionally used when intubating children younger than 8 years. In the event you encounter an endotracheal tube with a cuff in smaller sizes (designed for specialty and veterinary purposes), resist the temptation to inflate the cuff by cutting the inflation port from the tube. In cases in which the chosen tube is too small for the child, slight inflation of the cuff to seal the airway may be necessary. Be sure that this is the exception and not the rule, and monitor the amount and pressure of the air in the cuff.

Assemble the laryngoscope with the desired blade. For smaller infants and neonates, a No. 1 Miller is the preferred blade (MacIntosh blades are contraindicated due to anatomic differences in a child's upper airway). Ensure that the bulb is tight in the blade. Check the brightness of the bulb. A bright white light is best for all intubations. A yellow or dull light will cause the tissues of the hypopharynx to take on similar color schemes and result in difficulties visualizing landmarks and the vocal cords. Make sure the light is turned off until the laryngoscope is placed in the child's mouth.

Choosing the Right-Sized Tube and Blade						
	Premature	Newborn	6 months	1-3 years	3-6 years	6-12 years
Tube size	2.5 mm	3-3.5 mm	3.5-4 mm	4-5 mm	5-5.5 mm	5.5-6.5 mm
Blade size	0	0-1	1	1-2	2	2-3

Finally, always ensure that suction is available and working before beginning intubation. Both a rigid suction tip and a flexible catheter, appropriate for the size of the endotracheal tube, should be available.

▼

Step 9 **Place child in neutral or sniffing position, placing pad under child's torso.**

Gently extend the child's neck so that the head is positioned with the facial plane approximately 25° to 30° from the floor (just slightly extended from the neutral position). Place a 1″ pad beneath the shoulders of the child.

▼

Step **10** Insert blade while displacing tongue, lift mandible, and visualize larynx without using teeth as a fulcrum.

Carefully insert the blade of the laryngoscope into the child's mouth to the depth of the uvula. Using a sweeping motion, move the child's tongue to the left as you lift at a 45° angle along the facial plane to lift the mandible, keeping the laryngoscope off of the teeth.

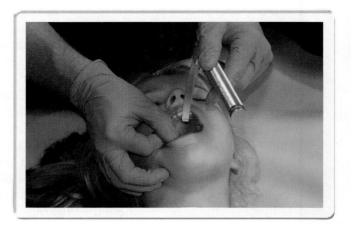

Step **11** Introduce the endotracheal tube and advance it to the proper depth.

Upon visualization of the vocal cords, pass the tube through the cords and into the trachea.

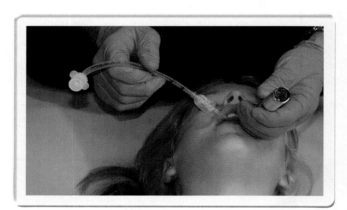

As the eye of the tube passes the cords, stop the insertion process and maintain its position as you remove the laryngoscope. Many smaller diameter tubes have a black line that indicates the position of the vocal cords. Be sure to document the position of the tube relative to the teeth.

If after two attempts you are not able to achieve endotracheal intubation, consider allowing another practitioner to perform the procedure or consider immediate transport without a secure airway.

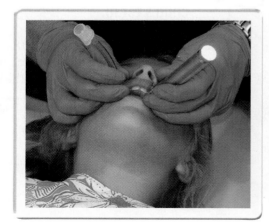

Remove the laryngoscope from the child's mouth and remove the stylet from the endotracheal tube.

Remove the laryngoscope from the child's mouth.
   If used, remove the stylet from the endotracheal tube.

▼

  Attach a colorimetric end-tidal carbon dioxide detector.

Attach a colorimetric end-tidal carbon dioxide detector to the endotracheal tube.

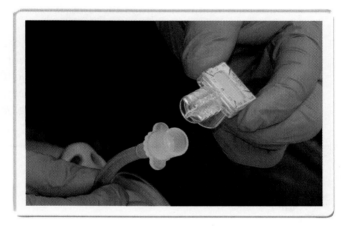

▼

 Direct ventilation of the child.

While still holding the tube in place, have your partner attach the bag-mask device to the endotracheal tube and begin ventilations. Instruct your partner to deliver breaths as you move your stethoscope over the patient's abdomen and chest.

▼

Confirm proper placement by auscultation over the epigastrium and bilaterally over each lung.

Auscultate the abdomen and the chest to determine the correct tube placement. The preferred sequence is to listen over the gastric region first, and then over the lower left, upper left, upper right, and finally the lower right chest. By using this sequence, you can determine incorrect placement with a minimal amount of unnecessary ventilations.

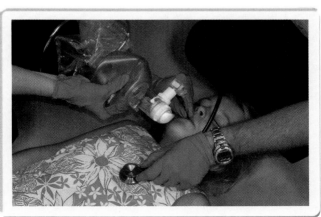

 Safety Tips

Neonate and Infant Intubation
In neonates and smaller infants, right mainstem intubations can cause pneumothoraces to develop. Be alert for a tension pneumothorax to develop and inform the receiving physician of the initial right mainstem intubation.

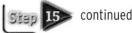 **Step 15** continued

In infants and small children, return the patient's head and neck to a neutral position and reassess the breath sounds. Be aware that any extension of the neck can reposition the tube into a right mainstem intubation, while a flexion of the neck can pull the tube out of the larynx. After confirming placement, move to the next step.

If air is heard over the epigastric region, remove the tube and begin ventilating the patient with a bag-mask device. Some practitioners prefer to leave endotracheal tubes in the esophagus upon finding a missed intubation, preferring instead to intubate around this first tube. *This should never be performed in a pediatric patient.*

Absent breath sounds on the left are an indication of right mainstem intubation. Gently and carefully pull back on the endotracheal tube until breath sounds are heard over the left chest. In neonates and smaller infants, right mainstem intubations can cause pneumothoraces to develop. Be alert for a tension pneumothorax to develop, and inform the receiving physician of the initial right mainstem intubation.

Safety Tips

Securing the Endotracheal Tube

In-hospital surgical and anesthesia personnel may apply tape only to the side of the patient's cheek when securing an endotracheal tube. This is a poor practice for prehospital intubations. While patients in the operating room are intubated briefly and are moved very little, patients who are intubated in the prehospital setting will be lifted, pulled and pushed, transported at high speed, wheeled on a stretcher, and face the miscommunications of movement attempts. Taping the endotracheal tube circumferentially around the face and neck is preferred. Even small lateral movements can easily dislodge a properly placed tube.

 Step 16 **Secure the endotracheal tube.**

Note the placement of the distance marker at the child's teeth or gums. Maintaining a hold on the tube, encircle the tube with tape at the level of the child's gums.

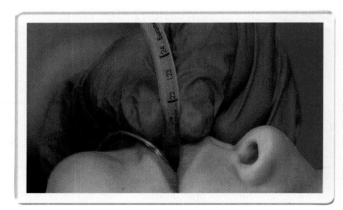

Wrap the tape around the child's neck, and again encircle the tape around the tube at the level of the child's gums. Ensure that you have not placed undue pressure on the vessels of the neck by placing the tape over the prominence of the anterior mandible.

Step 17 ▶ Ensure tube placement by additional means and apply extrication collar.

Reassess tube placement through assessment of gastric and breath sounds. At least two additional means of ensuring tube placement should be used. These include the following:

- Visualization of the tube passing between the cords
- End-tidal carbon dioxide meters (pediatric size)
- Fogging of the endotracheal tube
- Capnographic monitors

Finally, when placement is ensured, an appropriately sized extrication collar should be applied to maintain the position of the head and neck and thus the airway.

All findings should be verbalized so that all members of the team are aware of the child's airway status.

Even though the tube's placement has been ensured, continual reassessment should occur. This should be performed any time the patient is moved or defibrillated. Also, always ensure and document the tube placement before turning the child over to the receiving facility or to a transport team.

12 Introducer-Assisted Intubation

Performance Objective

Given an adult patient and appropriate equipment, the candidate shall insert an endotracheal tube with the assistance of a gum elastic bougie and verify proper placement using criteria herein prescribed, in 6 minutes or less.

Equipment

The following equipment is required to perform this skill:
- Appropriate body substance isolation/personal protective equipment
- Oxygen cylinder, regulator, and key
- Oxygen delivery device (appropriate to patient)
  - Bag-mask device
- Oropharyngeal airway (adult sized)
- Laryngoscope handle and blades (straight and curved)
- Endotracheal tubes, cuffed (6.0 to 9.0)
- Malleable intubation stylet (appropriate size for endotracheal tube)
- Gum elastic bougie (introducer) ■ Towel or other padding
- Water-soluble lubricant
- Syringes (10 mL, 20 mL) ■ Endotracheal tube holder or tape
- Stethoscope ■ Suction device and tubing
- Colorimetric end-tidal carbon dioxide detector
- Suction catheter
  - Rigid wand (Yankauer type) • Flexible catheter

Equipment that may be helpful:
- Pulse oximeter ■ Spare bulb, batteries
- End-tidal carbon dioxide meter

Indications

- Inability to visualize vocal cords
- Inability to intubate using standard visualization and placement techniques

Contraindications

- Patients younger than 14 years of age
- Small airways that do not permit placement of the introducer through the lumen of the endotracheal tube

Complications

- Damage to the trachea or esophagus
- Sore throat or hoarseness
- Trauma to the arytenoid cartilages

Procedures

Note: This procedure is usually performed *after* standard intubation attempts have failed but may be an initial means of intubation in some patients. In either case, it is assumed that proper airway and ventilation procedures and patient preparation have already been performed.

 Step 1 ▶ Ensure body substance isolation before beginning procedures.

Prior to beginning patient care, appropriate body substance isolation procedures should be employed.

▼

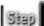 **Step 2** ▶ Prepare introducer and endotracheal tube.

Remove the gum elastic bougie (introducer) from the package. Place a new (sterile) endotracheal tube, cuffed end first, over the straight end of the introducer.

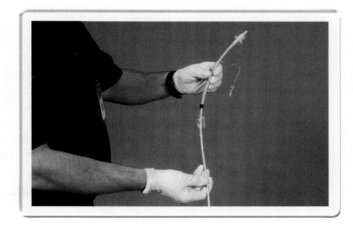

Because laryngeal edema may exist, it is recommended to use an endotracheal tube that is a half- to a full-size smaller than would normally be used in the patient.

▼

In the Field

Digital
Intubation
Because the
gum elastic bougie is thin-
ner and more maneuverable
than an endotracheal tube, it
is ideal for use during digital
intubation. Using the same
procedures for digital intubation, place the introducer and
then, following the procedures
for introducer-assisted intubation, complete the placement
of the endotracheal tube.

 Position the patient's head.

Have your partner stop ventilations and remove the mask from the bag-mask device. You will now have only 20 to 30 seconds to position the patient, place the endotracheal tube, and reestablish ventilations. Should you fail to intubate the patient, your partner should quickly place the mask back on the bag-mask device and begin hyperventilating the patient.

Remove the oropharyngeal airway and place it next to the patient's head or other readily available location. It will be necessary to replace this airway upon successful intubation or in the event the patient is unable to be intubated.

Gently extend the patient's neck so that the head is positioned with the chin and forehead approximately 45° from the floor. In the event the patient has had an injury to the neck or for other reasons cannot be hyperextended, refer to the procedures for In-Line Endotracheal Intubation (Skill 15).

▼

 Insert blade while displacing tongue, lift mandible, and visualize larynx without using teeth as a fulcrum.

Carefully insert the blade of the laryngoscope into the patient's mouth to the depth of the uvula. Using a sweeping motion, move the patient's tongue to the left as you lift at a 45° angle along the facial plane, elevating the mandible with the laryngoscope, keeping the laryngoscope off of the teeth.

Lifting should be performed with a free hand. The habit of resting or placing the left forearm against the patient's forehead frequently causes prying and can be a dangerous practice. Placing the forearm in this position greatly limits and po-tentially eliminates the ability to lift the patient's lower jaw and tongue. In effect, it promotes the use of the teeth as a fulcrum as the only lifting option.

▼

5 Insert gum elastic bougie and advance to proper depth.

Upon visualization of the vocal cords, pass the introducer through the cords and into the trachea. The introducer should be inserted with the J tip pointing up (anterior). As the tip slides into the trachea and slides against the tracheal cartilages, a slight clicking sensation should be felt. This is the proper depth.

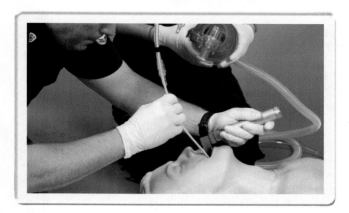

 6 Slide the endotracheal tube down the gum elastic bougie through the vocal cords.

Carefully holding the introducer in place, slide the endotracheal tube down and into the oropharynx. Rotate the tube 90° counterclockwise to position the bevel down (this will reduce damage to the arytenoid cartilages). Continue to advance the tube through the cords and into the larynx. Advance the tube until it measures 22 to 24 cm at the teeth (or three times the diameter of the tube).

While holding the endotracheal tube securely in place, remove the introducer.

7 Ventilate, confirm, and secure the endotracheal tube.

Ventilate, confirm, and secure the endotracheal tube as appropriate for standard intubation.

Nasotracheal Intubation

Performance Objective

Given an adult patient and appropriate equipment, the candidate shall insert an endotracheal tube through the nasal route and verify proper placement using criteria herein prescribed, in 8 minutes or less.

Equipment

The following equipment is required to perform this skill:
- Appropriate body substance isolation/personal protective equipment
- Oxygen cylinder, regulator, and key
- Oxygen delivery device (appropriate to patient)
  • Bag-mask device
- Endotracheal tubes, cuffed (6.0 to 9.0)
- Water-soluble lubricant   ■ Towel or other padding
- Colorimetric end-tidal carbon dioxide detector
- Syringes (10 mL, 20 mL)
- Endotracheal tube holder or tape
- Stethoscope   ■ Suction device and tubing
- Suction catheter
  • Rigid wand (Yankauer type)   • Flexible catheter

Equipment that may be helpful:
- Pulse oximeter   ■ Spare bulb, batteries
- End-tidal carbon dioxide meter

Indications

- Conscious, breathing patients or patients with an intact gag reflex

Contraindications

- Nonbreathing patients or patients with poor ventilatory effort
- Facial trauma or head injuries with evidence of nasal bleeding or discharge

Complications

- Nasal bleeding is a frequent and expected complication. This is not, however, an indication to discontinue the procedure.
- Unrecognized esophageal or right mainstem intubations will have serious or fatal effects.

Procedures

 Ensure body substance isolation before beginning procedures.

Prior to beginning patient care, appropriate body substance isolation procedures should be employed.

▼

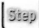 Place patient on high-flow oxygen by nonrebreathing mask.

Assess the adequacy of the patient's ventilations. Place the patient on high-flow oxygen by nonrebreathing mask. Explain the procedure to the patient and inquire about nasal surgery or injury.

▼

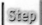 Select and check equipment.

Gather and assemble the endotracheal tube (sized for the patient's nares), water-soluble jelly, bag-mask device with appropriate mask, oxygen delivery system, suction unit with catheters, spare endotracheal tube, laryngoscope handle, and laryngoscope blade. Check that all equipment is in working order.

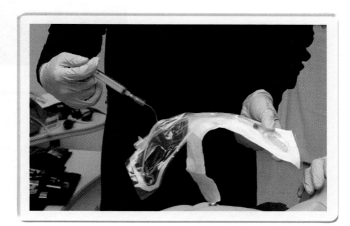

Consider the administration of phenylephrine into each naris to lessen the possibility of bleeding.

▼

Remove oxygen mask and keep patient's neck in a neutral position.

Remove the oxygen mask from the patient and keep the patient's neck in a neutral position.

▼

 Insert endotracheal tube into naris.

With water-soluble jelly applied to the end of the endotracheal tube, carefully insert it into the naris. The bevel of the tube should be placed against the patient's septum and inserted straight down (perpendicular to the face) into the nasal cavity. A slight twisting motion will facilitate the entry. If the entry is difficult, remove and reattempt on the opposite side. When the tube is through the nasopharynx, the sound of air movement should be heard through the tube.

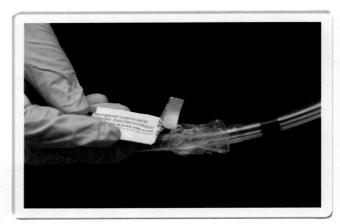

▼

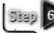

Step 6 Listen to the air movement through tube and place the tube through the cords.

Listening to the air movement through the tube, establish the respiratory rhythm. As the patient takes a breath (telling the patient to take a deep breath is often helpful), quickly insert the tube through the cords. A slight cough should be felt. The tube should rest with the hub at the nose.

Commercially made whistle devices are available to assist in hearing the patient's ventilations. If a whistle is used, it must be removed quickly after the tube is placed in the trachea.

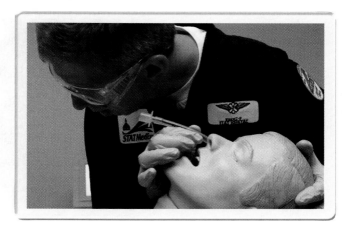

Step 7 Inflate cuff to the proper pressure and immediately disconnect syringe.

Inflate the distal cuff of the endotracheal tube with 5 to 10 mL of air. Most patients will need less than the full 10 mL to fill the cuff. Remove the syringe from the inflation port.

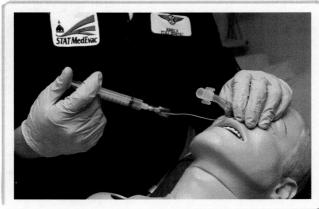

Step 8 ▷ **Confirm tube placement by auscultation.**

Auscultate the movement of air through the tube. The use of an end-tidal carbon dioxide meter is often helpful. Because this is a breathing patient, ventilation may not be necessary to assess breath sounds because air movement though the tube is evidence of passing the tube through the cords. Auscultation will determine the proper depth and confirm that the right bronchus is not intubated.

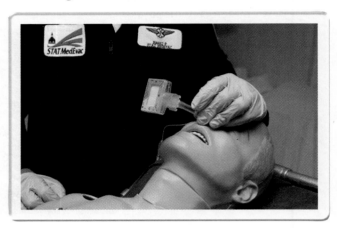

▼

Step 9 ▷ **Secure the endotracheal tube.**

Using tape or umbilical cord tape, secure the tube to the patient. The proper depth should be ensured by taping or tying the tube at the level of the naris.

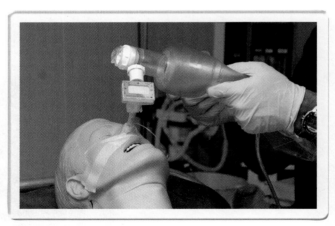

▼

Step 10 Ensure tube placement by additional means and apply extrication collar.

Reassess tube placement through assessment of gastric and breath sounds. At least two additional means of ensuring tube placement should be used. These include:

- End-tidal carbon dioxide meters
- Fogging of the endotracheal tube
- Esophageal detectors
- Capnographic monitors

Finally, when placement is ensured, an appropriately sized extrication collar should be applied to maintain the position of the head and neck and thus the airway.

All findings should be verbalized so that all members of the team are aware of the airway status.

Even though the tube's placement has been ensured, continual reassessment should occur. This should be performed any time the patient is moved or defibrillated. Also, always ensure and document the tube placement before turning over patient care at the receiving facility or to a transport team.

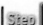 **Step 11 Assess ventilatory effort and provide assistance as needed.**

Assess the patient to determine if his or her own ventilatory effort is sufficient. As long as the patient can breathe at a consistent rate and volume without increased effort, there is no need for assisted ventilations. Additional oxygen can be delivered by attaching a T-bar. If the patient is having difficulty with ventilatory effort or if ventilatory effort is slow or absent, attach a bag-mask device and begin assisted ventilations at a rate and depth appropriate for the patient.

In the Field

Inhaling the Tube

Nasal intubation requires that the patient be breathing with an adequate volume. Although it is the paramedic who wields the endotracheal tube, it is the patient who actually places the tube. Through the patient's own breathing action, the tube is literally inhaled into the trachea. Obviously, the more effective, deep, and frequent the patient's breaths, the easier the process of nasotracheal intubation.

Laryngoscopy and Use of Magill Forceps

Performance Objective

Given an adult patient and appropriate equipment, the candidate shall apply direct laryngoscopy to visualize a foreign object in the airway and remove the foreign object using Magill forceps using the criteria herein prescribed, in 2 minutes or less.

Equipment

The following equipment is required to perform this skill:
- Appropriate body substance isolation/personal protective equipment
- Oxygen cylinder, regulator, and key
- Oxygen delivery device (appropriate to patient)
  - Bag-mask device
- Oropharyngeal airway (adult sized)
- Laryngoscope handle and blades (straight and curved)
- Magill forceps
- Endotracheal tubes, cuffed (6.0 to 9.0)
- Malleable intubation stylet (appropriate size for endotracheal tube)
- Water-soluble lubricant
- Towel or other padding
- Colorimetric end-tidal carbon dioxide detector
- Syringes (10 mL, 20 mL)
- Endotracheal tube holder or tape
- Stethoscope
- Suction device and tubing
- Suction catheter
  - Rigid wand (Yankauer type)
  - Flexible catheter

Equipment that may be helpful:
- Pulse oximeter
- Spare bulb, batteries
- End-tidal carbon dioxide meter

Indications

- Foreign body airway obstruction
- Foreign object removal from hypopharynx

Contraindications

- None

Complications

- Damage to hypopharynx or larynx
- Delays in removal may lead to anoxic injury

Procedures

Note: This procedure is usually performed as a part of standard intubation or when a known foreign body airway obstruction is highly suspected. In either case, it is assumed that proper airway and ventilation procedures and patient preparation have already been performed.

  Ensure body substance isolation before beginning procedures.

Prior to beginning patient care, appropriate body substance isolation procedures should be employed.

▼

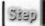 **Position head properly.**

Gently extend the patient's neck so that the head is positioned with the chin and forehead approximately 45° from the floor.

▼

  Insert blade while displacing tongue, lift mandible, and visualize larynx without using teeth as a fulcrum.

Carefully insert the blade of the laryngoscope into the patient's mouth to the depth of the uvula. Using a sweeping motion, move the patient's tongue to the left as you lift at a 45° angle along the facial plane to lift the mandible, keeping the laryngoscope off of the teeth.

Lifting should be performed with a free hand. The habit of resting or placing the left forearm against the patient's forehead frequently causes prying and can be a dangerous practice. Placing the forearm in this position greatly limits and potentially eliminates the ability to lift the patient's lower jaw and tongue. In effect, it promotes the use of the teeth as a fulcrum as the only lifting option.

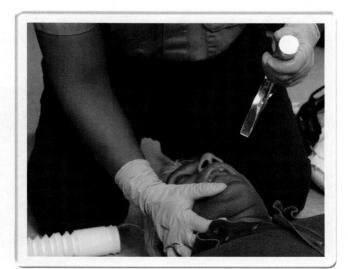

▼

Step **4** ▶ Visualize the foreign object and grasp using the Magill forceps.

Visualize the foreign object in the hypopharynx. With the Magill forceps in the right hand, reach into the patient's mouth to grasp the foreign object.

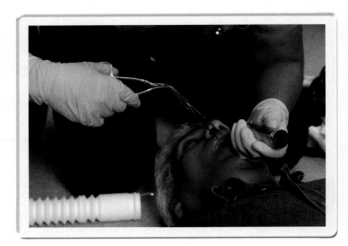

Occasionally the object is found past the vocal cords. In these cases extreme caution should be used to reach past the vocal cords to grasp the object. This is an extremely risky procedure and should be weighed against the possibility to perform a cricothyrotomy. As you make this decision, remember that the cricothyroid membrane is just below the vocal cords. There is a possibility that the object may interfere with the procedure.

▼

Step **5** ▶ Remove the object with Magill forceps.

With the foreign object held firmly in the Magill forceps, carefully pull the object from the hypopharynx. It may be necessary to rotate the object if resistance is felt or if the object has passed through the vocal cords.

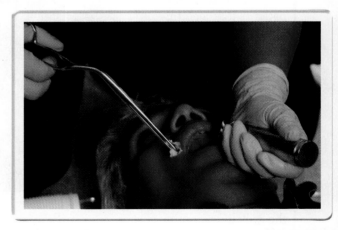

▼

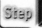 **6** **Visualize hypopharynx.**

With the laryngoscope still in place, visualize the hypopharynx to ensure that all pieces of the foreign object have been removed. Small pieces of the foreign object ventilated into the patient can cause complications later on. Removal of the remaining pieces of the foreign object may require you to use the Magill forceps or a rigid suction catheter.

▼

7 **Attempt ventilation of the patient.**

Following standard procedures of bag-mask ventilation, attempt to ventilate the patient. If the patient can be ventilated, continue ventilating the patient at the appropriate rate and depth while further assessment is performed.

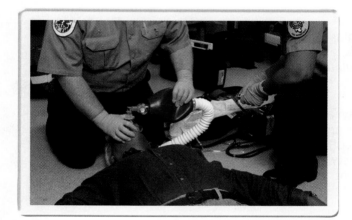

In-Line Endotracheal Intubation

Performance Objective

Given an adult patient with the potential for cervical spine injury and appropriate equipment, the candidate shall insert an endotracheal tube using in-line stabilization and verify proper placement using criteria herein prescribed, in 8 minutes or less.

Equipment

The following equipment is required to perform this skill:
- Appropriate body substance isolation/personal protective equipment
- Oxygen cylinder, regulator, and key
- Oxygen delivery device (appropriate to patient)
  - Bag-mask device
- Oropharyngeal airway (adult sized)
- Laryngoscope handle and blades (straight and curved)
- Endotracheal tubes, cuffed (6.0 to 9.0)
- Malleable intubation stylet (appropriate size for endotracheal tube)
- Water-soluble lubricant   ■ Towel or other padding
- Colorimetric end-tidal carbon dioxide detector
- Syringes (10 mL, 20 mL)
- Endotracheal tube holder or tape
- Stethoscope   ■ Suction device and tubing
- Suction catheter
  - Rigid wand (Yankauer type)   • Flexible catheter

Equipment that may be helpful:
- Pulse oximeter   ■ Spare bulb, batteries
- End-tidal carbon dioxide meter

Indications

- Ensure definitive airway in the patient with known or suspected cervical spine injury

Contraindications

- None

Complications

- Unrecognized and uncorrected esophageal intubation
- Right mainstem bronchial intubation
- Laryngeal injury   ■ Dental injury
- Injury to the cervical spine/paralysis

Procedures

 Step 1 ▶ **Ensure body substance isolation before beginning procedures.**

Prior to beginning patient care, appropriate body substance isolation procedures should be employed.

▼

 Step 2 ▶ **Open the airway manually.**

Open the airway using a jaw-thrust maneuver (see Skill 1). In the event that the airway cannot be opened using the jaw-thrust maneuver, open the patient's airway by performing the head tilt–chin lift maneuver (see Skill 3). Remember that it is more important for the patient to have an airway than for the patient to have a straight neck. In many cases, it is appropriate to apply an extrication collar.

▼

 Step 3 ▶ **Elevate the patient's tongue and appropriately insert simple adjunct (see Skill 7).**

Measuring from the corner of the mouth to the base of the earlobe, choose the correct-sized airway for your patient.

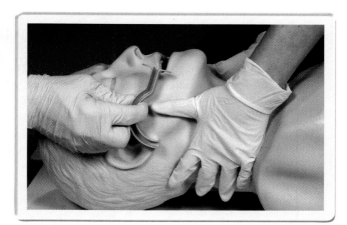

Open the mouth using the jaw-thrust or cross-finger technique. Insert the airway in front of the mouth with its tip pointed toward the roof of the mouth, or insert it from the side of the mouth with its tip toward the inside of the cheek.

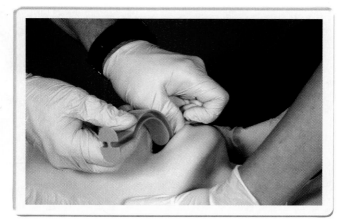

In the Field

Effectiveness of In-Line Intubation

This technique represents one of several techniques that have been introduced in the prehospital environment for the purpose of intubating the patient with a potential cervical spine injury. Practitioners may prefer one technique to others, some of which require extreme acrobatics and balance. It is important to be aware that *none* of the techniques have been proven to prevent the movement of the cervical spine. Each person who performs this or other techniques should take extreme care to limit the movement of the cervical spine.

Step **3** continued

Rotate the airway as it is inserted until the flange rests on the patient's lips.

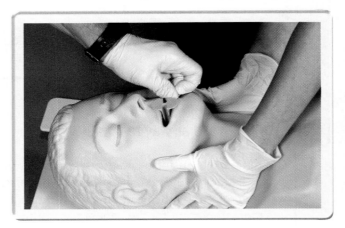

A tongue depressor can be used to hold the tongue inferior and the airway inserted tip down. If the patient starts to gag, remove the airway by pulling the flange anterior and inferior.

Step **4** Ventilate the patient immediately with bag-mask device.

Begin ventilations immediately with a bag-mask device. If the bag-mask device is not already attached to oxygen, begin ventilations with room air.

Select the appropriate-sized bag for the patient. Bag and mask sizes are normally listed as adult, child, and infant. These sizes are adequate for the average-sized person who meets the age definition criteria. However, large children will require a bag that will deliver the appropriate volume. Likewise, pediatric bags may be appropriate for small adults or adults where overpressurization can cause pulmonary damage. Masks should be chosen to fit the patient without air leakage.

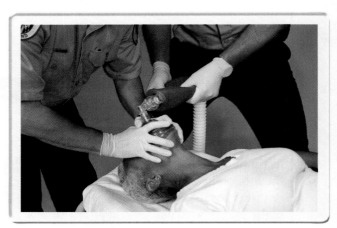

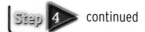 **Step 4** continued

Position the mask with the apex over the bridge of the nose and the base between the lower lip and the prominence of the chin. Begin ventilations as soon as the mask is sealed, and assess the mask for air leakage.

Begin ventilations at a rate of 10 to 12 breaths/min, with a tidal volume that achieves chest rise. Pay close attention to ensure that each ventilation is of the appropriate volume and of a consistent rate. Allow adequate exhalation between each breath.

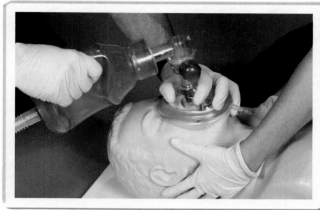

Effective ventilations are those breaths that cause the chest to rise adequately for the size of the patient. Be cautious not to overventilate. Each ventilation should be delivered slowly and easily, lasting approximately 1 second. Fast and high-pressure ventilations can cause air to enter the stomach, increasing the risk of vomiting.

If a second rescuer is available, the Sellick maneuver (cricoid pressure) may be applied. Assisting personnel can also attach a pulse oximeter.

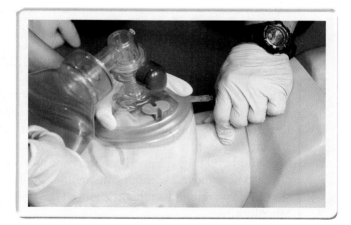

Although it will be necessary to stop ventilations for assessment and other procedures, you should never allow a nonbreathing patient to go without ventilations for more than 30 seconds.

Step 5 ▶ **Attach oxygen reservoir and connect to high-flow oxygen regulator.**

If not previously performed, attach oxygen tubing to the inlet on the bag-mask device and to the oxygen source. Open the cylinder valve and adjust the liter flow between 12 and 15 L/min (see Skill 4).

▼

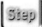 **Step 6** ▶ **Ventilate patient at a rate of 10 to 12 breaths/min with appropriate volumes.**

Continue ventilations at a rate of 10 to 12 breaths/min, and ensure adequate chest rise with each ventilation.

Ventilations should be associated with capnometry. The rate of ventilation should be adjusted to achieve a capnometry reading of between 35 and 45 mm Hg. In patients with head injuries, the reading should be 35 to 39 mm Hg. To drive the patient's carbon dioxide level, follow the reading. If the end-tidal carbon dioxide is too high, ventilate faster. If the reading is too low, ventilate slower.

Consider checking breath sounds. Knowing the status of breath sounds before tube placement can be helpful when determining the correct position.

▼

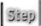 **Step 7** ▶ **Direct assistant to take over ventilations.**

Direct a qualified assistant to take over ventilations at a rate of 10 to 12 breaths/min with appropriate volumes, and ensure adequate chest rise with each ventilation.

▼

 Step 8 ▶ **Select, check, and prepare the equipment.**

While the patient is being ventilated, the person responsible for the intubation must ensure that all the necessary equipment is available and in working order. Ensure that the endotracheal tube is the proper size for the patient.

Using an aseptic technique, insert an intubation stylet into the endotracheal tube and bend it into a gentle curve. A properly curved stylet will allow the stylet to be removed without causing the tip of the tube to move. The stylet should be positioned so that the end of the stylet does not extend past the Murphy's eye.

Assemble the laryngoscope with the desired blade and check the brightness of the bulb. A bright white light is best for all intubations. A yellow or dull light will cause the tissues of the hypopharynx to take on similar color schemes and result in difficulties visualizing landmarks and the vocal cords. Make sure the light is turned off until the laryngoscope is placed in the patient's mouth.

Attach a 10-mL syringe to the endotracheal tube cuff port, and inflate it until the balloon is tight (this may take less than 10 mL of air) and check for leaks. Remove the air from the cuff and remove the syringe. Place the syringe next to

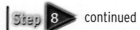
continued

the patient's head. Leaving the syringe attached to the endotracheal tube can cause tearing and detachment of the balloon tubing, resulting in leaks from the cuff. There is also the possibility that the syringe may slip off and become lost. It is better to get in the habit of always removing the syringe and placing it at the patient's head.

Prepare for the intubation by placing a 1″ pad under the patient's head. This will assist in lining up the three planes of the patient's airway. Although this step will make intubation easier, it is not required and is often difficult to accomplish in the prehospital setting. It is a good practice to learn to intubate both with and without the 1″ pad.

Finally, always ensure that suction is available and working before beginning intubation. Both a rigid suction tip and a flexible catheter, appropriate for the size of the endotracheal tube, should be available.

▼

 Hold the patient's neck and direct partner to manually maintain neutral position.

Kneeling or sitting at the patient's head, place your thighs in position to hold the patient's head while you intubate. Your thighs will be used to control the movement of the patient's cervical spine.

Instruct your partner to stop ventilating and remove the mask from the bag-mask device. Your partner should then hold the patient's head and neck in a neutral position.

Remove the oral airway from the patient and place it within reach. Be prepared to reinsert it as a bite block at the end of this procedure.

▼

Step 10 ▶ **Insert blade while displacing tongue, lift mandible, and visualize larynx without using teeth as a fulcrum.**

Carefully insert the blade of the laryngoscope into the patient's mouth to the depth of the uvula. Using a sweeping motion, move the patient's tongue to the left as you lift at a 45° angle along the facial plane to lift the mandible, keeping the laryngoscope off of the teeth.

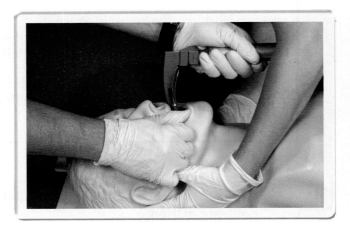

Lifting should be performed by leaning backward. With your thighs holding the patient's neck, leaning backward will give a clear view of the hypopharynx and the vocal cords.

▼

Step 11 Introduce the endotracheal tube and advance it to the proper depth.

Upon visualization of the vocal cords, pass the tube through the cords and into the trachea. As the cuff of the tube passes the cords, stop the insertion process and maintain its position. Usually this will place the tube at a depth of 22 to 24 cm at the patient's teeth. This is roughly three times the diameter of the tube. Be sure to document the position of the tube relative to the teeth.

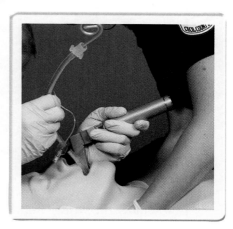

If after two attempts you are unable to perform endotracheal intubation, strongly consider using an alternative airway device or procedure.

▼

 Step 12 Remove the laryngoscope from the patient's mouth and remove the stylet from the endotracheal tube.

Remove the laryngoscope from the patient's mouth. Remove the stylet from the endotracheal tube.

▼

Step 13 ▶ **Inflate the distal cuff to proper pressure and immediately disconnect the syringe.**

Inflate the distal cuff of the endotracheal tube with 5 to 10 mL of air. Most patients will need less than the full 10 mL to fill the cuff.

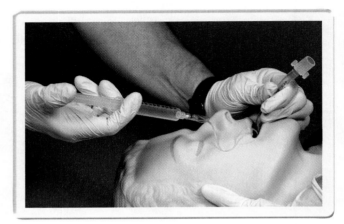

Remove the syringe from the inflation port.

▼

Step 14 ▶ **Attach a colorimetric end-tidal carbon dioxide detector.**

Attach a colorimetric end-tidal carbon dioxide detector to the endotracheal tube.

▼

Step 15 ▶ **Direct ventilation of the patient.**

While still holding the tube in place, have your partner attach the bag-mask device to the endotracheal tube and begin ventilations. Instruct your partner to deliver breaths as you move your stethoscope over the patient's abdomen and chest.

▼

16 **Confirm proper placement by auscultation over the epigastrium and bilaterally over each lung.**

Auscultate the abdomen and the chest to determine the correct tube placement. The preferred sequence is to listen over the gastric region first, then over the lower left, upper left, upper right, and finally the lower right chest. By using this sequence, you can determine incorrect placement with a minimal amount of unnecessary ventilations. After confirming the placement, move to the next step.

If air is heard over the epigastric region, remove the tube and begin ventilating the patient with a bag-mask device. Some practitioners prefer to leave endotracheal tubes in the esophagus upon finding missed intubation, preferring instead to intubate around this first tube. Their philosophy is that this reduces the chances of missing a second time. However, this may confuse the landmarks and definitely limits the visibility in the hypopharynx. A problem of inefficient ventilations is also created.

Absent breath sounds on the left are an indication of right mainstem intubation. Deflate the cuff. Gently and carefully pull back on the endotracheal tube until breath sounds are heard over the left chest. Reinflate the cuff. Note and document the tube's position in relation to the teeth.

▼

 17 **Secure the endotracheal tube.**

Maintaining a hold on the tube, attach a commercially made endotracheal tube holder. Commercially made devices are preferred over other techniques because they provide the most effective control of the airway. These devices also eliminate the need for an oral airway because they include a bite block.

If a commercially made device is not available, secure the endotracheal tube using tape. Begin by encircling the tube with tape at the level of the patient's teeth. Wrap the tape around the patient's neck, and again encircle the tape around the tube at the level of the patient's teeth. Ensure that you have not placed undue pressure on the vessels of the neck by placing the tape over the prominence of the anterior mandible. Insert an oropharyngeal airway to prevent the patient from biting the tube (see Skill 7).

In-hospital surgical and anesthesia personnel may apply tape only to the side of the patient's cheek. This is a poor practice for prehospital intubations. Patients in the operating room are intubated briefly and are moved very little. Because patients who are intubated in the prehospital setting will be lifted, pulled and pushed, transported at high speed, wheeled on a stretcher, and face the miscommunications of movement attempts, this technique is not recommended.

▼

Step **Ensure placement by additional means and apply an extrication collar.**

Reassess the tube placement through assessment of gastric and breath sounds. At least two additional means of ensuring tube placement should be used. These include the following:

- Visualization of the tube passing between the cords
- End-tidal carbon dioxide meters
- Fogging of the endotracheal tube
- Esophageal detectors
- Capnographic monitors

When proper placement is ensured, an appropriately sized extrication collar should be applied to maintain the position of the head and neck and thus the airway.

All findings should be verbalized so that all members of the team are aware of the patient's airway status.

Even though the tube's placement has been ensured, continual reassessment should occur. This should be performed any time the patient is moved or defibrillated. Also, always ensure and document the tube placement before turning over patient care at the receiving facility or to a transport team.

Digital Intubation

Performance Objective

Given an adult patient and appropriate equipment, the candidate shall insert an endotracheal tube and verify proper placement using criteria herein prescribed, in 8 minutes or less using a digital procedure.

Equipment

The following equipment is required to perform this skill:
- Appropriate body substance isolation/personal protective equipment
- Oxygen cylinder, regulator, and key
- Oxygen delivery device (appropriate to patient)
  - Bag-mask device
- Oropharyngeal airway (adult sized)
- Endotracheal tubes, cuffed (6.0 to 9.0)
- Malleable intubation stylet (appropriate size for endotracheal tube)
- Water-soluble lubricant
- Towel or other padding
- Colorimetric end-tidal carbon dioxide detector
- Syringes (10 mL, 20 mL)
- Endotracheal tube holder or tape
- Stethoscope
- Suction device and tubing
- Suction catheter
  - Rigid wand (Yankauer type)   • Flexible catheter

Equipment that may be helpful:
- Pulse oximeter   ■ Spare bulb, batteries
- End-tidal carbon dioxide meter

Indications

- Physical environment precludes the use of standard laryngoscopy

Contraindications

- Gag reflex
- Any condition above total unresponsiveness

Complications

- Oropharyngeal and hypopharyngeal trauma

Procedures

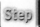 **Ensure body substance isolation before beginning procedures.**

Prior to beginning patient care, appropriate body substance isolation procedures should be employed.

▼

 Open the airway manually.

Before opening the airway, consider the possibility of cervical spine injury. If spinal injury is suspected, use a jaw-thrust maneuver to open the airway (see Skill 1). If no spinal cord injury is suspected, open the patient's airway by performing the head tilt–chin lift maneuver (see Skill 3).

▼

 **Elevate the patient's tongue and appropriately insert simple adjunct (see Skill 7).**

Measuring from the corner of the mouth to the base of the earlobe, choose the correct-sized airway for your patient.

Open the mouth using the jaw-thrust or cross-finger technique. Insert the airway in front of the mouth with its tip pointed toward the roof of the mouth, or insert it from the side of the mouth with its tip toward the inside of the cheek; rotate the airway as it is inserted until the flange rests on the patient's lips.

A tongue depressor can be used to hold the tongue inferior and the airway inserted tip down. If the patient starts to gag, remove the airway by pulling the flange anterior and inferior.

▼

Ventilate the patient immediately with bag-mask device.

Begin ventilations immediately with a bag-mask device. If the bag-mask device is not already attached to oxygen, begin ventilations with room air.

Select the appropriate-sized bag for the patient. Bag and mask sizes are normally listed as adult, child, and infant. These sizes are adequate for the average-sized person who meets the age definition criteria. However, large children will require a bag that will deliver the appropriate volume. Likewise, pediatric bags may be appropriate for small adults or adults where overpressurization can cause pulmonary damage. Masks should be chosen to fit the patient without air leakage.

Position the mask with the apex over the bridge of the nose and the base between the lower lip and the prominence of the chin. Begin ventilations as soon as the mask is sealed, and assess the mask for air leakage.

Begin ventilations at a rate of 10 to 12 breaths/min, with a tidal volume that achieves chest rise. Pay close attention to ensure that each ventilation is of the appropriate volume and of a consistent rate. Allow adequate exhalation between each breath.

Effective ventilations are those breaths that cause the chest to rise adequately for the size of the patient. Be cautious not to overventilate. Each ventilation should be delivered slowly and easily, lasting approximately 1 second. Fast and high-pressure ventilations can cause air to enter the stomach, increasing the risk of vomiting.

If a second rescuer is available, the Sellick maneuver (cricoid pressure) may be applied. Assisting personnel can also attach a pulse oximeter.

Although it will be necessary to stop ventilations for assessment and other procedures, you should never allow a nonbreathing patient to go without ventilations for longer than 30 seconds.

▼

 Attach oxygen reservoir and connect to high-flow oxygen regulator.

If not previously performed, attach oxygen tubing to the inlet on the bag-mask device and to the oxygen source. Open the cylinder valve and adjust liter flow to between 12 and 15 L/min (see Skill 4).

▼

Step 6 ▶ Ventilate the patient at a rate of 10 to 12 breaths/min with appropriate volumes.

Continue ventilations at a rate of 10 to 12 breaths/min, and ensure adequate chest rise with each ventilation.

Ventilations should be associated with capnometry. The rate of ventilation should be adjusted to achieve a capnometry reading of between 35 and 45 mm Hg. In patients with head injuries, the reading should be 35 to 39 mm Hg. To drive the patient's carbon dioxide level, follow the reading. If the end-tidal carbon dioxide is too high, ventilate faster. If the reading is too low, ventilate slower.

Consider checking breath sounds. Knowing the status of breath sounds before tube placement can be helpful when determining the correct position.

▼

Step 7 ▶ Direct assistant to take over ventilations.

Direct a qualified assistant to take over ventilations at a rate of 10 to 12 breaths/min with appropriate volumes, and ensure adequate chest rise with each ventilation.

▼

Step 8 ▶ Select, check, and prepare the equipment.

While the patient is being ventilated, the person responsible for the intubation must ensure that all the necessary equipment is available and in working order. Ensure that the endotracheal tube is the proper size for the patient.

Using an aseptic technique, insert an intubation stylet into the endotracheal tube and bend into a gentle curve. A properly curved stylet will allow the stylet to be removed without causing the tip of the tube to move. The stylet should be positioned so that the end of the stylet does not extend past the Murphy's eye. Form the endotracheal tube into a J by grasping the lower one third and folding the rest over the top of the hand. The top third should then be bent sideways to form a handle.

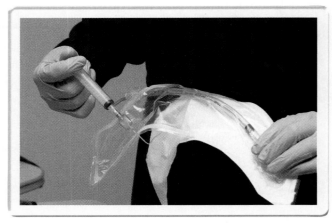

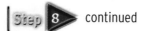 **8** continued

Attach a 10-mL syringe to the endotracheal tube cuff port and inflate until the balloon is tight (this may take less than 10 mL) and check for leaks. Remove the air from the cuff and remove the syringe. Place the syringe next to the patient's head. Leaving the syringe attached to the endotracheal tube can cause tearing and detachment of the balloon tubing, resulting in leaks from the cuff. There is also the possibility that the syringe may slip off and become lost. It is better to get in the habit of always removing the syringe and placing it at the patient's head.

If the patient is dehydrated, has been down a long time, or is otherwise dry, lubricating jelly may be applied to the end of the endotracheal tube.

Finally, always ensure that suction is available and working before beginning intubation. Both a rigid suction tip and a flexible catheter, appropriate for the size of the endotracheal tube, should be available.

▼

Step 9 Position the patient's head properly.

Have your assistant stop ventilations and remove the mask from the bag-mask device. You will now have only 20 to 30 seconds to position the patient, place the endotracheal tube, and reestablish ventilations. Should you fail to intubate the patient, your assistant should quickly place the mask back on the bag-mask device and begin ventilating the patient.

Gently extend the patient's neck so that the head is positioned with the chin and forehead approximately 45° from the floor. In the event the patient has had an injury to the neck or for other reasons cannot be hyperextended, refer to the procedures for in-line endotracheal intubation (Skill 15). For your own safety, it is best to place a bite block between the patient's molars. This will prevent the patient from biting during awakening or during a seizure.

▼

Step **Insert fingers and locate epiglottis.**

Place the first two fingers of your left hand into the patient's mouth. Locate the epiglottis with your middle finger. Your index finger will be used to guide the endotracheal tube into the larynx.

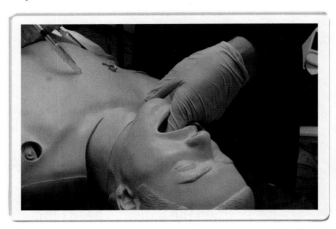

Step **Introduce endotracheal tube and advance it to the proper depth.**

Place the endotracheal tube into the patient's mouth and guide it into the hypopharynx using a hooking motion. With your index finger, guide the end of the endotracheal tube through the vocal cords and advance it into the trachea. When properly seated, gently straighten the endotracheal tube and remove the stylet.

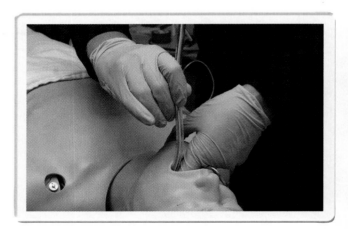

Advance the endotracheal tube so it rests at the appropriate depth. Usually this will place the tube at a depth of 22 to 24 cm at the patient's teeth. This is roughly three times the diameter of the tube.

Step 12 ▶ **Inflate cuff to proper pressure and immediately disconnect syringe.**

Attach a 10-mL syringe to the cuff port and inflate until the balloon is firm or a maximum of 10 mL has been placed. Most patients will need less than the full 10 mL to fill the cuff. Remove the syringe from the port.

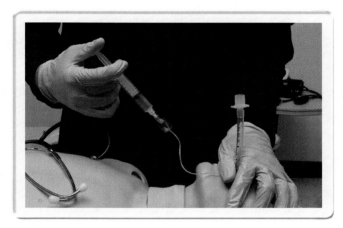

▼

 Step 13 ▶ **Attach a colorimetric end-tidal carbon dioxide detector.**

Attach a colorimetric end-tidal carbon dioxide detector to the endotracheal tube.

▼

 Step 14 ▶ **Direct ventilation of the patient.**

While still holding the tube in place, have your partner attach the bag-mask device to the endotracheal tube and begin ventilations. Instruct your partner to deliver breaths as you move your stethoscope over the patient's abdomen and chest.

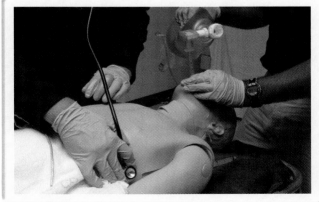

▼

Confirm proper placement by auscultation over the epigastrium and bilaterally over each lung.

Auscultate the abdomen and the chest to determine correct tube placement. The preferred sequence is to listen over the gastric region first, then over the lower left, upper left, upper right, and finally the lower right chest. By using this sequence, you can determine incorrect placement with a minimal amount of unnecessary and useless ventilations. After confirming placement, move to the next step.

If air is heard over the epigastric region, remove the tube and begin ventilating the patient with a bag-mask device. Some practitioners prefer to leave endotracheal tubes in the esophagus upon finding missed intubation, preferring instead to intubate around this first tube. Their philosophy is that this reduces the chances of missing a second time. However, this may confuse the landmarks and definitely limits the visibility in the hypopharynx. A problem of inefficient ventilations is also created.

Absent breath sounds on the left are an indication of right mainstem intubation. Deflate the cuff. Gently and carefully pull back on the endotracheal tube until breath sounds are heard over the left chest. Reinflate the cuff. Note and document the tube's placement in relation to the teeth.

Step 16 Secure the endotracheal tube.

Maintaining a hold on the tube, attach a commercially made endotracheal tube holder. Commercially made devices are preferred over other techniques because they provide the most effective control of the airway. These devices also eliminate the need for an oral airway because they include a bite block.

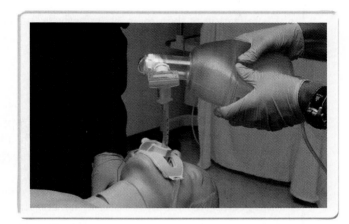

If a commercially made device is not available, secure the endotracheal tube using tape. If you have secured the endotracheal tube using tape, place a bite block in the patient's mouth. Begin by encircling the tube with tape at the level of the patient's teeth. Wrap the tape around the patient's neck, and again encircle the tape around the tube at the level of the patient's teeth. Ensure that you have not placed undue pressure on the vessels of the neck by placing the tape over the prominence of the anterior mandible. Insert an oropharyngeal airway to prevent the patient from biting the tube.

In-hospital surgical and anesthesia personnel may apply tape only to the side of the patient's cheek to secure the endotracheal tube. This is a poor practice for prehospital intubations. Patients in the operating room are intubated briefly and are moved very little. Because patients who are intubated in the prehospital setting will be lifted, pulled and pushed, transported at high speed, wheeled on a stretcher, and face the miscommunications of movement attempts, this technique is not recommended.

▼

 **Ensure placement by additional means and apply an extrication collar.**

Reassess tube placement through assessment of gastric and breath sounds. At least two additional means of ensuring tube placement should be used. These include:

- Visualization of the tube passing between the cords
- End-tidal carbon dioxide meters
- Fogging of the endotracheal tube
- Esophageal detectors
- Capnographic monitors

Finally, when placement is ensured, an appropriately sized extrication collar should be applied to maintain position of the head and neck and thus the airway.

All findings should be verbalized so that all members of the team are aware of the airway status.

Even though the tube's placement has been ensured, continual reassessment should occur. This should be performed any time the patient is moved or defibrillated. Also, always ensure and document the tube placement before turning over patient care at the receiving facility or to a transport team.

Dual-Lumen Airway Devices

Performance Objective

Given an adult patient and appropriate equipment, the candidate shall insert a dual-lumen airway and verify proper placement using criteria herein prescribed, in 6 minutes or less.

Equipment

The following equipment is required to perform this skill:
- Appropriate body substance isolation/personal protective equipment
- Oxygen cylinder, regulator, and key
- Oxygen delivery device (appropriate to patient)
  - Bag-mask device
- Oropharyngeal airway (adult sizes)   ■ Water-soluble lubricant
- Dual-lumen airway
  - Combitube   • KING LT-D*
  - Pharyngeotracheal lumen (PtL) airway
- Syringes (sizes 20 mL to 100 mL; usually included in kit with airway)
- Endotracheal tube holder or tape
- Suction device and tubing   ■ Stethoscope
- Colorimetric end-tidal carbon dioxide detector
- Suction catheter
  - Rigid wand (Yankauer type)   • Flexible catheter

Equipment that may be helpful:
- Pulse oximeter   ■ End-tidal carbon dioxide meter

*The KING LT-D airway is not dual-lumen. However, it is included here because it is an alternative airway device with similar placement and procedures to true dual-lumen airways.

Indications

- Failed attempt at endotracheal intubation or difficult anatomy
- Confined space airway control
- Advanced airway care not immediately available

Contraindications

- Intact gag reflex
- Esophageal disease
- Ingestion of caustic (acid/alkali) substance
- Patients with laryngeal edema from anaphylaxis, respiratory burns, or other causes

Complications

- Sore throat
- Dysphagia
- Laryngeal occlusion (if airway is placed too deep)
- Esophageal hemorrhage/rupture
- Upper airway bleeding

Procedures

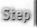 **Ensure body substance isolation before beginning procedures.**

Prior to beginning patient care, appropriate body substance isolation procedures should be employed.

 **Open the airway manually.**

Before opening the airway, consider the possibility of cervical spine injury. If spinal injury is suspected, use a jaw-thrust maneuver to open the airway (see Skill 1).

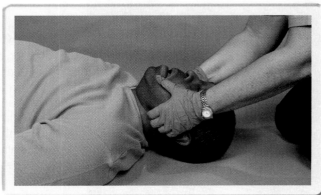

If no spinal cord injury is suspected, open the patient's airway by performing the head tilt–chin lift maneuver (see Skill 3).

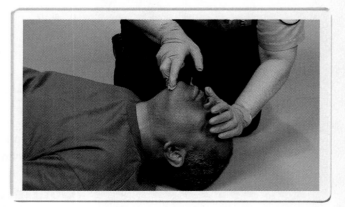

Step 3 Elevate tongue and appropriately insert simple adjunct (see Skill 7).

Measuring from the corner of the mouth to the base of the earlobe, choose the correct-sized airway for your patient. Open the mouth using the jaw-thrust or cross-finger technique. Insert the airway in the front of the mouth with the tip pointed toward the roof of the mouth, or insert the airway from the side of the mouth with the tip toward the inside of the cheek. A tongue depressor can be used to hold the tongue inferior and the airway inserted tip down. If the patient starts to gag, remove the airway by pulling the flange anterior and inferior. If a gag reflex remains, dual-lumen placement is contraindicated.

▼

Step 4 Ventilate the patient immediately with bag-mask device.

Begin ventilations immediately with a bag-mask device. If the bag-mask device is not already attached to oxygen, begin ventilations with room air.

Select the appropriate-sized bag for the patient. Bag and mask sizes are normally listed as adult, child, and infant. These sizes are adequate for the average-sized person who meets the age definition criteria. However, large children will require a bag that will deliver the appropriate volume. Likewise, pediatric bags may be appropriate for small adults or adults in whom overpressurization could cause pulmonary damage. Masks should be chosen to fit the patient without air leakage.

Position the mask with the apex over the bridge of the nose and the base between the lower lip and the prominence of the chin. Begin ventilations as soon as the mask is sealed, and assess the mask for air leakage.

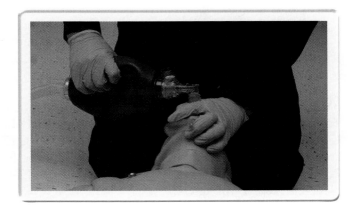

Begin ventilations at a rate of 10 to 12 breaths/min with a tidal volume that achieves chest rise. Pay close attention to ensure that each ventilation is of the appropriate volume and of a consistent rate. Allow adequate exhalation between each breath.

Effective ventilations are those breaths that cause the chest to rise adequately for the size of the patient. In addition to assessing chest rise, consider checking breath sounds. Be cautious not to overventilate. Each ventilation should be delivered slowly and easily, lasting approximately 1 second. Fast and high-pressure ventilations can cause air to enter the stomach, increasing the risk of vomiting.

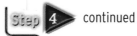 continued

If a second rescuer is available, the Sellick maneuver (cricoid pressure) may be applied. Assisting personnel can also attach a pulse oximeter.

Although it will be necessary to stop ventilations for assessment and other procedures, you should never allow a nonbreathing patient to go without ventilations for longer than 30 seconds.

▼

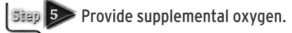

Step 5 Provide supplemental oxygen.

If not previously performed, attach oxygen tubing to the inlet on the bag-mask device and to the oxygen source. Open the cylinder valve and adjust liter flow to between 12 and 15 L/min (see Skill 4).

▼

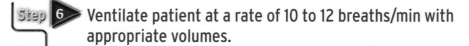

Step 6 Ventilate patient at a rate of 10 to 12 breaths/min with appropriate volumes.

Continue ventilations at a rate of 10 to 12 breaths/min, and ensure adequate chest rise with each ventilation.

Ventilations should be associated with capnometry. The rate of ventilation should be adjusted to achieve a capnometry reading of between 35 and 45 mm Hg. In patients with head injuries, the reading should be 35 to 39 mm Hg. To drive the patient's carbon dioxide level, follow the reading. If the end-tidal carbon dioxide is too high, ventilate faster. If the reading is too low, ventilate slower.

Consider checking breath sounds. Knowing the status of breath sounds before tube placement can be helpful when determining the correct position.

▼

Combitube, PtL, and KING LT-D

This skill describes steps for placement and removal of three different types of airways: Combitube, pharyngeotracheal lumen (PtL), and KING LT-D. The steps for the placement and removal of the Combitube begin below. The steps for placement and removal of the PtL begin on page 103, and the steps for the KING LT-D begin on page 107. Be sure to complete Steps 1 through 6 first.

Placement of Combitube

Step 7 **Direct assistant to take over ventilations.**

Direct a qualified assistant to take over ventilations.

▼

Step 8 **Select, check, and prepare the Combitube.**

While the patient is being ventilated, the person responsible for the intubation must ensure that all the necessary equipment is available and in working order. Two sizes of Combitube are available. Check to ensure that the correct tube is used from the following chart. Each tube will require a different amount of air in the esophageal cuffs. Choose the correct-sized Combitube for the patient.

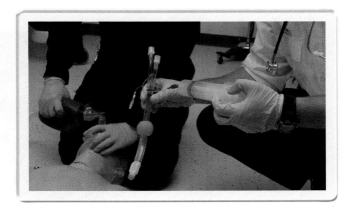

	Combitube	Combitube SA (small adult)
Intended patient height	5' and taller (caution over 6' 8")	4' to 5' 6"
Pharyngeal cuff–volume of air	100 mL	85 mL
Esophageal cuff–volume of air	15 mL	12 mL

Each kit comes complete with appropriately sized syringes, preloaded with the correct amount of air. Check these to ensure that the proper level has been set, and test the inflation of each cuff by inflating to the level indicated on the color-coded inflation ports. Refill each syringe to the proper volume of air. The Combitube kit also includes a nonsterile 10F suction catheter and a fluid deflector elbow. It is advisable to place the deflector on the end of the white tube before inserting the airway, aimed to deflect fluids toward the patient's side and away from active rescuers.

Additionally, always ensure that suction is available and working before beginning intubation. Both a rigid suction tip and a flexible catheter, appropriate for the size of the endotracheal tube, should be available.

▼

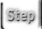 **Lubricate distal tip of the Combitube.**

The Combitube will pass in most patients with the natural lubrication of oral fluids. However, in patients who are dry, adding a water-soluble lubricant may be helpful.

▼

 Position patient's head properly.

Have your assistant stop ventilations, remove the oral airway, and remove the mask from the bag-mask device. You will now have only 30 seconds to position the patient, place the Combitube airway, and reestablish ventilations. Should you fail to intubate the patient, your assistant should quickly place the mask back on the bag-mask device and begin hyperventilating the patient. Gently return the patient's neck to a neutral or slightly flexed position.

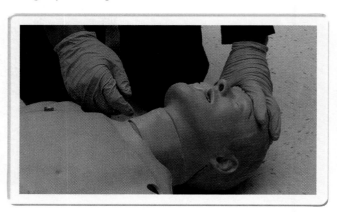

▼

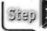

Step 11 Insert the Combitube midline and to a depth such that the printed ring is at the level of the teeth.

Place your thumb into the patient's mouth and lift the tongue and lower jaw anterior and inferior (tongue-jaw lift maneuver). Insert the Combitube and gently guide it straight down the center of the oral cavity into the hypopharynx. Stop advancing the tube when the patient's teeth are between the two black reference lines.

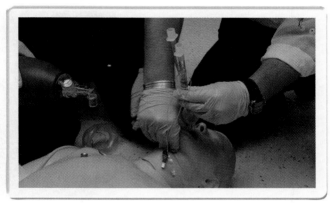

Step 12 Inflate the pharyngeal cuff with the proper volume of air and remove the syringe.

Inflate the pharyngeal cuff first through the *blue* pilot balloon port, using the prescribed amount of air (100 mL for Combitube, 85 mL for Combitube SA). Remove syringe and check pressure in the pilot balloon.

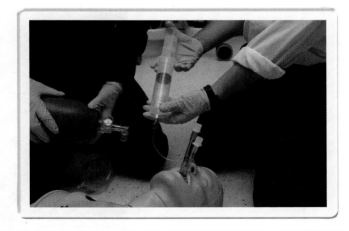

Step 13 Inflate the distal cuff with the proper volume and remove the syringe.

Inflate the esophageal cuff next through the *white* pilot balloon port, using the prescribed amount of air (15 mL for Combitube, 12 mL for Combitube SA). Remove the syringe and check pressure in the pilot balloon. Should either balloon show signs of insufficient volume, add air as needed.

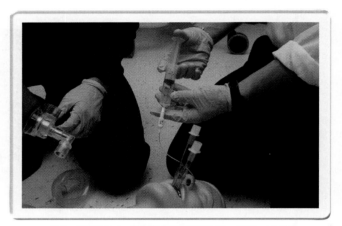

Step 14 Attach or direct attachment of bag-mask device to the first (pharyngeal placement) lumen and ventilate.

Attach bag-mask device to the *blue* tube and assess position by listening to abdominal and breath sounds.

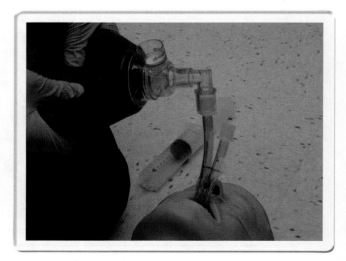

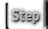

 Step 15 Confirm placement and ventilation through correct lumen by observing chest rise, auscultation over the epigastrium, and auscultation bilaterally over each lung.

Listen first over the patient's gastric region. With absent abdominal sounds, listen over the lung fields to assess the quality of ventilation. The presence of abdominal sounds is an indication of tracheal placement of the Combitube. Remove the fluid diverter elbow from the *white* tube, attach the bag-mask device, and reassess abdominal and breath sounds. If sounds are not heard in either location, reposition the Combitube slightly before complete removal. To reposition the tube, deflate both cuffs and pull the Combitube back 2 to 3 cm, reinflate the cuffs, and reassess. If sounds are still not heard, remove the Combitube and consider alternative airway procedures.

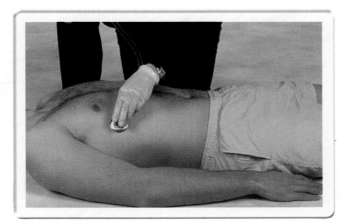

Step 16 Secure Combitube and confirm that the device remains properly secured.

Securing of the Combitube is not suggested by the manufacturer. However, applying tape similar to the method of securing an endotracheal tube may be extremely helpful, especially if the Combitube is located in the trachea.

Removal of the Combitube (from esophageal placement)

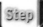 **Suction down gastric tube.**

Remove the fluid diverter elbow and, using the 10F catheter supplied, suction down the *white* tube of the Combitube. For thick emesis, a slightly larger suction catheter or nasal gastric tube may be required.

  Deflate cuffs.

Deflate the *blue* cuff first, followed quickly by the *white* cuff.

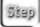 **Pull Combitube out.**

With suction ready and the patient's head in a neutral position, pull the Combitube straight out.

Step 20   **Turn patient's head to side and suction.**

Turn the patient's head to the side (unless contraindicated by trauma) and suction any emesis present.
   Note: For tracheal placement of the dual-lumen airway, *do not suction* prior to removal. Deflate the cuffs and pull the airway. Suction may be required as the dual-lumen airway is withdrawn.

Intubation Around Combitube (for esophageal placement)

  Suction down gastric tube.

Remove the fluid diverter elbow and, using the 10F catheter supplied, suction down the *white* tube of the Combitube. For thick emesis, a slightly larger suction catheter or nasal gastric tube may be required.

Step 22 **Deflate large cuff.**

Attach the large syringe and deflate the *blue* cuff. Leave the *white* cuff inflated until you are ready to remove the Combitube.

▼

Step 23 **Place laryngoscope and visualize cords.**

With your finger, push the Combitube over to the left side of the patient's mouth. Using a MacIntosh blade, visualize the vocal cords while holding the Combitube to the left. A Miller or straight blade may be used if necessary, but it will not directly hold the Combitube in position.

▼

Step 24 **Place endotracheal tube.**

Pass the appropriate-sized endotracheal tube through the vocal cords and into the trachea. Establish proper placement and secure the tube as described in the endotracheal intubation skills found in this review manual.

▼

Placement of Pharyngeotracheal Lumen Airway (PtL)

Step 7 **Direct assistant to take over ventilations.**

Direct a qualified assistant to take over ventilations.

▼

Step 8 **Check and prepare PtL.**

While the patient is being ventilated, the person responsible for the intubation must ensure that all the necessary equipment is available and in working order.

Additionally, always ensure that suction is available and working before beginning intubation. Both a rigid suction tip and a flexible catheter, appropriate for the size of the endotracheal tube, should be available.

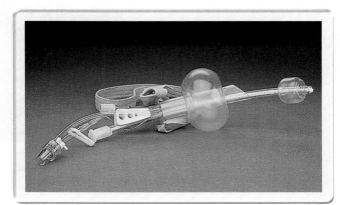

▼

Step **Lubricate distal tip of the PtL.**

Lubricate the distal tip of the PtL to ease placement into the patient.

▼

Step 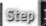 **Position patient's head properly.**

Have your assistant stop ventilations, remove the oral airway, and remove the mask from the bag-mask device. You will now have only 30 seconds to position the patient, place the esophageal airway, and reestablish ventilations. Should you fail to intubate the patient, your assistant should quickly place the mask back on the bag-mask device and begin hyperventilating the patient. Gently return the patient's neck to a neutral or slightly flexed position.

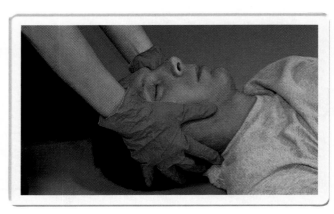

▼

Step **Insert PtL midline and to a depth such that the strap is at the level of the teeth.**

Place your thumb into the patient's mouth and lift the tongue and lower jaw anterior and inferior (tongue-jaw lift maneuver). Insert the PtL so the curvature of the tube is aligned with the natural curvature of the airway.

Apply gentle downward pressure to advance the tube until the teeth strap touches the patient's teeth or gums. Slight resistance is expected as the tube passes the back of the oropharynx. *Do not* force the airway. If the PtL does not advance easily, either redirect the tube by slightly adjusting the airway or withdraw the tube and start over.

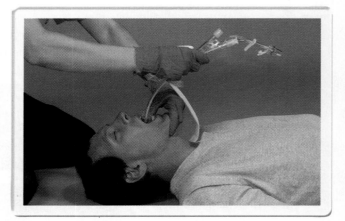

▼

Step 12 ▶ **Secure PtL.**

Position the neck strap around the patient's neck and attach it to the tube using the fastening system.

▼

Step 13 ▶ **Inflate cuffs with proper volume.**

Inflate the cuffs of the PtL by placing the ventilation port of a bag-mask device against the inflation valve (labeled tube 1). Ensure that the white cap is closed to prevent leakage.

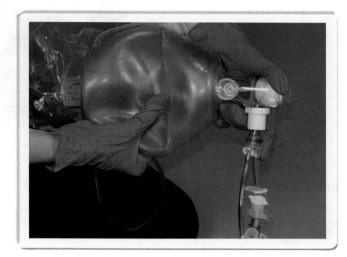

▼

Step 14 ▶ **Attach or direct attachment of the bag-mask device to tube 2 (the short green tube) and assess placement.**

Attach the bag-mask device to the short green tube (labeled tube 2) and assess its position by observing chest rise and listening to abdominal and breath sounds. If the chest rises, tube 3 is in the esophagus. Continue ventilating through tube 2.

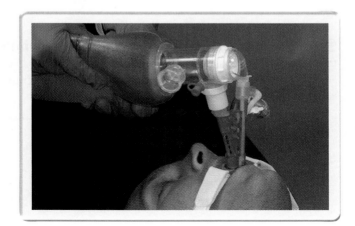

Step 14 continued

If the chest does not rise, tube 3 may be in the trachea. Remove the stylet from the long clear tube (labeled tube 3). Attach the bag-mask device and ventilate through the clear tube. Assess its position by observing chest rise and listening to abdominal and breath sounds.

Continue ventilation through the appropriate tube.

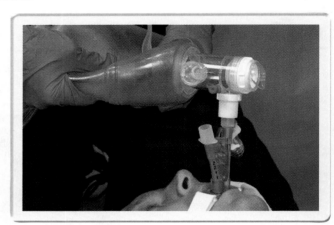

Removal of the PtL (from esophageal placement)

Step 15 **Deflate both cuffs.**

Open the white cap on tube 1 and allow air to escape from both tubes.

Step 16 **Pull PtL out.**

With suction ready and the patient's head in a neutral position, pull the PtL straight out.

Step 17 **Turn patient's head to side and suction.**

Turn the patient's head to the side (unless contraindicated by trauma) and suction any emesis present.

Placement of KING LT-D

The KING LT-D is a single-lumen airway. Unlike the Combitube, PtL, or other dual-lumen airways, the KING LT-D is only effective when it is placed in the esophagus. Because the KING LT-D is not a dual-lumen airway, inadvertent intubation of the trachea must be recognized and corrected as soon as possible. Failure to recognize tracheal intubation can have fatal consequences.

 Direct assistant to take over ventilations.

Direct a qualified assistant to take over ventilations.

 Check and prepare KING LT-D.

While the patient is being ventilated, the person responsible for the intubation must ensure that all the necessary equipment is available and in working order. Three sizes of KING LT-D airways are available. Check to ensure that the correct tube is used from the following chart. Each tube will require a different amount of air in the esophageal cuffs. Choose the correct-sized KING LT-D airway for the patient.

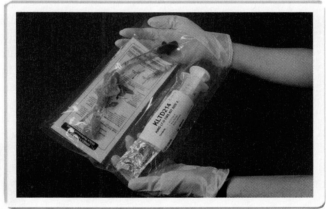

	KING LT-D (Size 3)	KING LT-D (Size 4)	KING LT-D (Size 5)
Intended patient heights	4' to 5'	5' to 6'	> 6'
Connector color	Yellow	Red	Purple
Inflation volume	45-60 mL	60-80 mL	70-90 mL

Test the cuff and the inflation system for leaks by placing the maximum recommended volume into the cuff. Before inserting the airway, remove all air from the cuffs.

The manufacturer advises you to have a spare KING LT-D ready and prepared for immediate use. Additionally, always ensure that suction is available and working before beginning intubation. Both a rigid suction tip and a flexible catheter, appropriate for the size of the tube, should be available.

Step 9 Lubricate distal tip of the KING LT-D.

Using water-soluble jelly, lubricate the distal tip and posterior aspects of the tube. *Do not* apply lubricant in or near the ventilatory openings.

▼

 Step 10 Position patient's head properly.

Have your assistant stop ventilations, remove the oral airway, and remove the mask from the bag-mask device. You will now have only 30 seconds to position the patient, place the esophageal airway, and reestablish ventilations. Should you fail to intubate the patient, your assistant should quickly place the mask back on the bag-mask device and begin hyperventilating the patient.

Gently return the patient's neck to a neutral or slightly flexed position.

▼

 Step 11 Insert the KING LT-D midline and to a depth at which the base of the connector is properly aligned.

Place your thumb into the patient's mouth and lift the tongue and lower jaw anterior and inferior (tongue-jaw lift maneuver). With the KING LT-D rotated so the blue line is touching the corner of the mouth, insert the tip into the mouth and behind the tongue. Rotate the tube as the tip passes under the tongue so that the blue line faces the chin. Advance the tube until the base of the connector is aligned with the teeth or gums.

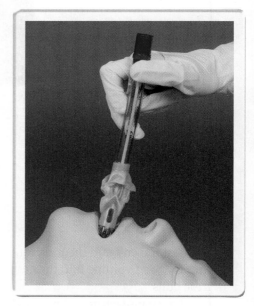

▼

Step 12 **Inflate cuffs with proper volume and remove syringe.**

Using the syringe provided in the KING LT-D kit, inflate the cuffs with the appropriate volume: approximately 50 mL for size 3, 70 mL for size 4, and 80 mL for size 5.

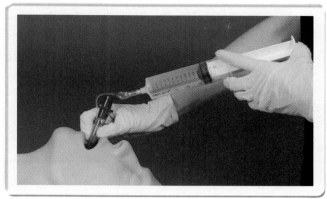

Remove the syringe from the inflation port.

 Step 13 **Attach or direct the attachment of the bag-mask device to the airway lumen and ventilate.**

Attach the bag-mask device to the 15-mm connector and begin gentle ventilation.

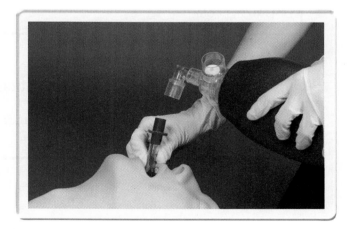

Assess breath and abdominal sounds while simultaneously pulling back on the KING LT-D until ventilation becomes easy. Withdrawing the tube with the cuffs inflated retracts the surrounding tissues and aids in the securing of a patent airway. Ventilations should deliver large tidal volumes with minimal airway pressure when properly positioned.

Secure the KING LT-D and confirm that the device remains properly secured.

Secure the KING LT-D using tape or a commercially made tube holder. If tape is used, consider inserting an oropharyngeal airway as a bite block.

▼

Removal of the KING LT-D (from esophageal placement)

 Prepare for removal.

Suction equipment should be present and in working order.

▼

 Deflate cuffs.

Remove all air from both cuffs. It may take more than one filling of the syringe to completely remove the air.

▼

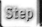 **Pull KING LT-D out.**

With suction ready and the patient's head in a neutral position, pull the KING LT-D straight out.

▼

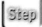 **Turn patient's head to side and suction.**

Turn the patient's head to the side (unless contraindicated by trauma) and suction any emesis present.

Laryngeal Mask Airways

Performance Objective

Given an adult patient and appropriate equipment, the candidate shall insert a laryngeal mask airway (LMA) and verify proper placement, using criteria herein prescribed, in 6 minutes or less.

Equipment

The following equipment is required to perform this skill:
- Appropriate body substance isolation/personal protective equipment
- Oxygen cylinder, regulator, and key
- Oxygen delivery device (appropriate to patient)
- Oropharyngeal airway (adult sized)
- Laryngeal mask airway (LMA); appropriate size for patient
- Water-soluble lubricant
- Towel or other padding
- Colorimetric end-tidal carbon dioxide detector
- Syringes (10 mL, 20 mL)
- Endotracheal tube holder or tape
- Stethoscope
- Suction device and tubing
- Suction catheter
  - Rigid wand (Yankauer type)
  - Flexible catheter

Equipment that may be helpful:
- Pulse oximeter
- Spare bulb, batteries
- End-tidal carbon dioxide meter

Indications

- Secondary airway device, used when the patient can be easily ventilated by bag-mask device, but endotracheal intubation is not necessary

Contraindications

- Patients who have eaten in the last 8 to 12 hours
- Morbid obesity
- Laryngeal edema
- Obstruction of the airway

Complications

- Inability to ventilate patients with obstructive airway disease
- Unrecognized aspiration of stomach contents

Procedures

 Ensure body substance isolation before beginning procedures.

Prior to beginning patient care, appropriate body substance isolation procedures should be employed.

▼

 **Open the airway manually.**

Before opening the airway, consider the possibility of cervical spine injury. If spinal injury is suspected, use a jaw-thrust maneuver to open the airway (see Skill 1). If no spinal cord injury is suspected, open the patient's airway by performing the head tilt–chin lift maneuver (see Skill 3).

▼

 Elevate tongue, appropriately insert simple adjunct.

Measuring from the corner of the mouth to the base of the earlobe, choose the correct size airway for your patient. Open the mouth using the jaw-thrust or cross-finger technique. Insert in front of mouth with tip pointed toward roof, or insert from side of mouth with tip toward inside of cheek. A tongue depressor can be used to hold the tongue inferior and the airway inserted tip down. If the patient starts to gag, remove the airway by pulling the flange anterior and inferior.

▼

Ventilate patient immediately with bag-mask device.

Begin ventilations immediately with a bag-mask device. If the bag-mask device is not already attached to oxygen, begin ventilations with room air.

Select the appropriate-sized bag for the patient. Bag and mask sizes are normally listed as adult, child, and infant. These sizes are adequate for the average size person who meets the age definition criteria. However, large children will require a bag that will deliver the appropriate volume. Likewise, pediatric bags may be appropriate for small adults or adults where overpressurization can cause pulmonary damage. Masks should be chosen to fit the patient without air leakage.

Position the mask with the apex over the bridge of the nose and the base between the lower lip and the prominence of the chin. Begin ventilations as soon as the mask is sealed, and assess the mask for air leakage.

Begin ventilations at a rate of 10 to 12 breaths/min, with a tidal volume that achieves chest rise. Pay close attention to ensure that each ventilation is of the appropriate volume and of a consistent rate. Allow adequate exhalation between each breath.

Effective ventilations, those breaths that cause the chest to rise adequately for the size of the patient, must be started within 30 seconds. Be cautious not to overventilate. Each ventilation should be delivered slow and easy, lasting approximately 1 second. Fast and high pressure ventilations can cause air to enter the stomach, increasing the risk of vomiting. If a second rescuer is available, the Sellick maneuver (cricoid pressure) may be applied. Although it will be necessary to stop ventilations for assessment and other procedures, you should never allow a nonbreathing patient to go without ventilations for more than 30 seconds.

 Attach oxygen reservoir and connect to high-flow oxygen regulator.

If not previously performed, attach oxygen tubing to the inlet on the bag-mask device and to the oxygen source. Open the cylinder valve and adjust the liter flow to between 12 and 15 L/min.

Ventilate patient at a rate of 10 to 12 breaths/min with appropriate volumes.

Continue ventilations at a rate of 10 to 12 breaths/min, and ensure adequate chest rise with each.

Ventilations should be associated with capnometry. The rate of ventilation should be adjusted to achieve a capnometry reading of between 35 and 45 mm Hg. In patients with head injuries, the reading should be 35 to 39 mm Hg. To drive the patient's carbon dioxide level, follow the reading. If the end-tidal carbon dioxide is too high, ventilate faster. If the reading is too low, ventilate slower.

Consider checking breath sounds. Knowing the status of breath sounds before tube placement can be helpful when determining the correct position.

Placement of Laryngeal Mask Airway (LMA)

 Direct assistant to begin ventilations.

To prepare for the placement of the endotracheal tube, direct a qualified assistant to take over ventilations.

 Check and prepare airway device.

While patient is being ventilated, the person responsible for the placement of the LMA must ensure that all the necessary equipment is available and in working order. The LMA comes in several sizes, and each tube will require a different amount of air in the mask. Choose the correct sized LMA based on the patient's weight from the following chart.

Patient Size	LMA Size	Proper Inflation
Under 5 kg (11 lb)	1	4
5 to 10 kg (11–22 lb)	1.5	7
10 to 20 kg (22–44 lb)	2	10
20 to 30 kg (44–66 lb)	2.5	14
30 kg to small adult	3	20
Adult	4	30
Large adult or poor seal with size 4	5	40

Examine the LMA to ensure it is free of tears or other abnormalities. Inspect the tube to be sure it is free from blockage or loose particles.

The LMA comes with the mask loosely inflated. Attach a syringe to the inflation port and deflate the cuff. Observe for signs that the mask will not maintain a vacuum. Reinflate the cuff to ensure that it does not leak.

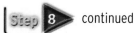 continued

Carefully deflate the cuff to form a smooth wedge that will pass into the hypopharynx without difficulty.

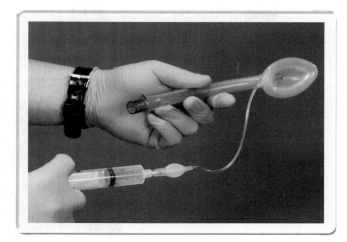

Additionally, always ensure that suction is available and working before beginning intubation. Both a rigid suction tip and a flexible catheter, appropriate for the size of the endotracheal tube, should be available.

▼

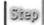 **Lubricate the mask.**

Using water-soluble jelly, ensure that the mask is well lubricated. Be sure to lubricate the ring of the mask and the posterior surface. Use caution that the anterior surface and bowl are minimally lubricated to avoid airway obstruction.

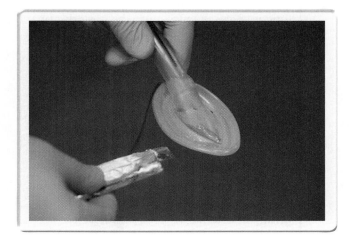

▼

Step **10** ▶ **Position the patient and visualize the posterior oropharynx.**

Have your assistant stop ventilations, remove the oral airway, and remove the mask from the bag-mask device. You will now have only 20 to 30 seconds to position the patient, place the LMA, and reestablish ventilations. Should you fail to properly place the device in the patient, your assistant should quickly place the mask back on the bag-mask device and begin ventilating the patient.

Position the patient with the head extended and the neck flexed. Your assistant should place his or her thumb into the mouth and pull the lower jaw downward.

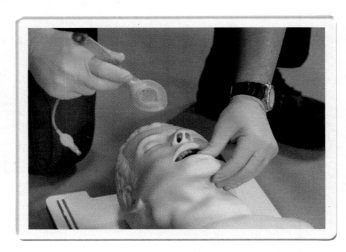

Step **11** ▶ **Insert the LMA.**

Grasp the tube of the LMA as near as possible to the mask end, holding it like a pen. Place the tip of the airway against the inner surface of the patient's upper teeth. Flatten out the mask by pressing the tip upward against the hard palate. Under direct vision, using your index finger, keep pressing upward as you advance the mask into the pharynx to ensure the tip remains flattened and avoids the tongue. Press the mask into the posterior pharyngeal wall using your index finger.

Continue pushing the mask with your index finger and guide downward into position. With the other hand, grasp the tube firmly while withdrawing your index finger. Gently press the mask downward into position to ensure the mask is fully inserted.

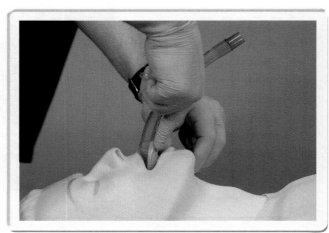

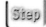
Safety Tips

Problems Associated With LMA Insertion

Failure to press the deflated mask up against the hard palate, inadequate lubrication, or deflation can lead to the mask tip folding back on itself.

When the mask tip has started to fold over, this may progress, pushing the epiglottis into its down-folded position, causing mechanical obstruction. If the mask tip is deflated forward, it can push down the epiglottis, causing obstruction. If the mask is inadequately deflated, it may either push down the epiglottis or penetrate the glottis.

Step **Inflate the mask.**

Inflate the mask with the recommended volume of air. *Do not* overinflate. While inflating, *do not* touch the LMA tube unless the position is obviously unstable. It is normal for the mask to rise slightly out of the hypopharynx as it is inflated and finds its correct position.

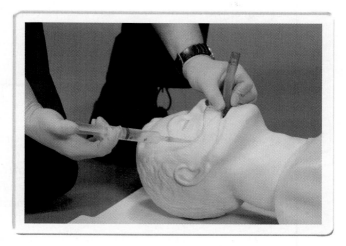

Step **Direct ventilation of the patient.**

While still holding the tube in place, attach the bag-mask device to the LMA tube and begin ventilations. Instruct your partner to deliver breaths as you move your stethoscope over the patient's abdomen and chest.

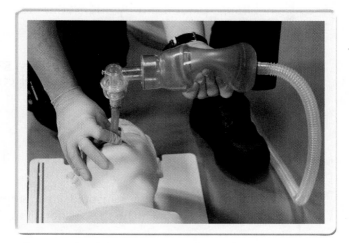

Step 14 Confirm proper placement by auscultation over the epigastrium and bilaterally over each lung.

Auscultate the abdomen and the chest to determine the correct tube placement. The preferred sequence is to listen over the gastric region first, then over the lower left, upper left, upper right, and finally the lower right chest. By using this sequence, you can determine incorrect placement with a minimal amount of unnecessary ventilations.

If you hear air over the epigastric region, remove the air from the LMA, reposition, reinflate, and assess placement again.

▼

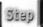 **Step 15** Secure the LMA tube.

Maintaining a hold on the tube, attach a commercially made endotracheal tube holder. However, unlike endotracheal tubes, it is important to keep the LMA tube centered in the mouth. Allowing the tube to move toward either side can cause displacement of the mask.

If a commercial device is not available, adhesive tape can be used. Begin by encircling the tube with tape at the level of the patient's teeth. Wrap the tape around the patient's neck and again encircle the tape around the tube at the level of the patient's teeth. Ensure that you have not placed undue pressure on the vessels of the neck by placing the tape over the prominence of the anterior mandible. Insert a bite block to prevent the patient from biting the tube.

▼

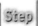 **Step 16** Ensure placement by additional means and apply an extrication collar.

Reassess tube placement through assessment of gastric and breath sounds. At least two additional means of ensuring tube placement should be used. These include:

- End-tidal carbon dioxide meters
- Fogging of the endotracheal tube
- Capnographic monitors

Finally, when placement is ensured, an appropriately sized extrication collar should be applied to maintain the position of the head and neck and thus the airway.

All findings should be verbalized so that all members of the team are aware of the airway status.

Even though tube placement has been ensured, continual reassessment should occur. This should be performed any time the patient is moved or defibrillated. Also, always ensure and document the tube placement before turning over patient care at the receiving facility or to a transport team.

Needle Cricothyrotomy

Performance Objective

Given a patient who meets the criteria for creating an artificial airway and appropriate equipment, the candidate shall demonstrate the procedures for needle cricothyrotomy using the criteria herein prescribed, in 3 minutes or less.

Equipment

The following equipment is required to perform this skill:
- Appropriate body substance isolation/personal protective equipment
- Oxygen cylinder, regulator, and key
- Oxygen delivery device (appropriate to patient)
  - Bag-mask device
- Povidone-iodine swabs
- Chlorhexidine
- 14-gauge or larger IV catheter
- 3.0 endotracheal tube (you will need the 15-mm adapter)
- 10-mL syringe
- Alcohol swabs
- 4" × 4" gauze sponges
- Stethoscope

Equipment that may be helpful:
- Pulse oximeter

Indications

- Inability to adequately ventilate a patient following unsuccessful attempts at intubation
- Children younger than 12 years of age

Contraindications

- Any patient who can be adequately ventilated with a bag-mask device and no threat to losing the airway exists

Complications

- Puncture/laceration of the thyroid gland
- Subcutaneous emphysema
- Puncture of a carotid artery or jugular vein
- Failure to enter the larynx by misplacement into surrounding tissue or advancement into the esophagus

Procedures

 Step 1 Ensure body substance isolation before beginning procedures.

Prior to beginning patient care, appropriate body substance isolation procedures should be employed.

▼

 **Step 2** Maintain sterility and safety throughout.

Ensure that all sterile equipment and the aseptic field are not contaminated. Maintain safety with needles, and use body substance isolation appropriately.

▼

 Step 3 Select, check, and prepare equipment.

Gather the necessary equipment for the needle cricothyrotomy. The required equipment will vary based on the method of cricothyrotomy performed, but all steps will require povidone-iodine swabs, alcohol swabs, or chlorhexidine, and 4″ × 4″ gauze sponges.

You will need a 14-gauge or larger IV catheter, a 3.0 endotracheal tube, and a bag-mask device with supplemental oxygen. Remove the tube from the 15-mm adapter of the 3.0 endotracheal tube. The 15-mm adapter will be attached to the end of the IV catheter and used to ventilate the patient.

▼

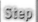 **Step 4** Locate and prepare the site.

If possible, place the patient's head and neck in a neutral position. Palpate the patient's neck and locate the thyroid cartilage. With a finger on the center of the thryroid cartilage, follow the ridge toward the chest until you locate the space between the thyroid and cricoid cartilages. This is the cricothyroid membrane.

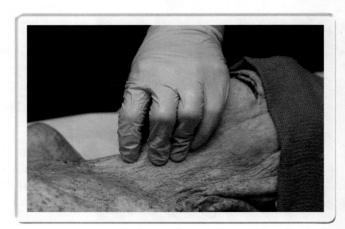

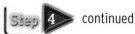

Step 4 continued

Prepare the insertion site by cleaning it with an antiseptic/antimicrobial agent. A 30-second vigorous scrub using chlorhexidine will kill 99.9% of all colonizing microbes when the solution is dry. Chlorhexidine is safe for adults and children, but because of skin sensitivity, it should not be used on neonates.

If chlorhexidine is not available, povidone-iodine is an acceptable alternative. It is important to allow the povidone-iodine solution to dry completely before injecting the site. Alcohol may be used when the povidone-iodine is dry to clean the dye and improve visualization of the injection site.

For years alcohol has been the used as the traditional injecting preparation. Because of its limited ability to kill microbial agents, it should be avoided in all cases unless the patient is allergic to both chlorhexidine and povidone-iodine (persons with shellfish allergies are allergic to iodine). Alcohol alone, as a prep for IV or hypodermic injection, should be considered below the standard of care.

Cleanse the site by applying the solution in a circular motion, starting in the center and working out. It is best not to reenter the clean area after it is cleaned.

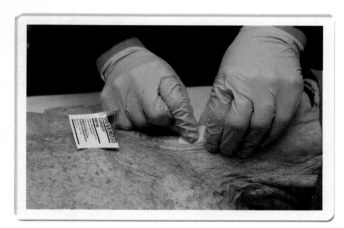

Step 5 **Insert the needle into the cricothyroid membrane.**

With your nondominant hand, stabilize the larynx by pulling the skin down, toward the back of the neck. Insert the needle through the skin and into the cricothyroid membrane at a 90° angle to the trachea. Advance the needle catheter only ½ to ¾ of an inch into the larynx, then angle the needle toward the chest.

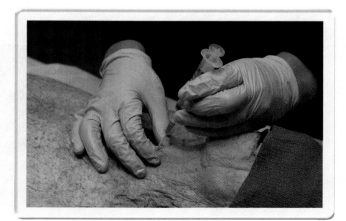

In the Field

Modified Jet Insufflation

This technique uses an IV catheter and high-flow oxygen to fill the lungs with oxygen rather than actually ventilating the patient. You will need a 14-gauge or larger IV catheter, a 10F suction catheter, and oxygen connective tubing. Remove the suction catheter from the thumb control port and attach the port to the free end of the oxygen connective tubing. This will be attached to the IV catheter, and it forms a thumb control for the oxygen administration.

Replace Steps 7 and 8 with the following steps to use an IV catheter and high-flow oxygen to fill the lungs with oxygen:

Step 7 **Attach oxygen tubing to IV catheter and attach at high flow.**

Attach the oxygen tubing, with the suction thumb port already attached, onto the IV catheter. Secure with a slight twist. Turn the oxygen on to the highest possible flow available through the regulator. Be careful to watch the pressure in the oxygen cylinder because this will rapidly drain the remaining volume.

Step 8 **Provide oxygen.**

Place your thumb over the thumb port and give a 1-second blast of oxygen. Remove your thumb and wait 4 seconds before repeating the 1-second blast. Continue this process until a large surgical airway can be established.

Step 6 **Advance the catheter and remove the needle stylet.**

Angle the needle 45° toward the patient's chest, and push the catheter into the trachea while holding the needle in place. When the catheter is fully inserted, remove the needle stylet. Dispose of the needle stylet in an approved sharps container.

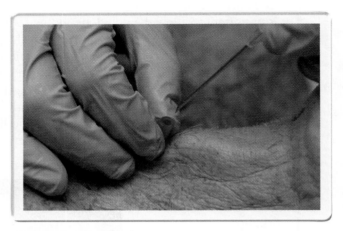

▼

Step 7 **Attach a 3.0 endotracheal tube adapter.**

Attach the 3.0 endotracheal tube adapter to the IV catheter and secure it with a slight twist.

▼

Step 8  **Ventilate the patient.**

Attach the bag-mask device to the adapter and begin ventilating. Each breath will be very firm, and subsequent breaths may become difficult if complete exhalation is prevented. Remember that most ventilations from a bag-mask device are relatively easy. When ventilating through a catheter, the resistance will be extremely high, and ventilations will be much more difficult.

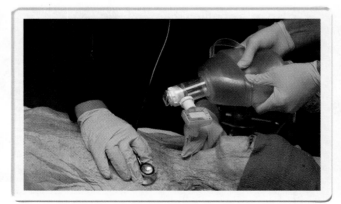

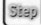 **Reassess the patient.**

Reassess the patient. Use of a pulse oximeter to determine the efficacy of the cricothyrotomy is recommended. Because of the limited amount of air delivered, chest expansion will be minimal, if noticeable at all. Breath sounds may be difficult or impossible to hear due to the small volume administered at any one time. Pupillary response, tissue color, and level of consciousness along with pulse oximetry readings are the best indicators of effective oxygenation.

▼

 Properly dispose of contaminated equipment.

Dispose of needles and all sharp instruments with blood or body fluid contamination in puncture-resistant sharps containers. Other materials that have been contaminated by blood or body fluids should be disposed of in biohazard bags. Waste materials that are not contaminated by blood or body fluids can be disposed of in normal trash receptacles.

Surgical Cricothyrotomy

Performance Objective

Given a patient who meets the criteria for creating an artificial airway and appropriate equipment, the candidate shall demonstrate the procedures for performing a surgical cricothyrotomy, in 3 minutes or less.

Equipment

The following equipment is required to perform this skill:
- Appropriate body substance isolation/personal protective equipment
- Oxygen cylinder, regulator, and key
- Oxygen delivery device (appropriate to patient)
  • Bag-mask device
- Povidone-iodine swabs
- Chlorhexidine
- Petroleum gauze
- Alcohol swabs
- 4″ × 4″ gauze sponges
- Scalpel with No. 10 blade
- A form of spreaders (curved hemostats, Magill forceps, cricothyroid spreaders, the blunt end of a scalpel, tracheal hook, or finger)
- Endotracheal tubes, cuffed (5.0 to 6.0)
- 10-mL syringe
- Tape
- Water-soluble lubricant

Equipment that may be helpful:
- Pulse oximeter

Indications

- Inability to adequately ventilate a patient after several unsuccessful attempts at intubation or other alternative airways

Contraindications

- Any patient who can be adequately ventilated with a bag-mask device, and no threat to losing the airway exists
- Children younger than 12 years of age

Complications

- Separation of the trachea from the larynx and resulting loss of the trachea into the chest
- Laceration of the trachea, larynx, or vocal cords
- Puncture/laceration of the thyroid gland
- Subcutaneous emphysema
- Puncture of a carotid artery or jugular vein
- Excessive hemorrhage
- Failure to enter the larynx by misplacement into surrounding tissue or advancement into the esophagus

Procedures

 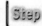 **Ensure body substance isolation before beginning procedures.**

Prior to beginning patient care, appropriate body substance isolation procedures should be employed.

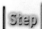 **Maintain sterility and safety throughout.**

Ensure that all sterile equipment and the aseptic field are not contaminated. Maintain safety with needles, and use body substance isolation appropriately.

Step 3 Select, check, and prepare equipment.

Gather the necessary equipment for the cricothyrotomy. The required equipment includes povidone-iodine swabs or alcohol swabs, 4″ × 4″ gauze sponges, petroleum gauze, a scalpel, a form of spreaders (curved hemostats, Magill forceps, cricothyroid spreaders, the blunt end of a scalpel, tracheal hook, or finger), a 5.0 to 6.0 cuffed endotracheal tube, 10-mL syringe, water-soluble lubricant, tape, and a bag-mask device.

Apply the water-soluble lubricant to the end of the endotracheal tube. Because this procedure will probably be performed on an apneic patient in which ventilations may not be possible, do not take the time to check the cuff of the endotracheal tube or to perform further equipment preparation.

  Locate and prepare the site.

If possible, place the patient's head and neck in a neutral position. Palpate the patient's neck and locate the thyroid cartilage. With a finger on the center of the thryroid cartilage, follow the ridge toward the chest until you locate the space between the thyroid and cricoid cartilages. This is the cricothyroid membrane.

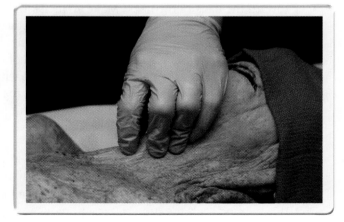

In the Field

Needle Cricothyrotomy or Surgical Cricothyrotomy

Surgical cricothyrotomy is *highly superior* to needle cricothyrotomy in almost every way. The surgical technique allows for the placement of a larger airway and allows effective ventilation without question. Needle cricothyrotomy is less than effective in many ways and serves only as a last ditch effort to provide minimal ventilation or oxygenation. Only in children should needle cricothyrotomy be considered definitive airway management.

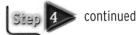 **Step 4** continued

Prepare the insertion site by cleaning it with an antiseptic/antimicrobial agent. A 30-second vigorous scrub using chlorhexidine will kill 99.9% of all colonizing microbes when the solution is dry. Chlorhexidine is safe for adults and children, but because of skin sensitivity, it should not be used on neonates.

If chlorhexidine is not available, povidone-iodine is an acceptable alternative. It is important to allow the povidone-iodine solution to dry completely before injecting the site. Alcohol may be used when the povidone-iodine is dry to clean the dye and improve visualization of the injection site.

For years alcohol has been the used as the traditional injecting preparation. Because of its limited ability to kill microbial agents, it should be avoided in all cases unless the patient is allergic to both chlorhexidine and povidone-iodine (persons with shellfish allergies are allergic to iodine). Alcohol alone, as a prep for IV or hypodermic injection, should be considered below the standard of care.

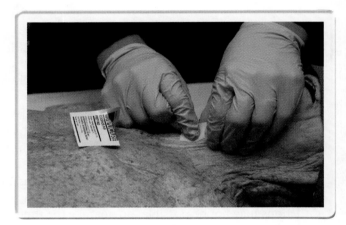

Cleanse the site by applying the solution in a circular motion, starting in the center and working out. It is best not to reenter the clean area after it is cleaned.

 Step 5 **Make incision through the cricothyroid membrane.**

With your nondominant hand, stabilize the larynx by pulling the skin down, toward the back of the neck. Make an incision through the skin of the neck and cricothyroid membrane. There are two methods to perform this procedure. Both are acceptable in the prehospital setting, and neither is free from complication (the most common complication is laceration of the thyroid gland).

The first method is a straightforward approach that calls for a controlled stab through the skin and the cricothyroid membrane in one move. Holding the scalpel in line with the cricothyroid membrane, cut through the skin and membrane. Insert the blade with a shallow puncture. Leave the scalpel in the incision until the spreaders are in place.

The second method cuts the skin and cricothyroid membrane separately. Many physicians prefer this method because it allows better visualization of the thyroid gland and a more controlled cut of the membrane. It is also believed that this method seals the tube better and reduces subcutaneous emphysema of the

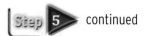

Step 5 continued

neck. Begin by making a 2- to 3-cm superficial, vertical incision into the skin along the midline of the larynx, over the cricothyroid membrane. Using your finger, separate the tissues and locate the cricothyroid membrane. When it is located, use the scalpel to cut the cricothyroid membrane 1 cm in each direction from the midline.

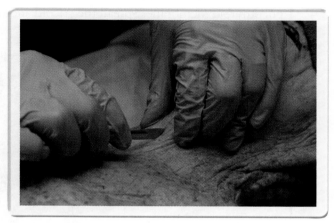

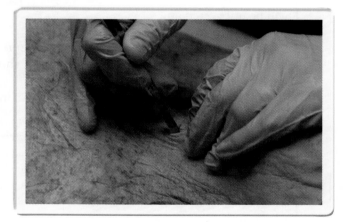

Dispose of the scalpel in a sharps container. Again, use your finger or spreaders to open and spread the cricoid cartilage.

In both cases, prepare for a considerable amount of bleeding. Always manage the airway first and control the bleeding second.

Step **6** ▶ **Spread the cricoid cartilage.**

Spreading the cricoid cartilage can be performed in various ways. The simplest and safest method is to use your finger. Insert your finger into the incision and work the fingertip into the cricothyroid membrane.

Other techniques include using curved Kelly clamps or hemostats as a spreader. With the scalpel remaining in the incision, insert the tips of the clamp into the cricothyroid membrane. Spread the cricoid and the thyroid cartilages apart by opening the clamp.

As a last resort, the handle of the scalpel can be used to spread the cartilage. Simply lift the blade from the incision, turn the scalpel blade up, and insert the handle into the incision. Rotate the handle 90° to spread the cartilages. Because the blade of the scalpel will be uncovered and standing straight up into the area where you will be working, extreme caution must be taken to avoid being stabbed. For this reason, this technique should be reserved for only the most extreme cases.

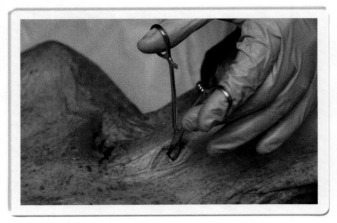

When you are finished with the scalpel, be sure to place it in a puncture-resistant container.

▼

Step **7** ▶ **Insert endotracheal tube.**

Insert the endotracheal tube into the incision and advance it until the cuff is in the trachea. A twisting motion is helpful. It may be necessary to manipulate the spreader slightly to prevent tearing of the cuff on the endotracheal tube. If spreaders were used to hold the insertion open, do not remove the spreader until the endotracheal tube is in place.

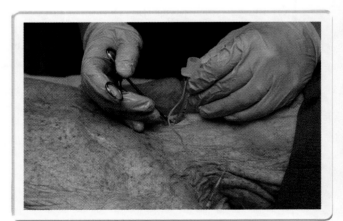

▼

8 Ventilate the patient.

Attach the bag-mask device to the end of the endotracheal tube and begin ventilating the patient. Attach supplemental oxygen at a high liter flow.

▼

 9 Reassess the patient.

Reassess the patient. Use of a pulse oximeter and capnography to determine the efficacy of the cricothyrotomy is recommended. Because of the volume of air delivered, breath sounds should be audible, and you should see chest expansion. Still, pupillary response, tissue color, and level of consciousness, along with pulse oximetry and capnography readings, are the best indicators of effective ventilations and oxygenation.

▼

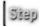 **10 Inflate the cuff.**

Inflate the cuff with sufficient air to achieve a firm balloon, to a maximum of 10 mL. Be sure not to overinflate the cuff. Remove the syringe from the inflation port.

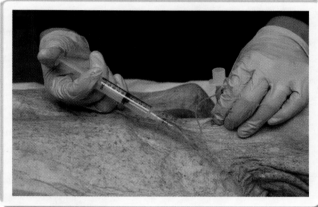

▼

Step 11 ▶ **Assess breath sounds.**

Assess the breath sounds, comparing the right and left sides of the chest. Assess abdominal sounds to ensure the endotracheal tube has not been passed through the trachea into the esophagus.

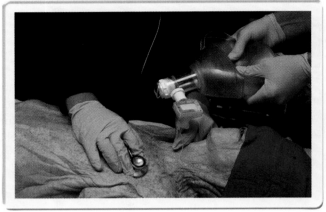

▼

Step 12 ▶ **Dress and bandage the incision.**

Apply a dressing around the endotracheal tube, and secure the bandage with tape.

▼

Step 13 ▶ **Secure the endotracheal tube.**

Hold the endotracheal tube in place with tape. Be careful that circumferential taping does not occlude movement of blood through the carotid arteries or jugular veins. When the tube is secure, reassess its placement by assessing breath sounds and capnography.

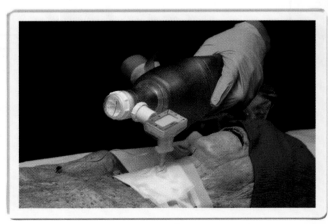

▼

Step 14 **Properly dispose of contaminated equipment.**

Dispose of the scalpel and all sharp instruments with blood or body fluid contamination in puncture-resistant sharps containers. Other material that has been contaminated by blood or body fluids should be disposed of in biohazard bags. Waste materials that are not contaminated by blood or body fluids can be disposed of in normal trash receptacles.

SKILL 21 Pharmacologically Assisted Intubation

Performance Objective

Given an adult patient and all appropriate equipment, the candidate shall administer sedative and paralytic medications to insert an endotracheal tube, assessing proper placement as required, in 8 minutes or less.

Equipment

The following equipment is required to perform this skill:
- Appropriate body substance isolation/personal protective equipment
- Oxygen cylinder, regulator, and key
- Oxygen delivery device (appropriate to patient)
- Bag-mask device
- Oropharyngeal airway (adult sized)
- Laryngoscope handle and blades (straight and curved)
- Endotracheal tubes, cuffed (6.0 to 9.0)
- Malleable intubation stylet (appropriate size for endotracheal tube)
- Water-soluble lubricant
- Towel or other padding
- Colorimetric end-tidal carbon dioxide detector
- Selection of syringes (3 mL, 5 mL, 10 mL, 20 mL)
- Selection of needles
- Medications
  - Chosen sedative (diazepam, etomidate, lorazepam, midazolam)
  - Chosen paralytic (rocuronium, succinylcholine, vecuronium)
  - Pain management (fentanyl, hydromorphone, meperidine, morphine)
  - For head injuries (lidocaine)
  - For pediatrics or mucus drying (atropine)
- Endotracheal tube holder or tape
- Stethoscope
- Suction device and tubing
- Suction catheter
  - Rigid wand (Yankauer type)
  - Flexible catheter

Equipment that may be helpful:
- Pulse oximeter
- Spare bulb, batteries
- End-tidal carbon dioxide meter

Indications

- Combative patients with potential head injury
- Active seizures
- Muscle rigidity
- Gag reflex in compromised patient

Contraindications

- Obstacles to success such as laryngeal edema (anaphylaxis, burns) or laryngeal trauma

Complications

- Unrecognized and uncorrected esophageal intubation
- Laryngeal injury
- Right mainstem bronchial intubation
- Dental injury
- Complications of medication (allergic reactions, adverse reactions)

Procedures

 Ensure body substance isolation before beginning procedures.

Prior to beginning patient care, appropriate body substance isolation procedures should be employed.

▼

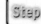 **Direct assistant to begin ventilations.**

When the need to intubate has been established, the patient should be ventilated for at least 2 minutes. This is best performed by an assistant rather than by the person who is responsible for the actual intubation. In many cases, the patient will have been ventilated at a standard rate for several minutes, and possibly longer, prior to the decision to intubate. This does not supersede or replace the need to hyperventilate. Ventilation should be performed at a rate of 10 to 12 breaths/min. If an oropharyngeal airway has not yet been placed, one should be inserted at this time (see Skill 7).

▼

 Evaluate the need for pharmacologically assisted intubation.

The need for pharmacologically assisted intubation is determined by the patient's *need* for immediate intubation. This is determined through several factors, not the least of which is the patient's rapid decline from hypoventilation and respiratory insufficiency. Pharmacologically assisted intubation should be considered when oxygenation alone fails to bring about improvement in the patient's status. Additional considerations include those patients who are combative from closed head injuries. These patients need sedation and airway control to reduce the intracerebral pressures and prevent a worsening of the condition. Before deciding to perform paralysis on any patient, assess the risks of a failed intubation and the prospect of simple bag-mask ventilation.

▼

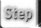 **Select, check, and prepare equipment, and draw up medications.**

While the patient is being ventilated, the person who is responsible for the intubation must ensure that all the necessary equipment is available and in working order. Ensure that the endotracheal tube is the proper size for the patient.

Using an aseptic technique, insert an intubation stylet into the endotracheal tube, and bend it into a gentle curve. A properly curved stylet will allow the stylet to be removed without causing the tip of the tube to move. The stylet should be positioned so that the end of the stylet does not extend past the Murphy eye.

Attach a 10-mL syringe to the endotracheal tube cuff port and inflate until the balloon is tight (this may take less than 10 mL of air) and check for leaks.

Pharmacologically Assisted Intubation Algorithm

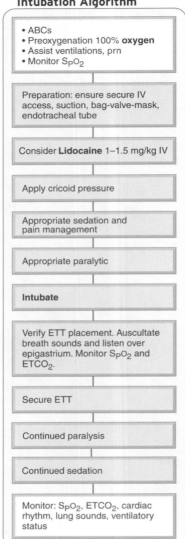

- ABCs
- Preoxygenation 100% **oxygen**
- Assist ventilations, prn
- Monitor S$_P$O$_2$

Preparation: ensure secure IV access, suction, bag-valve-mask, endotracheal tube

Consider **Lidocaine** 1–1.5 mg/kg IV

Apply cricoid pressure

Appropriate sedation and pain management

Appropriate paralytic

Intubate

Verify ETT placement. Auscultate breath sounds and listen over epigastrium. Monitor S$_P$O$_2$ and ETCO$_2$.

Secure ETT

Continued paralysis

Continued sedation

Monitor: S$_P$O$_2$, ETCO$_2$, cardiac rhythm, lung sounds, ventilatory status

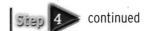

Step 4 continued

Remove the air from the cuff and remove the syringe. Place the syringe next to the patient's head. Leaving the syringe attached to the endotracheal tube can cause tearing and detachment of the balloon tubing, resulting in leaks from the cuff. There is also the possibility that the syringe may slip off and become lost. It is better to get in the habit of always removing the syringe and placing it at the patient's head. If the patient is dehydrated, has been down a long time, or is otherwise dry, lubricating jelly may be applied to the end of the endotracheal tube.

Assemble the laryngoscope with the desired blade and check the brightness of the bulb. A bright white light is best for all intubations. A yellow or dull light will cause the tissues of the hypopharynx to take on similar color schemes and result in difficulties visualizing landmarks and the vocal cords. Make sure the light is turned off until the laryngoscope is placed in the patient's mouth.

Prepare for the intubation by placing a 1″ pad under the patient's head. This will assist in lining up the three planes of the patient's airway. Although this step will make intubation easier, it is not required and is often difficult to accomplish in the prehospital setting. It is a good practice to learn to intubate both with and without the 1″ pad.

Prepare syringes with appropriate medications as listed in the Pharmacologically Assisted Intubation Algorithm or local protocol.

Syringes should be properly labeled to prevent medication errors.

Lastly, always ensure that suction is available and working before beginning intubation. Both a rigid suction tip and a flexible catheter, appropriate for the size of the endotracheal tube, should be available. Additionally, some protocols require an alternative airway to be available in case you are unable to obtain intubation.

Step **5**  **Preoxygenate and prepare patient.**

Ensure that the patient is adequately oxygenated prior to beginning pharmacologically assisted intubation. Patients with severe compromise should be oxygenated as well as can be expected. Cricoid pressure should be applied, and each ventilation should be slow and controlled, lasting 1 second per ventilation.
   Ensure patient IV access.

Step **6** **Premedicate the patient.**

Prior to administering paralytics, ensure that the patient is adequately sedated. This should be performed on all patients, regardless of perceived level of consciousness. Premedication should be aimed at five levels:

1. Sedation, to reduce anxiety in the paralyzed patient.
2. Pain management, because the patient will not be able to voice complaints.
3. Reduction of bradycardia in the pediatric patient.
4. Reduction of increased intracranial pressure in the brain-injured patient.
5. Defasciculation when succinylcholine will be given as a paralytic. Follow the Pharmacologically Assisted Intubation Algorithm on page 134 or local protocol as a guide to premedication.

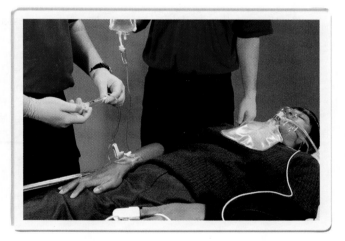

In the Field

Managing the Chemically Paralyzed Patient

Paralytics remove physical movement from the patient and present the illusion that the patient is asleep. The reality is that the patient's level of consciousness is unchanged from the time that paralytic medications were administered. Always assume that all chemically paralyzed patients are conscious and alert, fully aware of everything that is happening around them, and capable of feeling extreme pain. The use of long-term sedation, such as lorazepam, along with pain management should be maintained as long as the patient is paralyzed.

Also, remember that the patient is capable of having a seizure while under the paralytics, but the most obvious indicator, convulsions, have been eliminated. Watch for pupillary changes and tachycardia as indicators that the patient is experiencing a seizure. Benzodiazepine anticonvulsants may be used until the heart rate returns to normal.

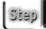 **7** ▶ **Paralyze.**

After 3 minutes (sooner if the patient loses consciousness) administer the paralytic.

Cricoid pressure should be maintained throughout the paralyzing process and intubation. Lack of eyelid flutter is an indication that the paralytics have taken control. Remember: Paralytics remove physical movement only. The patient's mental status has not changed. Many patients remain conscious and alert under the paralytic. Even with sedation and pain management, the patient's level of consciousness does not change when paralytics are applied.

▼

 8 ▶ **Position the patient's head properly.**

Have your assistant stop ventilations and remove the mask from the bag-mask device. You will now have only 20 to 30 seconds to position the patient, place the endotracheal tube, and reestablish ventilations. Should you fail to intubate the patient, your assistant should quickly place the mask back on the bag-mask device and begin hyperventilating the patient.

Remove the oropharyngeal airway and place it next to the patient's head or other readily available location. It will be necessary to replace this airway upon successful intubation or in the event the patient is unable to be intubated.

Gently extend the patient's neck so that the head is positioned with the chin and forehead approximately 45° from the floor (known as the sniffing position). In the event the patient has had an injury to the neck or for other reasons cannot be hyperextended, refer to the procedures for in-line endotracheal intubation (Skill 15).

▼

9 **Insert blade while displacing tongue, lift mandible, and visualize larynx without using teeth as a fulcrum.**

After paralytics have taken effect (approximately 30 seconds), carefully insert the blade of the laryngoscope into the patient's mouth to the depth of the uvula. Using a sweeping motion, move the patient's tongue to the left as you lift at a 45° angle along the facial plane to lift the mandible, keeping the laryngoscope off of the teeth.

Lifting should be performed with a free hand. The habit of resting or placing the left forearm against the patient's forehead frequently causes prying and can be a dangerous practice. Placing the forearm in this position greatly limits and potentially eliminates the ability to lift the patient's lower jaw and tongue. In effect, it promotes the use of the teeth as a fulcrum as the only lifting option.

▼

 10 **Introduce the endotracheal tube and advance it to the proper depth.**

Upon visualization of the vocal cords, pass the endotracheal tube through the cords and into the trachea. As the cuff of the tube passes the cords, stop the insertion process.

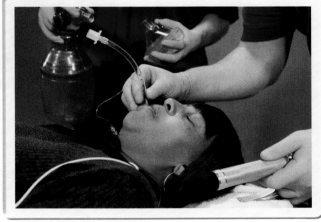

▼

 11 **Remove the laryngoscope from the patient's mouth and remove the stylet from the endotracheal tube.**

Remove the laryngoscope from the patient's mouth and remove the stylet from the endotracheal tube.

▼

Step 12 ▶ Inflate the distal cuff to proper pressure and immediately disconnect syringe.

Inflate the distal cuff of the endotracheal tube with 5 to 10 mL of air. Most patients will need less than the full 10 mL to fill the cuff. Remove the syringe from the inflation port.

▼

Step 13 ▶ Direct ventilation of the patient.

While still holding the tube in place, have your partner attach the bag-mask device to the endotracheal tube and begin ventilations. Instruct your partner to deliver breaths as you move your stethoscope over the patient's abdomen and chest.

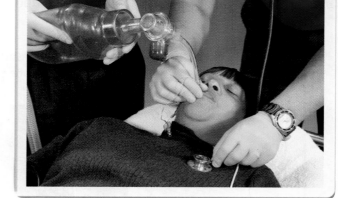

▼

Step 14 ▶ Confirm proper placement by auscultation over the epigastrium and bilaterally over each lung.

Auscultate the abdomen and the chest to determine the correct tube placement. The preferred sequence is to listen over the gastric region first, then over the lower left, upper left, upper right, and finally the lower right chest. By using this sequence, you can determine incorrect placement with a minimal amount of unnecessary ventilations. After confirming placement, move to the next step.

If you hear air over the epigastric region, remove the tube and begin ventilating the patient with a bag-mask device. Some practitioners prefer to leave endotracheal tubes in the esophagus upon finding missed intubation, preferring instead to intubate around this first tube. Their philosophy is that this reduces the chances of missing a second time. However, this may confuse the landmarks and definitely limits the visibility in the hypopharynx. A problem of inefficient ventilations is also created.

In the Field

RSI, RSI, or PAI: Which Is It Really?

RSI can be called either rapid sequence induction or rapid sequence intubation. *Induction* is actually correct for its original context and use, but *intubation* has become the prehospital adaptation. Induction is the process of inducing anesthesia and putting a patient to sleep for surgery and other therapies. Although many EMS agencies use paralytics to assist in intubation, the patient is not asleep, so we don't use induction. Rapid sequence intubation is also a poor term for EMS because there is nothing rapid about it. It is actually the slowest method of performing intubation used. The most accurate term for the use of drugs to aid the intubation process is pharmacologically assisted intubation (PAI). This term applies to all aspects and preferences, ranging from light sedation to full chemical paralysis.

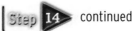 **continued**

Absent breath sounds on the left are an indication of right mainstem intubation. Deflate the cuff. Gently and carefully pull back on the endotracheal tube until you hear breath sounds over the left chest. Reinflate the cuff. Note and document the tube's position in relation to the teeth.

Step 15 Secure the endotracheal tube.

Maintaining a hold on the tube, attach a commercially made endotracheal tube holder. Commercially made devices are preferred over other techniques because they provide the most effective control of the airway. These devices also eliminate the need for an oral airway because they include a bite block.

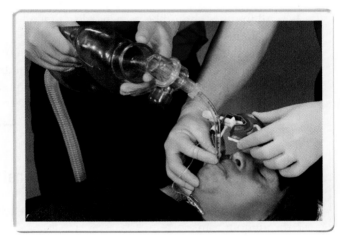

If a commercially made device is not available, secure the endotracheal tube using tape. If you have secured the endotracheal tube using tape, place a bite block in the patient's mouth.

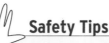

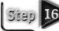 **16** Use three means to ensure tube placement and apply an extrication collar.

Reassess the tube placement through assessment of gastric and breath sounds. At least two additional means of ensuring tube placement should be used. These include:

- Visualization of the tube passing between the cords
- End-tidal carbon dioxide meters
- Fogging of the endotracheal tube
- Esophageal detectors
- Capnographic monitors

Lastly, when placement is ensured, an appropriately sized extrication collar should be applied to maintain the position of the head and neck and thus the airway.

All findings should be verbalized so that all members of the team are aware of the patient's airway status.

Even though the tube's placement has been ensured, continual reassessment should occur. This should be performed any time the patient is moved or defibrillated. Also, always ensure and document the tube placement before turning over patient care at the receiving facility or to a transport team.

 17 Maintain paralysis, sedation, and analgesia.

Following the standard recommendations for each drug used, maintain paralysis throughout transport.

Tracheal Suctioning

Performance Objective

Given an adult patient with an endotracheal tube in place and appropriate equipment, the candidate shall suction down the endotracheal tube, using sterile procedures, in 3 minutes or less.

Equipment

The following equipment is required to perform this skill:
- Appropriate body substance isolation/personal protection equipment
- Oxygen cylinder, regulator, and key
- Oxygen delivery device (appropriate to patient)
  - Bag-mask device
- Suction device and tubing
- Suction catheter
  - Rigid wand (Yankauer type)
  - Flexible catheter
- Sterile water

Indications

- Secretions in the endotracheal tube
- Removal of mucus plugs in patients with asthma

Contraindications

- Hypoxemia
- Atelectasis
- Cardiac arrhythmias
- Tracheobronchial trauma
- Increased intracranial pressure (from excessive cough reflex and agitation)

Complications

- Hypoxemia
- Atelectasis
- Cardiac arrhythmias
- Tracheobronchial trauma
- Increased intracranial pressure (from excessive cough reflex and agitation)

Procedures

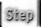 **Ensure body substance isolation before beginning procedures.**

Prior to beginning patient care, appropriate body substance isolation procedures should be employed. Gloves and eye protection are essential. Masks are highly recommended if the patient has any possibility of a respiratory disease. Because this is an aseptic procedure, sterile gloves will be worn. It is recommended that the sterile gloves be donned over nonsterile gloves for greater protection of the provider.

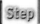 **Ensure sterility throughout the procedure.**

The suction catheter that is placed into the airway should be sterile when inserted. Maintenance of the sterile field through the use of sterile gloves and procedures is essential. Should the sterile field be contaminated, a fresh sterile field should be created to prevent respiratory infections.

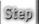 **Identify and select appropriate suction catheter.**

Endotracheal suctioning is performed using a flexible suction catheter. The size of the catheter is determined by the size of the internal diameter of the endotracheal tube (see the table below). The catheter should be small enough to pass the curves of the endotracheal tube and large enough to provide adequate suction. A catheter that is too small will have difficulty suctioning the entire airway and may not pick up thick secretions. This will reduce the efficiency of each suctioning attempt, prompting the practitioner to make repeated attempts to clear the airway and thus increasing the possibility of complications and injury.

Endotracheal Tube Size (Internal Diameter)	Catheter Size
8.0 mm	12F to 16F
7.0 mm	10F to 12F
6.0 mm	10F
5.0 mm	10F
4.0 mm	8F to 10F
3.0 mm	6F

Step 4 ▶ Prepare equipment.

Prepare the suctioning system to provide a negative pressure of 100 to 150 mm Hg. Using an aseptic technique, open the catheter package. Don the sterile glove on the dominant hand. Many suction packages come with a collapsed water cup. If this is present, open the cup with the sterile hand and have an assistant fill the cup with sterile water. If no assistant is available, you may fill the cup with sterile water using the nondominant hand. If the suction package does not have a water cup, open a bottle of sterile water and have it ready to clean the catheter as necessary.

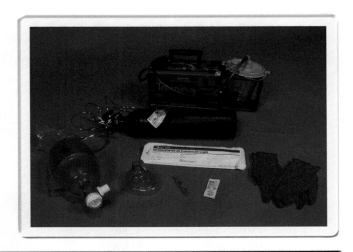

Step 5 ▶ Preoxygenate the patient.

Provide three to five quick breaths to hyperoxygenate the patient.

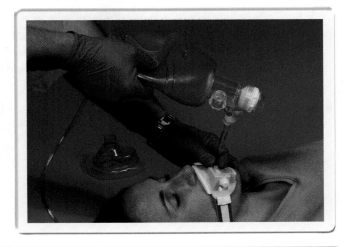

Step **6** ► **Mark maximum insertion length with thumb and forefinger.**

The catheter should be long enough to extend approximately 2″ past the end of the endotracheal tube in the adult patient and no more than 1″ in pediatric patients. Estimate this distance and mark the location by grasping the tube with the thumb and forefinger of your dominant hand. This will be your maximum insertion depth.

Most practitioners prefer to insert the catheter until resistance is felt. This is an accepted practice, and in many ways it is preferred.

Step **7** ► **Insert catheter into the endotracheal tube, leaving catheter port open.**

Using the nondominant hand, remove the bag-mask device from the endotracheal tube. Carefully, observing aseptic procedures, insert the catheter into the endotracheal tube. Continue to insert the catheter until resistance is felt or you have reached your predetermined maximum depth. For thick secretions, the instillation of up to 10 mL of normal saline down the endotracheal tube may be helpful.

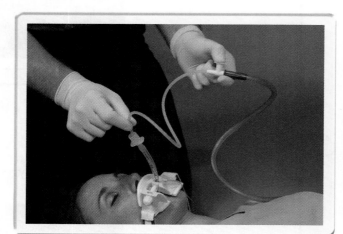

In the Field

Communication

Remember that you should be talking to your patient while performing procedures. Conscious and alert or not, it is good practice to tell the patient what is being done and what to expect during and after the procedure.

Step **8** **At proper insertion depth, cover the catheter port and apply suction while withdrawing the catheter.**

Pull the catheter back approximately 1 cm from the point where resistance is felt and apply suction by covering the catheter port with the thumb of the nondominant hand. Carefully suction while removing the catheter. A twisting motion that includes slight advancements back into the tube should be used. Limit suctioning to no more than 10 seconds while monitoring the patient for cardiac arrhythmias and drop in oxygen saturation. Use the dominant hand to guide the sterile portion of the catheter out of the tube. Keep it away from nonsterile surfaces. Wrapping the catheter in the dominant hand will help protect the sterile environment.

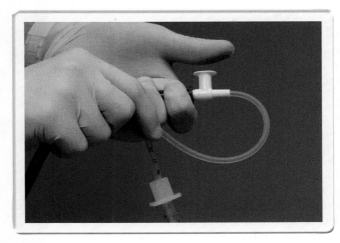

Step **9** **Ventilate or direct ventilation of the patient as the catheter is flushed with sterile water.**

Using the nondominant hand, reattach the bag-mask device and return to ventilation. Using the dominant hand, insert the suction catheter into the prepared sterile water and clean the tip by applying short periods of suction.

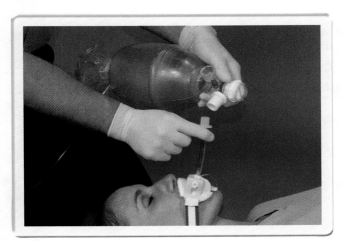

Step **10** **Repeat suction as necessary.**

Following the same procedures, continue to suction until the airway is clear.

Performance Objective

Given an adult patient and appropriate equipment, the candidate shall apply continuous positive airway pressure using criteria herein prescribed, in 3 minutes or less.

Equipment

The following equipment is required to perform this skill:
- Appropriate body substance isolation/personal protective equipment
- Oxygen cylinder, regulator, and key
- Oxygen delivery device (appropriate to patient)
- CPAP machine with required accessories that may include:
  - Face mask with straps appropriate for patient size
  - Corrugated tubing and circuit
  - Positive end-expiratory pressure (PEEP) valve
  - Bacteriostatic filter

Equipment that may be helpful:
- Pulse oximeter
- End-tidal carbon dioxide meter

Indications

- Dyspnea/hypoxia associated with congestive heart failure or pulmonary disease (emphysema, chronic bronchitis, asthma, pneumonia)

Contraindications

- Any patient unable to protect own airway
  - Loss of gag reflex
  - Unresponsiveness
  - Glasgow Coma Scale score of 10 or less
- Thoracic trauma
- Facial trauma or anomalies
- Gastrointestinal bleeding
- Nausea/vomiting
- Respiratory arrest

Complications

- Claustrophobic sensation with increased anxiety
- Increased intrathoracic pressure, resulting in:
  - Decreased venous return to the heart
  - Pneumothorax
  - Gastric distension
  - Sinusitis from poorly fitted mask
  - Conjunctivitis from poorly fitted mask
  - Aspiration pneumonia following vomiting in the mask

Procedures

 Step 1 ► Ensure body substance isolation before beginning procedures.

Prior to beginning patient care, appropriate body substance isolation procedures should be employed.

▼

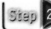 **Step 2 ► Assess patient for indications and contraindications.**

Perform patient assessment to ensure the patient is conscious and alert, can maintain her or his own airway, and has sufficient respiratory effort. Obtain baseline electrocardiogram and vital signs, including oxygen saturation (S_pO_2) and breath sounds to ensure that the patient does not have hypotension or a pneumothorax. Throughout the care of the patient, be sure to continue to reassess vital signs and breath sounds.

▼

 Step 3 ► Assemble the CPAP circuit and machine based on manufacturer's specifications.

CPAP machines and devices vary greatly between manufacturers.

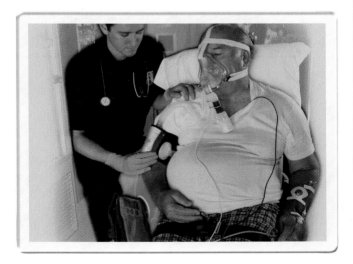

Despite the differences there are also many similarities. Those similarities include:

- Attach the device to an oxygen source. Most machines attach through a standard 50 pounds per square inch (psi) port. Some devices, however, operate by connection to a high-flow flowmeter. If using the flowmeter, ensure it has the ability to deliver 25 L/min.

In the Field

CPAP and BiPAP

CPAP, continuous positive airway pressure, and BiPAP, bi-phasic airway pressure, are similar procedures with one very simple difference. CPAP maintains the airway with *one* pressure, while BiPAP uses two airway pressures. In BiPAP, the inhalation pressure is higher than the exhalation pressure. While patients are usually more comfortable using the BiPAP devices, the machines are more complicated, more expensive, and require more power to operate, leaving them less suited to the prehospital setting—for now.

In the Field

Oxygen Hog

Most prehospital CPAP machines are operated by oxygen pressure. This makes them very inefficient when it comes to conserving oxygen in a portable cylinder. Depending on the amount of oxygen required to operate the device, a standard D cylinder will be drained in less than 5 minutes. This is an important consideration when it comes to moving the patient from his or her house to the ambulance and from the ambulance to the emergency department. It may be necessary to carry several cylinders. Also remember that when changing cylinders, it may be necessary to remove the mask from the patient or at least to remove the PEEP valve from the circuit.

 Step 3 continued

- A face mask and corrugated tubing must be assembled and attached to an outflow port on the machine.
- PEEP valves and bacteriostatic filters are often attached to the CPAP circuit.
- Some devices will begin to operate as soon as the oxygen begins to flow; others will require that an On or Power switch be activated.

▼

 Step 4 **Explain the procedure to the patient.**

Patients who have experienced CPAP in the past may actually ask for the device when you enter the room. If the procedure is new to a patient, you will need to explain the benefits and the sensation he or she is about to experience. Explain that the patient will experience an effect similar to sticking his or her head out of a moving car. The patient should be coached to breathe in through the nose and out through the mouth.

▼

 Step 5 **Seat and fit mask.**

Hold the mask up to the patient's face and ensure there is a tight seal. It may be more comfortable for the patient to hold the mask against her or his face until becoming accustomed to the pressure. When the patient has become accustomed to the face mask, attach the straps so the mask remains in place without being held.

▼

6 ► **Adjust pressure.**

Adjust the setting to deliver the proper pressure for the patient's needs. For most congestive heart failure and pulmonary edema patients, the pressure will be set to 10 cm of water (cm H_2O). For asthma, COPD, and other conditions, the pressure is set to 5 cm H_2O.

▼

 7 ► **Assess effects of therapy.**

Assess the patient to determine the effects of CPAP. Remember that the patient must be breathing with a sufficient effort for CPAP to be effective. CPAP aids in maintaining airway pressures but is not a ventilator. Should the patient's condition deteriorate, it will be necessary to support ventilations with a bag-mask device and consider the need for endotracheal intubation.

In the Field

Delivering Medications

It is important to note that the use of CPAP is an alleviating therapy, not a corrective therapy. Medications must be incorporated to remove the cause of the problem.

- For congestive heart failure it may be necessary to administer sublingual nitroglycerin. The initial therapy is easy to administer before the mask is attached to the patient. Repeated doses can be given by removing the mask just long enough to administer the nitroglycerin.
- Nebulized medications can be administered through the CPAP circuit. Many devices have a nebulizer port built into the system. If there is not a nebulizer port, one can be attached by simply cutting the corrugated tubing and placing the nebulizer into the existing line.

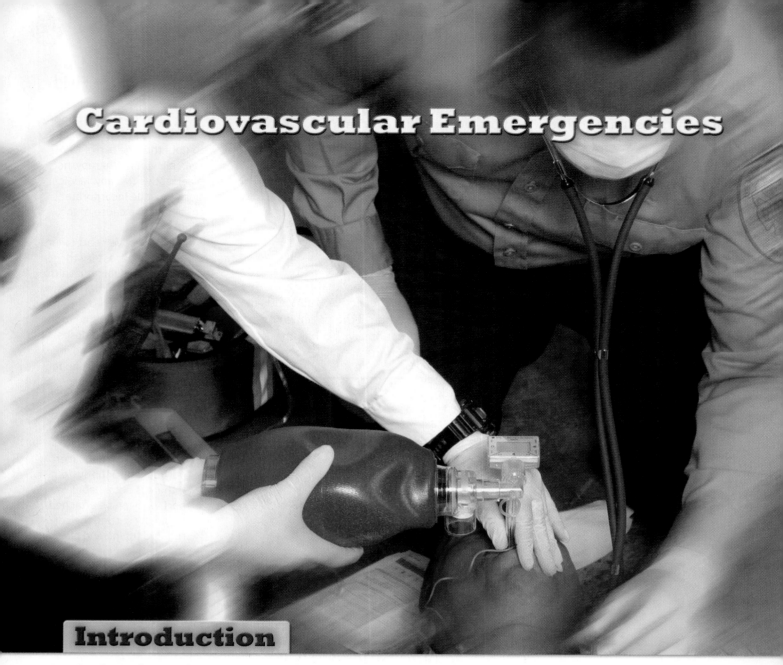

Cardiovascular Emergencies

Introduction

Cardiopulmonary resuscitation (CPR) is the process of using chest compression and ventilation to replace the patient's normal heart and lung functions. The process is intended to ensure minimal blood flow to the brain while other interventions work to return the patient's heartbeat.

Cardiopulmonary resuscitation standards are set by the International Liaison Committee on Resuscitation (ILCOR). The standards reflect the most current thinking and research available for the management of patients in cardiac arrest and in critical cardiac situations.

When assigned the task of performing chest compressions or ventilations, the rescuer must focus all of his or her attention and efforts on the task at hand. The application of electrical therapy in critical heart patients is an essential component in identifying and managing life-threatening arrhythmias. The skills in this section will assist you in performing resuscitation techniques for patients of all ages.

Performance Objective

Given an unconscious adolescent or adult patient, the candidate should assess of the need for CPR and proceed as indicated upon identifying cardiac arrest. The candidate shall perform the procedure for adult CPR in 5 minutes or less.

Equipment

The following equipment is required to perform this skill:
- Appropriate body substance isolation/personal protective equipment
- Pocket mask with
  - One-way valve
  - Oxygen connecting port
- Bag-mask device

Equipment that may be helpful:
- Oropharyngeal airways (various sizes)
- Nasopharyngeal airways (various sizes)
- Oxygen cylinder, regulator, and key
- Automated external defibrillator
- Suction device
- Pulse oximeter
- End-tidal carbon dioxide meter

Indications

- Cardiac arrest in adolescent (ie, displaying secondary sexual characteristics) and adult patients
- Severe bradycardia

Contraindications

- Obvious signs of death
- Valid, verifiable Do Not Resuscitate order

Complications

- Fractured ribs or sternum
- Lacerated liver from fracture of the xiphoid process

Procedures

 Step 1 ⟩ **Ensure body substance isolation before beginning procedures.**

Prior to beginning patient care, appropriate body substance isolation procedures should be employed.

▼

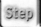 **Step 2** ⟩ **Assess level of consciousness.**

Grasp the patient's shoulders and gently shake. Firm, nonviolent action may be required to awaken a deeply sleeping or impaired patient. Shout "Are you OK?" or a similar question. If known, use the patient's name. It should take less than 10 seconds to arouse the patient. The patient can be assessed in any position; however, to assess the airway and, more important, to begin chest compressions, the patient should be positioned supine with a hard surface beneath the back.

▼

 Step 3 ⟩ **Open airway.**

Kneel beside the patient's shoulders and open the airway using the most appropriate method. Begin with the jaw-thrust maneuver until you are sure no cervical spine injury exists. Patients with stiff or large necks may also require a jaw thrust. Once a neck injury has been ruled out, the use of the head tilt–chin lift maneuver is recommended.

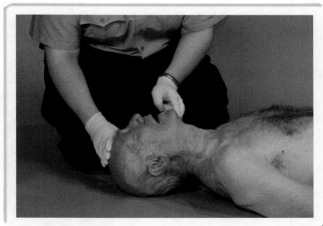

▼

 In the Field

The Lone Rescuer: Call for Help or Begin CPR?

As a professional rescuer working as a part of a fully equipped arriving EMS or First Response unit, there is no need to call for help. However, when encountering a patient while you're off duty or when you arrive alone, it is essential to call for help as soon as appropriate. The decision is based on the speed of the patient's collapse. Sudden collapse is most often the result of ventricular fibrillation. In these cases it is important to call for help immediately, because the patient's survival is dependent on early defibrillation. Leave the patient, call for help/defibrillation, and return for further assessment and care. In cases where the cause of collapse is hypoxia or asphyxia, ventilations are essential. Begin CPR and perform five cycles (2 minutes) of chest compressions and ventilations before calling for help.

Step **4** ► **Assessment: Determine breathlessness.**

While maintaining the open airway, place your ear approximately 1 inch above the patient's mouth. Face the patient's chest and look for chest rise.

This is known as the *look, listen, and feel* procedure: *Look* for chest rise, *listen* for air exchange, and *feel* for air against your cheek. If any of these are found, the patient is breathing and should be assessed for adequacy of ventilations and other concerns. A breathing patient is usually placed in the recovery position if no trauma is suspected. It

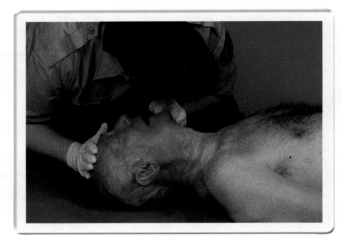

should take less than 10 seconds to determine breathlessness.

If the victim is breathing, place him or her in the recovery position and continue further assessment.

Step **5** ► **Begin effective ventilations.**

Properly position a pocket mask or other barrier device over the patient's face. Deliver two slow breaths, each over 1 full second, causing chest rise. Allow complete deflation of the chest between breaths. It is important to watch the patient's chest throughout the ventilation procedure.

 In the Field

Mouth-to-Mouth Ventilations

Although professional rescuers should possess the skills necessary to perform mouth-to-mouth resuscitation, it is not recommended. Instead, professional responders should use mouth-to-mask ventilations or other barrier devices when available.

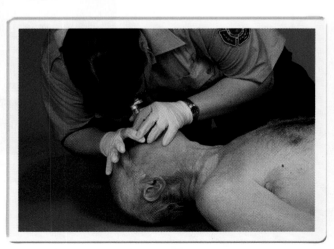

Step **6** **Assessment: Determine pulselessness.**

While maintaining an open airway, move your hand under the patient's chin down along the neck and feel for a carotid pulse. It should take less than 10 seconds to assess circulation. If after 10 seconds no definite pulse is felt, prepare to deliver chest compressions. It is very important not to focus on finding a pulse. Delaying the start of compressions can be fatal to the patient.

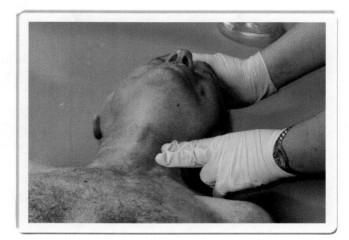

If a pulse is present but the victim is still not breathing, provide rescue breathing, one breath every 5 to 6 seconds. Recheck the victim's pulse about every 2 minutes.

▼

Step **7** **Use appropriate hand position for compressions.**

Place the heel of one hand over the lower half of the patient's sternum in the center of the chest, between the nipples. Place the heel of the other hand on top of the first.

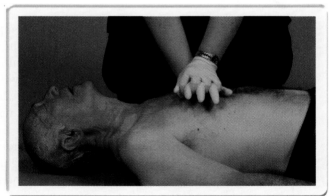

▼

Step **8** **Begin chest compressions.**

Compress the chest vertically 1.5 to 2 inches, keeping your elbows locked. The compressions should be smooth and even, equally up and down in a fluid motion. The end of the upstroke should allow the chest to return to the relaxed position without removing your hands from the chest. It is often helpful to count out a mnemonic to keep the rhythm.

▼

In the Field

Chest Compressions
Remember to "push hard and push fast." It is very important to the patient that the chest compressions be delivered with absolute effectiveness. Studies of both in-hospital and out-of-hospital compressions have found that 40% of delivered chest compressions are of insufficient depth to develop adequate blood flow. Close attention to the delivery of chest compressions will correct this devastating oversight.

 Step 9 **Performs Steps 1 to 8 in proper sequence.**

It is essential that these steps be performed in the proper sequence. Failure to do so may result in chest compressions being performed on an adequately perfusing patient, or ventilations on an adequately breathing patient. Both are embarrassing.

 Step 10 **Perform five cycles of 30 compressions and two ventilations at a rate of 100/min (5 compressions in 3 to 4 seconds).**

Chest compressions are delivered at a rate of 100/min. After each set of 30 compressions, stop, open the airway, and deliver two breaths exactly as described in Step 5. It is essential to relocate the proper hand position on the patient's chest each time chest compressions begin. Continue this sequence of 30 compressions to two ventilations for five cycles, and then stop and reassess the patient for perfusion.

 Step 11 **Assessment: Determine pulselessness.**

Check the pulse as described in Step 6, lasting less than 10 seconds.

 Step 12 **Continue CPR.**

If the patient is still pulseless, resume chest compressions. Relocate the proper hand placement and continue the compression/ventilation ratio of 30:2. Continue to check for signs of perfusion every 5 minutes.

If the patient's pulse returns, the probability that respirations will also return is initially low. Ventilations may need to continue for some time. If respirations do return to an adequate rate and no signs of trauma are found, place the patient in the recovery position and continue to monitor pulse and respirations.

CPR should be continued as long as any chance of survival exists. In advanced life support (ALS) systems, with electrocardiographic monitoring, defibrillation, and ALS capabilities, all resuscitative efforts should be performed at the scene. It should be understood that competent ALS care administered by paramedics in the field provides a greater chance of successful resuscitation than care of the patient transported to the hospital. Studies have shown that there is no chance that a hospital emergency department will be successful in reviving a patient that paramedics could not.

It is also important to accept death. In ALS systems, patients who have been adequately managed but remain in cardiac arrest should not be transported. These patients need resuscitative efforts stopped. However, before deciding to halt efforts, you must be prepared to inform the patient's family that the patient has died. This may be the most difficult step, but it is essential that paramedics learn how to deliver devastating news to a patient's family.

Adult Team CPR

Performance Objective

Given an unconscious adolescent or adult patient and a partner, candidates should assess of the need for CPR and proceed as indicated upon identifying cardiac arrest. The candidates shall perform the procedure for adult team CPR in 5 minutes or less.

Equipment

The following equipment is required to perform this skill:
- Appropriate body substance isolation/personal protective equipment
- Pocket mask with
  - One-way valve
  - Oxygen connecting port
- Bag-mask device

Equipment that may be helpful:
- Oropharyngeal airways (various sizes)
- Nasopharyngeal airways (various sizes)
- Oxygen cylinder, regulator, and key
- Automated external defibrillator
- Suction device
- Pulse oximeter
- End-tidal carbon dioxide meter

Indications

- Cardiac arrest in adolescent (ie, displaying secondary sexual characteristics) and adult patients
- Severe bradycardia

Contraindications

- Obvious signs of death
- Valid, verifiable Do Not Resuscitate order

Complications

- Fractured ribs or sternum
- Lacerated liver from fracture of the xiphoid process

Procedures

Rescuer One takes initial responsibility for patient assessment. Rescuer Two assists Rescuer One.

 Ensure body substance isolation before beginning procedures.

Prior to beginning patient care, appropriate body substance isolation procedures should be employed.

 Rescuer One: Assess patient.   **Rescuer Two: Prepare equipment.**

Following the procedures described in adult one-rescuer CPR (Skill 24), assess the patient's level of consciousness, airway, and ventilations.

Gather and prepare the equipment needed to care for a patient in cardiac arrest. This should include a pocket mask or bag-mask device and an automated external defibrillator (AED). Other equipment that may be helpful includes suction equipment, backboard, and automatic compression devices.

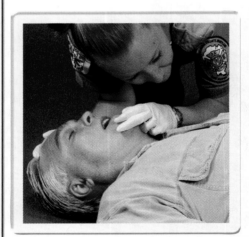

Step 3 **Rescuer One: Instruct partner to begin ventilations and check for pulse.**

Upon determining breathlessness, instruct your partner(s) to begin ventilations. Once ventilations have been delivered, assess the patient for the presence of a pulse. Check for a carotid pulse for no more than 10 seconds.

Rescuer Two: Ventilate the patient.

Using a pocket mask or bag-mask device, deliver two ventilations sufficient to cause chest rise. Ventilations should be given over 1 second.

To ensure proper ventilation using a bag-mask device, two rescuers should work together: one to achieve mask seal, the other to squeeze the bag. If a third person is available, cricoid pressure should be applied.

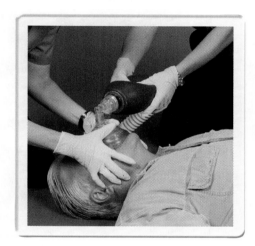

In the Field

Alternate Technique If only two rescuers are present, it may be more effective for the person at the head to create and hold a two-handed mask seal. The person giving chest compressions can then reach with one hand and deliver two breaths. This will improve ventilation quickly.

Rescuer One: Deliver chest compressions.

Locate the correct hand position on the patient's chest and deliver 30 compressions at a rate of 100/min. Repeat compressions after each set of two ventilations for a total of five cycles. In two-rescuer CPR, your hands should never leave the patient's chest, so relocating the correct position between ventilations is not necessary.

Rescuer Two: Ventilate after each set of 30 compressions. Attach defibrillator pads if available.

Continue to ventilate after each set of 30 compressions for a total of five cycles. Between sets of ventilations, attach defibrillator pads to the patient's chest if they are available.

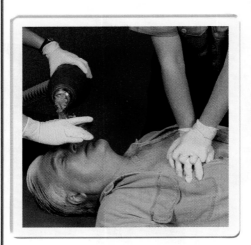

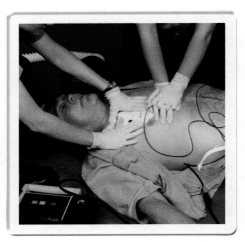

 Rescuer One: Reassess patient.

Immediately after giving the last set of chest compressions, reassess the patient for the presence of a pulse. If an AED or standard defibrillator is available, check for the presence of a shockable rhythm. If a shockable rhythm is identified, deliver the required energy level.

Rescuer Two: Move to chest.

Move to the patient's chest and prepare for chest compressions. If an AED or standard defibrillator has been attached, stand clear of the patient and avoid patient movement while the rhythm is being identified.

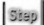 **6**

Rescuer One: Instruct partner to begin compressions.

Immediately after determining the absence of a pulse, or immediately after the defibrillator has delivered its shock, instruct your partner to begin chest compressions.

Rescuer Two: Begin chest compressions.

Locate the correct hand position on the patient's chest and deliver 30 compressions at a rate of 100/min.

7

Rescuer One: Ventilate the patient after each set of 30 compressions.

Continue to ventilate after each set of 30 compressions for a total of five cycles.

Rescuer Two: Repeat compressions for a total of five cycles.

Repeat compressions after each set of two ventilations for a total of five cycles. In two-rescuer CPR, your hands should never leave the patient's chest, so relocating the correct position between ventilations is not necessary.

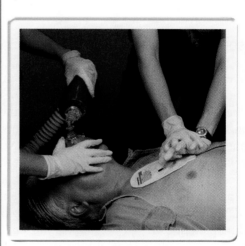

 In the Field

Adequate Ventilations Patients experiencing sudden cardiac arrest may display occasional gasps. These should not be considered adequate ventilations. Treat the patient with occasional gasps as if he or she were not breathing.

Special Populations

CPR Following Endotracheal Intubation

A patient who is intubated with a properly placed endotracheal tube can have chest compressions performed simultaneously with ventilations, removing the need to pause. The compression-to-ventilation ratio no longer exists. Chest compressions should be given uninterrupted at a rate of 100/min, while ventilations are given at a rate of 6 to 8 breaths/min. Remember to prevent compressor fatigue and a reduction in compression rate and depth by rotating the responsibilities every 2 minutes.

In the Field

Interposed Abdominal Compressions

If a third rescuer is available, interposed abdominal compressions can be delivered. This technique is an adjunct to chest compressions and is used to enhance venous return during CPR. The technique is performed by compressing the abdomen midway between the xiphoid process and the umbilicus during the relaxation phase of the chest compressions. Properly performed, the chest and abdominal compressions should function like a see-saw, with one up and one down at any one time.

Although there is little evidence to recommend abdominal compressions in the prehospital setting, there is no reason the technique should not be employed if the personnel are properly trained and it is approved by medical control.

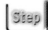 **Step 8** ▸ **Reassess patient.**

After each set of five cycles, assess the patient for the presence of a pulse. If an AED or standard defibrillator is available, assess the patient for a shockable rhythm. If a shockable rhythm is identified, deliver the required energy level.

An effective switch should have both rescuers repositioned and CPR reestablished in less than 10 seconds. It is always best, when possible, for rescuers to work on opposite sides of the patient. This allows rescuers to simply move up or down during the switch. However, in the back of an ambulance it may be necessary for the compressor to move forward into the door opening while the ventilator slides down to the chest. This allows for a smooth switch without crawling on top of each other.

▼

 Step 9 ▸ **Continue compressions and ventilations.**

Continue to deliver compressions and ventilations as a team. Remember to change responsibilities for chest compressions with each assessment of the patient.

▼

 Step 10 ▸ **Prepare patient for transport and advanced life support.**

While maintaining the sequence of chest compressions and ventilations, prepare the patient for transport. The decision of when and how to accomplish this move should not be taken lightly. Basic life support units should work toward transport from the first minute they arrive on scene. Advanced life support units should only transport after all initial patient care procedures and medications have been accomplished or when the patient will benefit more from rapid transport than from on-scene patient care. It is important to remember that CPR in the back of a moving ambulance, especially an ambulance that is being driven in an emergency mode, is less than optimal. CPR in the back of a moving ambulance is also hazardous to the personnel providing patient care.

When advanced life support is available, endotracheal intubation will be established in most cases (see Skill 10). Once the patient is intubated, chest compressions should be given at a rate of 100/min and without stopping for the ventilations. Ventilations will then be delivered at a rate of 6 to 8 breaths/min using a bag-mask device.

Adult Foreign Body Airway Obstruction

Performance Objective

Given a conscious adolescent or adult patient who appears to be choking, the candidate should assess the need for abdominal thrusts and proceed as indicated upon identifying an airway obstruction. The candidate shall perform the procedure for conscious adult foreign body airway obstruction in 3 minutes or less.

Equipment

The following equipment is required to perform this skill:
- Appropriate body substance isolation/personal protective equipment
- Pocket mask with
  - One-way valve
  - Oxygen connecting port

Equipment that may be helpful:
- Oropharyngeal airways (various sizes)
- Nasopharyngeal airways (various sizes)
- Bag-mask device
- Oxygen cylinder, regulator, and key
- Automated external defibrillator
- Suction device
- Pulse oximeter
- End-tidal carbon dioxide meter

Indications

- Foreign body airway obstruction in the adolescent (ie, displaying secondary sexual characteristics) or adult patient

Contraindications

- Patients who can speak or cough

Complications

- None if properly performed

Procedures

 Ensure body substance isolation before beginning procedures.

Prior to beginning patient care, appropriate body substance isolation procedures should be employed.

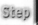 **Assess airway and breathing.**

Begin your assessment with the simple question "Are you choking?" If the patient nods "yes" or continues to grab his or her throat and does not speak, prepare to perform abdominal thrusts to remove the obstruction from the airway.

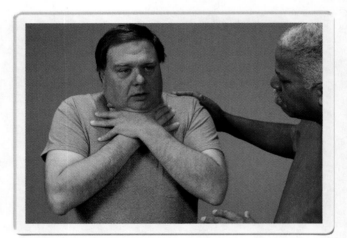

If the patient is able to breathe on his or her own and can speak, the patient is able to move air and does not need emergent assistance. Encourage the patient to cough. Inform the patient you are going to help him or her. Continue to talk to the patient and explain each step as you perform the procedure.

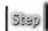 **3** ▶ **Stand behind the patient and position hands.**

Position yourself behind the patient. Reach around the patient's waist and make a fist with one hand.

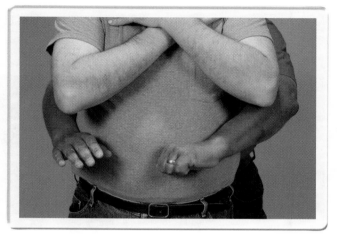

With the thumb side against the patient's abdomen, place the fist just above the umbilicus, but below the xiphoid process. Grasp your fist with your opposite hand.

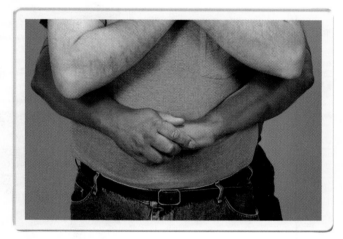

▼

 4 ▶ **Perform abdominal thrusts.**

With both hands in position, apply quick, upward thrusts into the patient's abdomen. Ensure each thrust is individual and distinct, allowing the abdomen to return to its original position.

▼

5 ▶ **Repeat abdominal thrusts.**

Repeat thrusts until the foreign body is expelled, the patient can breathe spontaneously, or the patient becomes unconscious.

If the patient becomes unconscious, guide the patient to the ground and call for help.

▼

Special Populations

Foreign Body Airway Maneuvers on Large Patients
Patients who are obese or pregnant, or who in general have a large abdominal mass, cannot have abdominal thrusts performed with success. In these patients you can achieve the same effect through the use of chest compressions. Chest compressions are delivered by standing behind the patient and placing your arms around his or her chest and delivering thrusts to the midsternum between the nipple line. If the patient is too large for you to reach around his or her chest, consider moving the patient against a wall and performing the compressions from the front. Remember to duck.

Deliver chest compressions (for unconscious patients or for patients who become unconscious while removing an airway obstruction).

Place the heel of one hand over the lower half of the patient's sternum in the center of the chest, between the nipples.

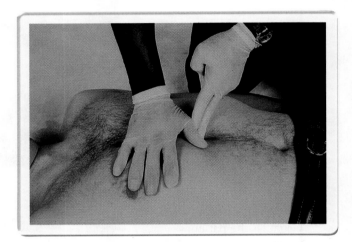

Place the heel of the other hand on top of the first.

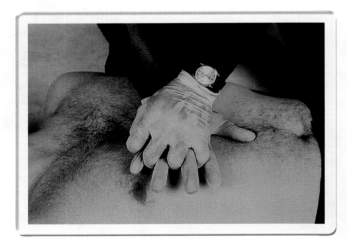

Compress the chest vertically 1.5 to 2 inches, keeping your elbows locked. The compressions should be smooth and even, equally up and down in a fluid motion. The end of the upstroke should allow the chest to return to the relaxed position without removing your hands from the chest. Deliver the full 30 compressions.

Step 7 Inspect the airway and assess for breathing.

After delivering 30 compressions, open the patient's mouth and look for the dislodged foreign object. If it is seen, perform a finger sweep to remove the object.

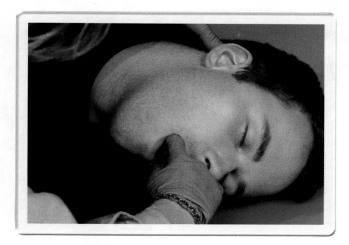

If the object cannot be removed, attempt to ventilate around it rather than waste time in recovery. If no object is seen, attempt to ventilate. If able to ventilate, give two breaths, each lasting 1 full second.

▼

Step 8 Repeat Steps 6 and 7 until successful.

Continue with chest compressions, inspection, and attempted ventilations until ventilations are effective. If the object is not able to be recovered, it may be necessary for a person with appropriate training to remove it with direct visualization and Magill forceps. This is an advanced procedure, but it is the definitive treatment.

Child CPR

Performance Objective

Given an unconscious child patient, the candidate should assess the need for CPR and proceed as indicated upon identifying cardiac arrest. The candidate shall perform the procedure for child CPR in 5 minutes or less.

Equipment

The following equipment is required to perform this skill:
- Appropriate body substance isolation/personal protective equipment

Equipment that may be helpful:
- Oropharyngeal airways (various sizes)
- Nasopharyngeal airways (various sizes)
- Bag-mask device
- Oxygen cylinder, regulator, and key
- Automated external defibrillator
- Suction device
- Pulse oximeter
- End-tidal carbon dioxide meter

Indications

- Cardiac arrest in children between the ages of 1 to adolescence (ie, displaying secondary sexual characteristics)
- Severe bradycardia

Contraindications

- Obvious signs of death
- Valid, verifiable Do Not Resuscitate order

Complications

- Fractured ribs or sternum
- Lacerated liver from fracture of the xiphoid process

Procedures

 1 **Ensure body substance isolation before beginning procedures.**

Prior to beginning patient care, appropriate body substance isolation procedures should be employed.

▼

 2 **Determine unresponsiveness and position patient.**

Grasp the child's shoulders and gently shake. Firm, nonviolent action may be required to awaken a deeply sleeping or impaired child. Shout "Are you OK?" or a similar question. If possible, use the child's name. It should take no more than 10 seconds to arouse the child. The child can be assessed in any position; however, to assess the airway and, more important, to begin chest compressions, the child should be positioned supine with a hard surface beneath the back.

▼

 3 **Open airway.**

Kneel beside the child's shoulders and open the airway using the most appropriate method. Children with potential cervical injury will require the use of a jaw-thrust maneuver, but in most circumstances the head tilt–chin lift maneuver is recommended. Position your hand nearest the child's head on the forehead. Place the fingers of your other hand on the underside of the chin. Pulling up on the chin and pushing down on the forehead will tilt the head back and open the airway. The head should rest between 45° and 60° back. Children will require less manipulation than adults.

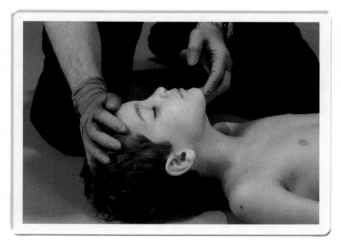

▼

 Special Populations

The Child Patient

For the purposes of basic cardiac life support, ILCOR recommends that professional health care providers consider a child any patient who is older than 1 year and has not developed secondary sexual characteristics. This extends the definition given to the lay rescuer from 8 to nearly 14 years of age.

 Special Populations

The Lone Rescuer: Call for Help or Begin CPR?

Unlike adults, children seldom experience ventricular fibrillation. Most cases of cardiac arrest are the result of a serious respiratory compromise. In most cases, children experience cardiac arrest following a hypoxic episode. It is important to administer CPR with five cycles (2 minutes) of compressions and ventilations before calling for help. When the cardiac arrest appears suddenly, it is important to call for help first, and then return to the patient and begin CPR.

Step 4 ▶ **Assessment: Determine breathlessness.**

While maintaining the open airway, place your ear approximately 1 inch above the child's mouth. Face the child's chest and look for chest rise. This is known as the *look, listen, and feel* procedure: *Look* for chest rise, *listen* for air exchange, and *feel* for air against your cheek. If any of these are found and no trauma is suspected, the child is breathing and should be placed in the recovery position and assessed for adequacy of ventilations and other concerns. It should take no more than 10 seconds to determine breathlessness. Remember that in children, small chest movement and more subtle breaths will be present. You must pay close attention to all signs.

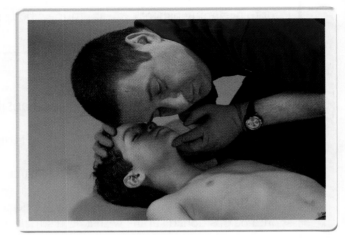

▼

Step 5 ▶ **Ventilate twice.**

While maintaining the open airway, pinch the child's nose and make a tight seal over the child's mouth with a barrier device.

In smaller children it may be possible, and necessary, to occlude the nose with your cheek. Deliver two gentle breaths, each lasting 1 second, to cause chest rise. Allow complete deflation of the chest between breaths. It is important to watch the child's chest throughout the ventilation procedure.

▼

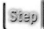

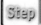 **Assessment: Determine pulselessness.**

Slide your hand under the chin down along the child's neck and feel for a carotid pulse. It should take no more than 10 seconds to assess circulation. If there are no signs of definitive circulation present after 10 seconds, prepare to deliver chest compressions. It is very important not to focus on finding a pulse. In a child who is not breathing, is unconscious, and not moving, consider the pulse to be absent. Delaying the start of compressions can be fatal to the child.

If a pulse is present but the child is still not breathing, provide rescue breathing, one breath every 3 to 5 seconds. Recheck the child's pulse about every 2 minutes.

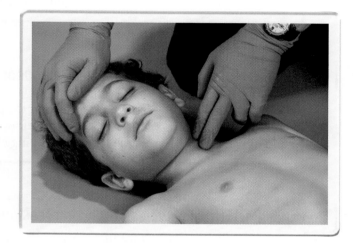

▼

Step 7 ▶ Use appropriate hand position for compressions.

Place the heel of your hand on the lower half of the child's sternum between the nipples. In larger children it may be necessary to use your second hand as you would on the adult patient.

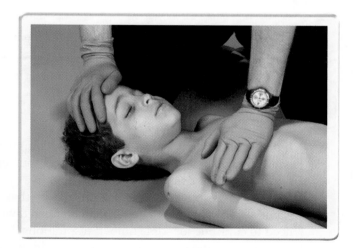

▼

Begin chest compressions.

Compress the chest vertically one third to one half the depth of the child's chest, keeping your elbow locked. The compressions should be smooth and even, equally up and down in a fluid motion. The end of the upstroke should allow the chest to return to the relaxed position without removing your hands from the chest. It is often helpful to count out a mnemonic to keep the rhythm.

▼

 Perform Steps 1 to 8 in proper sequence.

It is essential that these steps be performed in the proper sequence. Failure to do so may result in chest compressions being performed on an adequately perfusing child, or ventilations on an adequately breathing child.

▼

 Perform five cycles of 30 compressions and two ventilations at a rate of 100/min (5 compressions in 3 to 4 seconds).

Chest compressions are delivered at a rate of 100/min. After each set of 30 compressions, stop, open the airway, and deliver two breaths exactly as performed in Step 5. Continue this sequence of 30 compressions to two ventilations for five cycles, and then stop and reassess the child for perfusion.

▼

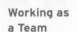

Working as a Team

When professional rescuers are working as a team in the care of a child or infant in cardiac arrest, it is recommended that 15 compressions be given for every two ventilations. Once the child has been intubated, no pause between compressions is necessary, but be sure to give compressions at a rate of 100/min and to ventilate at 12 to 20 breaths/min.

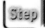 **Reassessment: Determine pulselessness.**

Check the pulse as described in Step 6, lasting no more than 10 seconds.

▼

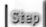 **Continue CPR.**

If the child is still pulseless, resume chest compressions. Relocate the proper hand placement and continue the compression/ventilation ratio of 30:2. Continue to check for signs of perfusion every five cycles.

If the child's pulse returns, the probability that respirations will also return is initially low, but much better than compared with an adult. Ventilations may need to continue for some time. If respirations do return to an adequate rate and no signs of trauma are found, place the child in the recovery position and continue to monitor pulse and respirations.

CPR should continue as long as any chance of survival exists. In advanced life support (ALS) systems, with electrocardiographic monitoring, defibrillation, and ALS capabilities, all resuscitative efforts should be performed at the scene. It should be understood that competent ALS care administered by paramedics

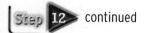

Step 12 continued

in the field provides a greater chance of successful resuscitation than care of the child transported to the hospital.

It is also important to accept death. In ALS systems, children who have been adequately managed but remain in cardiac arrest should not be transported. These children need resuscitative efforts stopped. However, before deciding to halt efforts, you must be prepared to inform the child's family that the child has died. This may be the most difficult step, but it is essential that paramedics learn how to deliver devastating news to a pediatric patient's family. If transport is determined to be necessary, it is important that a pediatric facility be considered rather than a local or regional hospital. Pediatric care is very specialized. Transporting to local hospitals is not in the child's best interest and in many ways could be considered negligence.

Child Foreign Body Airway Obstruction

Performance Objective

Given a conscious child patient who appears to be choking, the candidate begin assess the need to perform abdominal thrusts and proceed as indicated upon identifying an airway obstruction. The candidate shall perform the procedure for conscious child foreign body airway obstruction in 3 minutes or less.

Equipment

The following equipment is required to perform this skill:
- Appropriate body substance isolation/personal protective equipment

Equipment that may be helpful:
- Oropharyngeal airways (various sizes)
- Nasopharyngeal airways (various sizes)
- Bag-mask device
- Oxygen cylinder, regulator, and key
- Automated external defibrillator
- Suction device
- Pulse oximeter
- End-tidal carbon dioxide meter

Indications

- Foreign body airway obstruction in children between the ages of 1 to adolescence (ie, displaying secondary sexual characteristics)

Contraindications

- Patients who can speak or cough

Complications

- None if properly performed

Procedures

Step 1 ▶ Ensure body substance isolation before beginning procedures.

Prior to beginning patient care, appropriate body substance isolation procedures should be employed.

▼

Step 2 ▶ Assess airway and breathing.

Begin your assessment with the simple question "Are you choking?" If the child nods "yes" or continues to grab her or his throat and does not speak, prepare to perform abdominal thrusts to remove the obstruction from the airway.

   If the child is able to breathe on his or her own and can speak, the child is able to move air and does not need emergent assistance. Encourage the child to cough. Inform the child you are going to help him or her. Continue to talk to the child and explain each step as you perform the procedure.

▼

Step 3 ▶ Stand behind the child and position hands.

Position yourself behind the child. Reach around the child's waist and make a fist with one hand. With the thumb side against the child's abdomen, place the fist just above the umbilicus, but below the xiphoid process. Grasp your fist with your opposite hand.

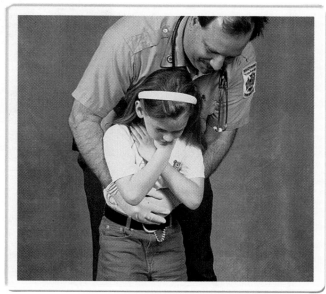

▼

Step 4 ▶ **Perform abdominal thrusts.**

With both hands in position, apply quick, upward thrusts into the child's abdomen. Ensure each thrust is individual and distinct, allowing the abdomen to return to its original position.

▼

Step 5 ▶ **Repeat abdominal thrusts.**

Repeat thrusts until the foreign body is expelled, the child can breathe spontaneously, or the child becomes unconscious.

If the child becomes unconscious, guide the child to the ground and call for help. Continue to Step 6.

▼

Step 6 ▶ **Start CPR (for unconscious children or for children who become unconscious while removing an airway obstruction).**

Attempt to ventilate the child. If unsuccessful, reopen the airway and attempt ventilation again. Perform chest compressions. Place the heel of your hand on the lower half of the child's sternum between the nipples. In larger children it may be necessary to use your second hand as you would on the adult patient.

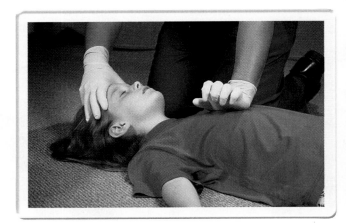

Compress the chest vertically one third to one half the depth of the child's chest, keeping your elbow locked. The compressions should be smooth and even, equally up and down in a fluid motion. The end of the upstroke should allow the chest to return to the relaxed position without removing your hands from the chest. Deliver the full 30 compressions.

▼

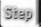 **Inspect the airway and assess for breathing.**

After delivering 30 compressions, open the child's mouth and look for the dislodged foreign object. If it is seen, perform a finger sweep to remove the object. If the object cannot be removed, attempt to ventilate around it rather than waste time in recovery. If no object is seen, attempt to ventilate. If able to ventilate, give two breaths, each lasting 1 full second.

▼

  Repeat Steps 6 and 7 until successful.

Continue with compressions, inspection, and attempted ventilations until ventilations are effective. If the object is not able to be recovered, it may be necessary for a person with appropriate training to remove it with direct visualization and Magill forceps. This is an advanced procedure, but it is the definitive treatment.

Performance Objective

Given an unconscious infant, the candidate should assess the need for CPR and proceed as indicated upon identifying cardiac arrest. The candidate shall perform the procedure for infant CPR in 5 minutes or less.

Equipment

The following equipment is required to perform this skill:
- Appropriate body substance isolation/personal protective equipment

Equipment that may be helpful:
- Oropharyngeal airways (various sizes)
- Nasopharyngeal airways (various sizes)
- Bag-mask device
- Oxygen cylinder, regulator, and key
- Suction device
- Pulse oximeter
- End-tidal carbon dioxide meter

Indications

- Cardiac arrest in patients younger than 1 year
- Bradycardia with associated poor perfusion

Contraindications

- Obvious signs of death
- Valid, verifiable Do Not Resuscitate order

Complications

- Fractured ribs or sternum
- Lacerated liver from fracture of the xiphoid process

Procedures

Step **1** Ensure body substance isolation before beginning procedures.

Prior to beginning patient care, appropriate body substance isolation procedures should be employed.

▼

Step **2** Determine unresponsiveness and position patient.

Gently grasp the victim and call out loudly, "Are you all right?" Tapping or flicking the infant's feet may also be used. Firm, nonviolent action may be required to awaken a deeply sleeping or impaired infant. If known, use the infant's name. It should take no more than 10 seconds to arouse the infant. The infant can be assessed in any position; however, to assess the airway and, more important, to begin chest compressions, the infant should be positioned supine with a hard surface beneath the back.

▼

Step **3** Open airway.

Open the airway using a head tilt–chin lift maneuver. An infant's airway is more pliable than that of adults; thus, less extension is needed. Overextension can actually occlude the airway. To maintain the open airway, it is helpful to place the rescuer's hand or a folded towel under the infant's upper back. This will allow the head to fall naturally and maintain the open airway.

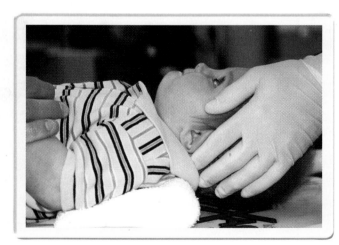

▼

Step **Assessment: Determine breathlessness.**

While maintaining the open airway, place your ear approximately 1 inch above the infant's mouth. Face the infant's chest and look for chest rise. This is known as the *look, listen, and feel* procedure: *Look* for chest rise, *listen* for air exchange, and *feel* for air against your cheek. If any of these are found, the infant is breathing and should be assessed for adequacy of ventilations and other concerns. It should take no more than 10 seconds to determine breathlessness. Remember that in infants and children, small chest movement and more subtle breaths will be present. You must pay close attention to all signs.

▼

Step 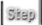 **Ventilate twice.**

While maintaining the open airway, cover both the infant's mouth and nose with your mouth. Deliver two slow breaths, each lasting 1 full second, causing adequate chest rise. Allow complete deflation of the chest between breaths. It is important to watch the infant's chest throughout the ventilation procedure.

▼

Step **Assessment: Determine pulselessness.**

While maintaining an open airway, move your hand from under the chin down along the infant's arm and feel for a brachial pulse.

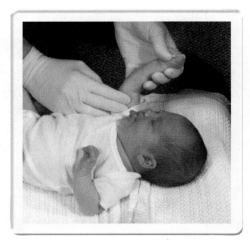

▼

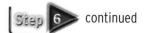
continued

It should take no more than 10 seconds to assess circulation. If after 10 seconds no signs of circulation are present, prepare to deliver chest compressions (see Steps 7 and 8). It is very important not to focus on finding a pulse. In an infant who is not breathing, not conscious, and not moving, consider the pulse to be absent. Delaying the start of compressions can be fatal to the infant.

If a pulse is present but the infant is still not breathing, provide rescue breathing, one breath every 3 to 5 seconds. Recheck the infant's pulse about every 2 minutes.

▼

 Use appropriate finger position for compressions.

With a firm surface, such as the rescuer's hand or a folded towel behind the infant's back, locate the correct position on the chest by placing two fingers just below the midnipple line. Many practitioners prefer to place the index finger on the nipple line, set the next two fingers on the chest, then lift the index finger.

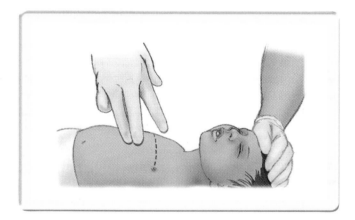

In larger infants, it may be necessary to use three fingers to adequately depress the sternum. When using three fingers, position the first two as just described and place the third finger at the midnipple line.

▼

Begin chest compressions.

Using the fingers, compress vertically one third to one half the depth of the chest. Make sure that you achieve equal compression and relaxation cycles. Without removing the fingers from the chest, allow complete chest relaxation on upstroke.

 Perform Steps 1 to 8 in proper sequence.

It is essential that these steps be performed in the proper sequence. Failure to do so may result in chest compressions being performed on an adequately perfusing infant, or ventilations on an adequately breathing infant.

 Perform five cycles of 30 compressions and two ventilations at a rate of at least 100/min.

Chest compressions are delivered at a rate of 100/min. After each set of 30 compressions, stop and deliver two breaths exactly as performed in Step 5. Since the fingers should never leave the infant's chest, it is not necessary to relocate the proper finger position each time chest compressions begin. Continue this sequence of 30 compressions to two ventilations for five cycles, and then stop and reassess the infant for perfusion.

In the Field

Team Infant CPR

When working as a team, infant CPR should be performed with one dedicated person performing chest compressions and a second person providing ventilations with a bag-mask device. When working together, the compression to ventilation ratio should be 15 compressions to two ventilations, and the person performing chest compressions should use the two thumb technique. This technique involves encircling the chest with both hands and placing the thumbs on the infant's sternum. Chest compressions are performed by pressing the thumbs against the sternum.

 Reassessment: Determine pulselessness.

Check the pulse as described in Step 6, lasting no more than 10 seconds.

 Continue CPR.

If the infant is still pulseless, resume chest compressions. Relocate the proper finger placement and continue the compression/ventilation ratio of 30:2. Continue to check for signs of perfusion every 5 minutes.

If the infant's pulse returns, the probability that respirations will also return is low initially, but much better than compared with an adult. Ventilations may need to continue for some time. If respirations return to an adequate rate and no signs of trauma are found, place the infant in the recovery position and continue to monitor pulse and respirations.

CPR should continue as long as any chance of survival exists. In advanced life support (ALS) systems, with electrocardiographic monitoring, defibrillation, and ALS capabilities, all resuscitative efforts should be performed at the scene.

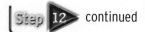 continued

It should be understood that competent ALS care administered by paramedics in the field provides a greater chance of successful resuscitation than care of the infant transported to the hospital.

It is also important to accept death. In ALS systems, infants who have been adequately managed but remain in cardiac arrest should not be transported. These infants need resuscitative efforts stopped. However, before deciding to halt efforts, you must be prepared to inform the infant's family that the infant has died. This may be the most difficult step, and it may be better to transport and have the news of death relayed by a physician. Almost all pediatric arrests are transported to an appropriate medical facility. It is important that a pediatric trauma center be considered rather than a local or regional hospital because pediatric care is very specialized. Stabilization at local hospitals is not possible in most cases.

Infant Foreign Body Airway Obstruction

Performance Objective

Given a conscious infant who appears to be choking, the candidate should assess the need to perform back slaps and chest thrusts, and proceed as indicated upon identifying an airway obstruction. The candidate shall perform the procedure for conscious infant foreign body airway obstruction in 3 minutes or less.

Equipment

The following equipment is required to perform this skill:
- Appropriate body substance isolation/personal protective equipment

Equipment that may be helpful:
- Oropharyngeal airways (various sizes)
- Nasopharyngeal airways (various sizes)
- Bag-mask device
- Oxygen cylinder, regulator, and key
- Suction device
- Pulse oximeter
- End-tidal carbon dioxide meter

Indications

- Foreign body airway obstruction in infants younger than 1 year

Contraindications

- Infants who can cry or cough

Complications

- None if properly performed

Procedures

Step **1** **Ensure body substance isolation before beginning procedures.**

Prior to beginning patient care, appropriate body substance isolation procedures should be employed.

▼

Step **2** **Assess airway and breathing.**

Assess the infant's ability to breathe on his or her own. An infant who can cry or cough is moving air and does not need emergent assistance. Back slaps may be useful to assist the infant to cough.

   If it appears that the infant cannot cry or cough, prepare to deliver back slaps and chest thrusts.

▼

Step **3** **Deliver back slaps.**

Supporting the head and neck, lift the infant and rotate face down onto your arm with the head lower than the trunk. Support your arm against your thigh if necessary. Deliver *five* upward, glancing back slaps between the shoulder blades using the heel of one hand. This procedure should occur quickly, in less than 3 to 5 seconds.

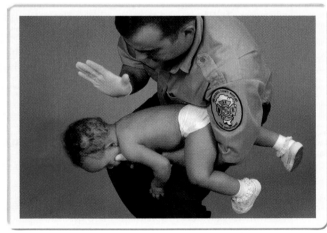

▼

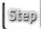

Step **4** ▶ **Deliver chest thrusts.**

Supporting the head and neck, rotate the infant face up, keeping the head lower than the trunk. Locate the midsternum by placing two fingers just below the nipple line. Deliver *five* chest thrusts, straight down to a depth one third to one half the depth of the chest. *Do not* use upward, glancing compressions.

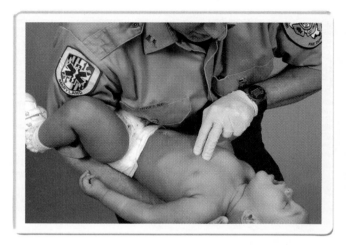

▼

  ▶ **Repeat back slaps and chest thrusts.**

Repeat back slaps and chest thrusts until the foreign body is expelled, the infant can breathe spontaneously, or he or she becomes unconscious. If the foreign body does not fall from the mouth, check the mouth to see if it is visible. If it is seen, perform a finger sweep to remove the object. Once the object has been expelled, assess the infant's ability to breathe on his or her own as described in Step 2.

If the infant becomes unconscious, call for help. Continue to Step 6.

 ▼

 ▶ **Deliver chest compressions (for unconscious infants or for infants who become unconscious while removing an airway obstruction).**

Locate the correct position on the chest by placing two fingers just below the midnipple line (see Step 4). Compress the chest vertically one third to one half the depth of the chest. The compressions should be smooth and even, equally up and down in a fluid motion. Deliver the full 30 compressions.

▼

Inspect the airway and assess for breathing.

After delivering 30 compressions, open the infant's mouth and look for the dislodged foreign object. If it is seen, perform a finger sweep to remove the object. If the object cannot be seen, do not perform a finger sweep. If no object is seen, attempt to ventilate. If able to ventilate, give two breaths, each lasting 1 full second.

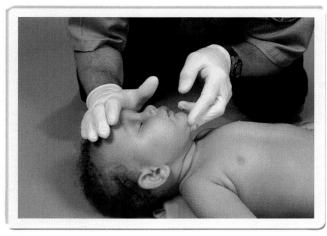

▼

 Repeat Steps 6 and 7 until successful.

Repeat the sequence of 30 compressions and two ventilations until the infant can be adequately ventilated. Remember to inspect the mouth to see if the foreign object can be seen before each set of ventilations. Once the airway has been cleared and the infant can be ventilated, assess the infant to determine the need for infant CPR.

Cardiac Arrest Management With an AED

Performance Objective

Given the proper equipment, the candidate shall demonstrate proper cardiac arrest management with an automated external defibrillator (AED), using the criteria herein prescribed, in 5 minutes or less.

Equipment

The following equipment is required to perform this skill:
- Appropriate body substance isolation/personal protective equipment
- Automated external defibrillator and pads
- Pocket mask with
  - One-way valve
  - Oxygen connecting port

Equipment that may be helpful:
- Oropharyngeal airways (various sizes)
- Nasopharyngeal airways (various sizes)
- Bag-mask device
- Oxygen cylinder, regulator, and key
- Suction device
- Pulse oximeter
- End-tidal carbon dioxide meter

Indications

- Ventricular fibrillation/nonperfusing ventricular tachycardia

Contraindications

- Infants

Complications

- Asystole

Procedures

 Step 1 Ensure body substance isolation before beginning procedures.

Prior to beginning patient care, appropriate body substance isolation procedures should be employed.

▼

 Step 2 Briefly question rescuers and witnesses about arrest events.

Before applying the AED, question initial rescuers and witnesses about the events leading to cardiac arrest. Specific questions should include the following:

- What time was the onset of the arrest?
- What care was provided before the arrival of rescuers (such as the determination of pulselessness and breathlessness and the initiation of CPR)?
- What was the patient doing before the arrest?
- Did the patient have any complaints before the arrest (such as chest pain or dyspnea)?
- (In some situations) Is there a Do Not Resuscitate order active for this patient?

▼

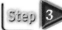 **Step 3** Direct rescuers to stop CPR.

Direct the rescuers performing CPR to stop compressions and ventilations.

▼

 Step 4 Verify absence of spontaneous pulse to verify the need to attach defibrillator.

Check the carotid pulse for the presence of a spontaneous pulse for up to 10 seconds. The absence of a pulse is an indication to attach the AED.

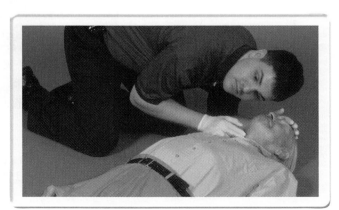

▼

 Special Populations

Pediatric AEDs

Newer models of AEDs have been designed with a high specificity in recognizing ventricular fibrillation and ventricular tachycardia in children. Some AEDs also have dose attenuating systems to reduce the energy delivered. These devices are intended for children 1 to 8 years of age. If these devices are available, they should be used when a pediatric patient is in a shockable rhythm. However, if no pediatric-specific AED is available, a standard adult AED should be used in pediatric cardiac arrests.

 In the Field

Immediate Defibrillation or Immediate CPR?

When an AED is immediately available, it should be used as soon as possible with a witnessed sudden onset of cardiac arrest. However, when the patient is found in cardiac arrest with a downtime reported or assumed to be over 4 minutes, perform CPR for five cycles (2 minutes) of compressions and ventilations before delivering the first shock.

5 Redirect rescuers to continue CPR.

After 10 seconds, if no definitive pulse is found, direct rescuers to continue CPR. Throughout the management of cardiac arrest, interruptions of CPR should be kept to a minimum and should last no longer than is absolutely necessary.

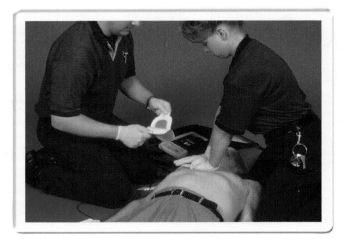

 6 Turn on defibrillator power.

Turn on power to the AED and wait for the computer to cycle. Pay attention to any written or verbal messages that occur.

 7 Attach automated defibrillator to patient.

Attach the patient pads to the defibrillator cables. If the cables have positive and negative leads, make sure the pads are attached to the correct lead.

Place one pad just to the right of the upper sternum below the right clavicle, and the other pad just below and to the left of the left nipple.

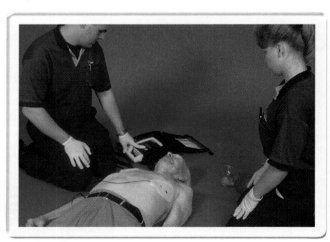

An alternative is to place one pad on the sternum, and the other pad on the patient's back directly posterior to the first pad. The determination of which position to use will be made by either protocol or manufacturer's specifications.

Ensure all individuals are standing clear of the patient.

Instruct personnel doing CPR to stop CPR after completing their fifth cycle of compressions and ventilations and to stand clear of the patient.

Explain to other rescuers that you are analyzing the rhythm and that patient motion will interfere with this process.

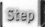 **Initiate analysis of rhythm.**

Press the Analyze button on the AED and stand clear of the patient, the AED, and the cables. Wait for the AED to analyze the need to defibrillate. All other resuscitative measures should be withheld while this step is in process to avoid delays or false analysis due to patient motion.

 Deliver shock.

When advised to defibrillate by the AED, instruct all other rescuers to stand clear. Visually confirm that *all* rescuers and bystanders are clear of the patient, bed, or conductive equipment attached to the patient.

Charge the defibrillator and deliver the shock as directed by the AED.

For monophasic defibrillators, the first and all subsequent shocks should be set at 360 J. For biphasic defibrillators, the energy should be set at the level recommended by the manufacturer. This will usually be between 120 J and 200 J.

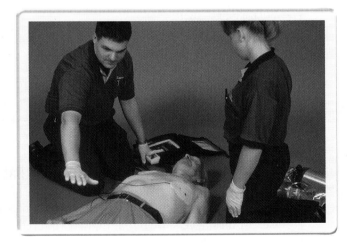

Step **11** ▶ **Immediately direct rescuers to continue CPR.**

CPR should be started immediately after the shock is delivered, without reassessment of the rhythm or the pulse.

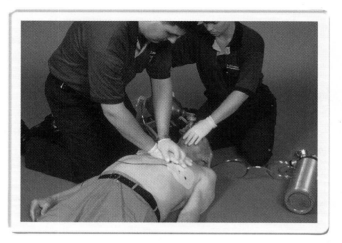

Step 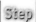 **12** ▶ **Gather additional information on the arrest event.**

Question witnesses, especially if they are family or close friends, about the patient's medical history. This should include the following:

- History of cardiovascular disease
- History of respiratory disease
- History of diabetes
- Presence of cardiac risk factors

In some arrest circumstances, especially those involving children and young adults, arrest is not caused by a preexisting cardiac event. Be sure to question witnesses about the possibility of trauma, drug use, and anaphylactic events.

Step **13** ▶ **Confirm effectiveness of CPR (ventilation and compressions).**

Traditionally, the effectiveness of CPR has been assessed by checking the carotid pulse. Studies have shown that jugular vein reflex waves have been misinterpreted as a pulse, making pulse assessment during chest compressions unreliable. Better means of identifying effective ventilations and compressions are improvement of pulse oximeter readings, improved end-tidal carbon dioxide readings, responsive pupils, and, occasionally, patient movement.

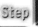 **Direct insertion of a simple airway adjunct (oropharyngeal or nasopharyngeal airway).**

Direct rescuers to insert an oropharyngeal airway (see Skill 7). Nasopharyngeal airways should be reserved for patients who have been revived and have a gag reflex (see Skill 9).

▼

 Direct ventilation of patient.

Confirm that ventilations are appropriate and effective. Proper rate and depths should be ensured. If initial ventilations were begun with mouth-to-mask resuscitation, direct rescuers to begin ventilations with a bag-mask device.

▼

 Ensure high concentration of oxygen connected to the ventilatory adjunct.

Direct rescuers to begin supplemental oxygen delivery to the bag-mask device. Oxygen should be administered at 15 L/min or greater.

▼

 Ensure CPR continues without unnecessary or prolonged interruption.

Ensure that compressions are delivered correctly. Depths and rate of compressions should be monitored. Interruptions should be avoided.

▼

 Reevaluate patient after five cycles of CPR.

At the completion of five cycles of 30 compressions and two ventilations, direct rescuers performing CPR to stop compressions and ventilations.

Check carotid pulse for presence of spontaneous pulse. Press the Analyze button on the AED and stand clear of the patient, the AED, and the cables. Wait for the AED to analyze the need to defibrillate. All other resuscitative measures should be withheld while this step is in process to avoid delays or false analysis due to patient motion.

▼

Repeat defibrillation sequence.

When advised to defibrillate by the AED, instruct the rescuers to continue CPR. With CPR in progress, charge the defibrillator.

When the AED is charged, instruct the rescuers to stop CPR and stand clear. Once you are sure no rescuers are in contact with the patient, deliver the shock as directed by the AED.

Immediately following the shock, direct the rescuers to continue CPR. After five more cycles of CPR, reassess the patient. Continue the sequence of defibrillation and CPR as needed.

▼

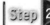 **Begin transportation of patient.**

The patient must be prepared for transport without unnecessarily interrupting CPR. The patient should be placed on a long backboard and secured, and then placed on the cot. Raise the cot only half way to allow for effective chest compression during movement. Carefully and *slowly* move the patient to the ambulance. Reassessment of the patient should be performed every five cycles of 30 compressions and two ventilations, with defibrillation delivered as indicated.

Defibrillation

Performance Objective

Given a patient whose condition meets criteria for defibrillation, the candidate shall demonstrate the proper technique for defibrillation using the criteria herein prescribed, in 5 minutes or less.

Equipment

The following equipment is required to perform this skill:
- Appropriate body substance isolation/personal protection equipment
- Manual or automated external defibrillator
- Defibrillator pads

Equipment that may be helpful:
- Oropharyngeal airways (various sizes)
- Nasopharyngeal airways (various sizes)
- Pocket mask with:
  - One-way valve
  - Oxygen connecting port
- Bag-mask device
- Oxygen cylinder, regulator, and key
- Suction device
- Pulse oximeter
- End-tidal carbon dioxide meter

Indications

- Ventricular fibrillation
- Pulseless ventricular tachycardia

Contraindications

- None

Complications

- Asystole

Procedures
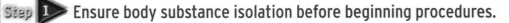

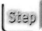**Step 1 Ensure body substance isolation before beginning procedures.**

Prior to beginning patient care, appropriate body substance isolation procedures should be employed.

▼

Step 2 Assess pulse, patient, and downtime; make shock first or compress first decision.

Assess the patient for the presence of a pulse. Check the carotid artery for no longer than 10 seconds.
    Upon failure to identify a definitive pulse, continue care by one of two options:

- **Witnessed arrest or downtime less than 4 minutes.** Proceed immediately to Step 3.
- **Downtime over 4 minutes or unknown.** Perform five cycles of 30 compressions and two ventilations before proceeding to Step 5. During this time perform Steps 3 and 4.

▼

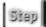**Step 3 Turn on the monitor and set it to the Paddles setting or the appropriate setting for hands-free defibrillation.**

Turn the monitor on and set the lead selector to the Paddles setting. If the patient was previously connected to an electrocardiogram (ECG) monitor, leave the lead selector in the monitoring lead and skip to Step 4. (Chest compressions and ventilations can be performed while accomplishing this step.)

▼

In the Field

Delayed Defibrillation
The traditional approach to the treatment of defibrillation has been to defibrillate as soon as possible after identifying the rhythm. Although defibrillation remains the most important single countermeasure to reverse fibrillation, immediate defibrillation may result in the less desirable asystole. Research on defibrillation effects show that when a patient has been in ventricular fibrillation for over 4 to 5 minutes, that the heart's internal environment becomes inhospitable and responds poorly to increased energy delivery. Remember that defibrillation does not "jump start" the heart, it stops it; we then hope that the hearts own inherent electrical network will pick up again at a normal rate. When the acid and electrolyte imbalances, and hypoxia of the long fibrillating heart are shocked, the heart stops, and frequently fails to return any electrical activity at all.

For the best patient outcome, immediate defibrillation should be reserved for witnessed or known short term durations of ventricular fibrillation. All other cases of ventricular fibrillation should receive five cycles (two minutes) of 30:2 chest compressions and ventilations.

Step 4 ▶ **Properly place pads/paddles on the patient.**

Pads are preferred to paddles for defibrillation and other electrical therapy because pads are placed once and allow for monitoring as well as pacing. They are also safer than paddles. Apply defibrillation pads to the patient or ECG gel to the paddles.

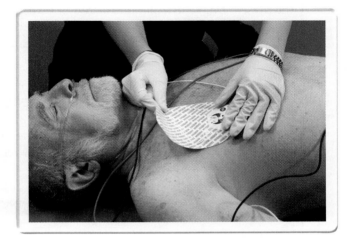

Place one ECG pad/paddle just to the right of the upper sternum below the right clavicle and the other pad/paddle just below and to the left of the left nipple. To properly monitor the patient's ECG rhythm, the left (sternum) pad/paddle should be negative and the right (apex) positive. Proper placement will allow you to properly monitor the patient's ECG rhythm.

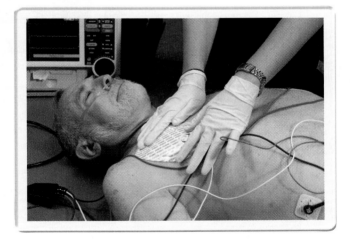

This will create a lead II tracing. However, for the identification of ventricular fibrillation or ventricular tachycardia, polarity is not a concern. (Chest compressions and ventilations can be performed while accomplishing this step.)

Defibrillation pads are available in adult and child sizes. Child pads should be used for patients who are younger than 8 years of age or less than 25 kg (55 lb). Defibrillation paddles also come in adult and infant sizes. Large paddles (8 to 10 cm) should be used on all patients over 10 kg (22 lb) in body weight (older than 1 year of age in most cases).

▼

5 **With proper pad/paddle placement, confirm rhythm by looking at the ECG monitor.**

Have all rescuers who are performing CPR or other tasks stand clear of the patient. Determine that the patient is a candidate for defibrillation by confirming the presence of ventricular fibrillation or ventricular tachycardia. Verbalization of this confirmation will allow all other responders to prepare for defibrillation.

▼

 6 **Set the defibrillator to the proper energy setting.**

Set the defibrillator to the proper energy setting for the patient, based on the type of defibrillator used. (Chest compressions and ventilations can be performed while accomplishing this step.)

 In the Field

Selecting the Energy Level

First shock:
- Monophasic defibrillator: 360 joules (J)
- Manual biphasic defibrillator: Use device-specific recommendation
  - Biphasic truncated exponential defibrillator: 150 J to 200 J
  - Biphasic rectilinear defibrillator: 120 J
  - Biphasic defibrillator of unknown type: 200 J

Second and subsequent shocks:
- Use the same energy setting or higher.
- Consider using the maximum setting for obese patients.

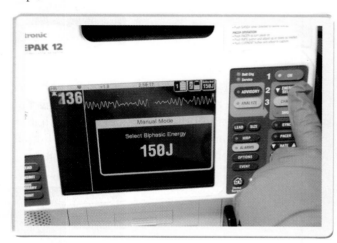

▼

 7 **Charge the defibrillator.**

Charge the defibrillator making sure the synchronizer is *off*. Continue CPR while defibrillator is charging. (Chest compressions and ventilations can be performed while accomplishing this step.)

▼

8 Instruct personnel to clear the area and confirm that personnel are clear.

Position the pad/paddle on the patient and check that you and all other personnel are clear of the patient and any conductive surfaces. Verbally clear yourself and all other personnel by stating, "I'm going to shock on three. One, I am clear. Two, you are clear. Three, everybody's clear."

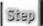 **9** Defibrillate the patient.

When you have ensured that all personnel are clear of the patient, depress the defibrillator button(s) and deliver the appropriate energy. When using the paddles, apply and hold 25 pounds of pressure to each paddle before depressing the defibrillator buttons.

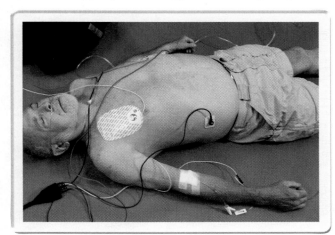

 In the Field

Defibrillating the Hypothermic Patient

Provide the initial shock, but withhold further defibrillations until the patient's core temperature exceeds 86°F.

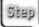 **10** Instruct personnel to begin chest compressions immediately.

Immediately following defibrillation, instruct other personnel to begin or resume chest compressions (five cycles of 30 compressions and two ventilations). Do not delay chest compressions to assess pulse or ECG rhythm. In most cases, even if the rhythm was converted from ventricular fibrillation to a normal tracing, chest compressions will be helpful to generate a blood pressure.

  After five cycles of 30 compressions and two ventilations, assess pulse and ECG rhythm.

Charge defibrillator as chest compressions are paused for assessment of ECG rhythm and perfusion. If rhythm remains ventricular fibrillation/nonperfusing ventricular tachycardia, prepare for immediate defibrillation without assessment of perfusion. Repeat Steps 5 through 11.

SKILL 33 Cardioversion

Performance Objective

Given a patient whose condition meets criteria for cardioversion, the candidate shall demonstrate the proper technique for synchronized cardioversion using the criteria herein prescribed, in 5 minutes or less.

Equipment

The following equipment is required to perform this skill:
- Appropriate body substance isolation/personal protection equipment
- Manual defibrillator
- Defibrillator pads/combination pads
- Electrocardiogram (ECG) cables
- ECG electrodes

Equipment that may be helpful:
- Equipment for the establishment of an intravenous line
- Equipment for the administration of sedative medications
- Sedative medications
- Equipment for delivering oxygen to the patient

Indications

- Extreme tachycardia with hemodynamic compromise

Contraindications

- None

Complications

- Asystole

Procedures

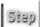 **Ensure body substance isolation before beginning procedures.**

Prior to beginning patient care, appropriate body substance isolation procedures should be employed.

▼

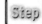 **Place ECG electrodes and lead wires.**

Place the ECG electrodes and lead wires in the following position:

White electrode: Right arm/shoulder (negative electrode in lead II)
Black electrode: Left arm/shoulder (ground electrode in lead II)
Red electrode: Left leg/lower chest (positive electrode in lead II)
Green electrode: Right leg/lower chest (not involved in lead II)

When the same electrode placements are to be used to obtain a 12-lead ECG, it is better to position the electrodes at the wrists and ankles rather than on the chest.

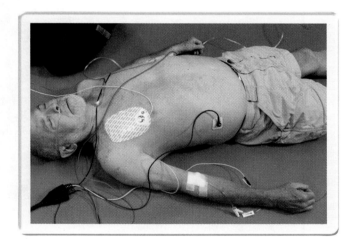

▼

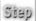 **Turn on monitor and set to Lead II.**

Turn the monitor on and set the lead selector to Lead II. Older monitors will offer only a choice between paddles and electrodes. Choose electrodes.

▼

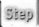 **Assess pulse.**

Check the patient's carotid pulse. If the pulse is absent, reevaluate the ECG rhythm and the need for other interventions. If a pulse is present, prepare to cardiovert.

▼

5 Confirm rhythm by looking at monitor.

Confirm the patient's ECG rhythm. It is best that this confirmation be made verbally so other caregivers are aware of the patient's situation.

▼

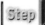 **6** Consider oxygen, IV access, and sedation.

If time and the patient's condition permit, consider basic patient care, such as oxygen administration and IV access. The need for sedation of the patient with benzodiazepines should also be considered.

▼

 7 Attach defibrillator pads or ECG gel to paddles.

Apply defibrillation pads to patient or ECG gel to paddles.

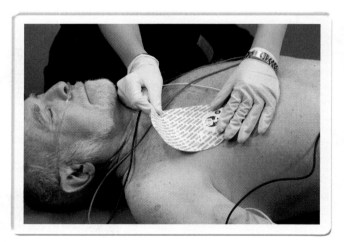

Place one ECG pad/paddle just to the right of the upper sternum below the right clavicle and the other pad/paddle just below and to the left of the left nipple. To properly monitor the patient's ECG rhythm, the left (sternum) pad/paddle should be negative and the right (apex) should be positive for lead II. However, determination of ventricular fibrillation or ventricular tachycardia polarity is not a concern.

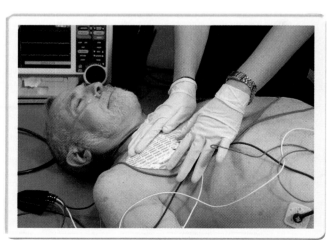

▼

Step 8 **Set defibrillator to the appropriate level for the first cardioversion.**

Set the defibrillator to the proper energy setting for the patient, based on the type of defibrillator used.

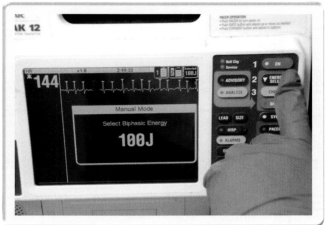

 In the Field

Selecting the Energy Level
Provide escalating energy as needed to convert the rhythm.

Ventricular tachycardia	100 J, 200 J, 300 J, 360 J
Paroxysmal supraventricular tachycardia	50 J, 100 J, 200 J, 300 J, 360 J
Atrial fibrillation	100 J, 200 J, 300 J, 360 J
Atrial flutter	50 J, 100 J, 200 J, 300 J, 360 J

These settings are for monophasic defibrillators. Clinically equivalent doses should be used for biphasic defibrillators.

 Step 9 **Activate synchronizer.**

Set the defibrillator to synchronize.

Charge the defibrillator.

Charge the defibrillator.

▼

 Perform Steps 1 through 9 before Step 10.

Before charging the defibrillator, ensure that all preparatory steps have been accomplished.

▼

 Instruct personnel to clear and confirm that personnel are clear.

Check that you and all other personnel are clear of the patient and any conductive surfaces. Verbally clear yourself and all other personnel by stating, "I'm going to shock on three. One, I am clear. Two, you are clear. Three, everybody's clear."

▼

 Reconfirm rhythm by looking at monitor and perform synchronized cardioversion.

Reconfirm that the rhythm still requires cardioversion. Turn your attention back to the paddles, quickly inspect that all personnel are clear, and shock.

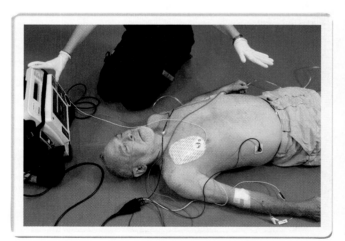

If the rhythm converts, either to a stable perfusing rhythm or nonperfusing rhythm, perform the necessary patient assessment and management as recommended by the International Liaison Committee on Resuscitation and local protocol.

▼

14 Confirm rhythm by looking at monitor.

Confirm the patient's ECG rhythm. Prepare to continue with cardioversion at the next appropriate energy level if the patient is still in an unstable rhythm.

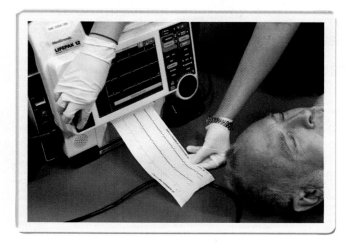

 15 Perform Steps 11 through 13 in proper order.

Ensure that the steps of paddle placement and personnel safety, rhythm reassessment, and cardioversion are completed in the proper order.

Step 16 Repeat as needed.

Repeat the preceding procedures following the recommended energy settings if needed.

Performance Objective

Given a patient who meets the criteria for transcutaneous pacing and appropriate equipment, the candidate shall apply pacing electrodes and begin pacing following the guidelines of the International Liaison Committee on Resuscitation, in 5 minutes or less from the time the need for pacing is determined.

Equipment

The following equipment is required to perform this skill:
- Appropriate body substance isolation/personal protection equipment
- Manual defibrillator
- Pacing pads/combination pads
- Electrocardiogram (ECG) cables
- ECG electrodes

Equipment that may be helpful:
- Equipment for the establishment of an intravenous line
- Equipment for the administration of sedative medications
- Sedative medications
- Equipment for delivery of oxygen to the patient

Indications

- Treatment of hemodynamically unstable bradycardia, including heart blocks
- Overdrive pacing in torsade de pointes

Contraindications

- None

Complications

- Skeletal muscle contraction and discomfort. Some patients can relieve the discomfort by simple deep breathing exercises. However, the use of sedatives such as diazepam (Valium), midazolam (Versed), or lorazepam (Ativan) are recommended if the patient complains of intense discomfort or pain. Analgesia may also be considered if the patient is stable enough to tolerate the depressant activity.

Procedures

 Ensure body substance isolation before beginning procedures.

Prior to beginning patient care, appropriate body substance isolation procedures should be employed.

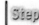 **Recognize/determine the need for pacing.**

After connecting the patient to the ECG monitor and assessing the initial vital signs, determine the need for transcutaneous pacing based on the indications previously listed. Remember that the use of other procedures or medication administration may supersede pacing. Refer to protocols or ACLS algorithms as appropriate.

 Obtain precapture strip.

Obtain a precapture strip of the ECG tracing for documentation.

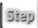 **Explain the need for transcutaneous pacing to the patient and the family.**

Explain to the patient and family why transcutaneous pacing is indicated and what can be expected. If the patient is coherent, explain that discomfort is expected and that deep breathing may help alleviate it.

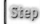 **Consider oxygen, IV access, and sedation.**

If time and the patient's condition permit, consider basic patient care, such as oxygen administration and IV access. The need for sedation of the patient with benzodiazepines should also be considered.

Step **Apply pacing electrodes and attach cables.**

Place the pacing electrodes on the patient's chest. The positive electrode is placed over the left-lateral sternum along the nipple line, and the negative electrode is placed just to the left of the spine along the midscapular line. Because this placement requires rolling the patient, it is best to attach the cables to the electrodes before placing them on the patient.

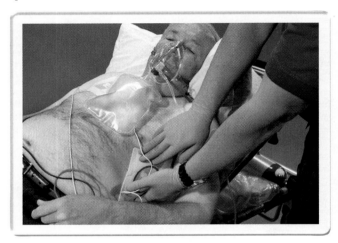

In the Field

Pads and Cables
Although the hands-free defibrillation pads can be used to monitor lead II rhythm tracings, they *cannot* monitor and pace at the same time. For a transcutaneous pacemaker to operate properly, it must be able to receive cardiac signals through the cables while pacing occurs through the pads. Both must be used to pace the patient.

Some patients or circumstances make placing a posterior electrode difficult or impossible. In these instances, the electrodes may be placed with an anterior approach similar to defibrillation. The positive electrode should be placed on the right chest just below the clavicle. The negative electrode is then positioned in the left midaxillary area even with the nipple line.

Attach the cables to the electrodes if not done previously.

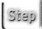 **7** ► **Turn pacing function on and adjust rate.**

Turn the pacemaker on and adjust for the desired rate. Usually a rate of 70 to 80 beats/min is appropriate.

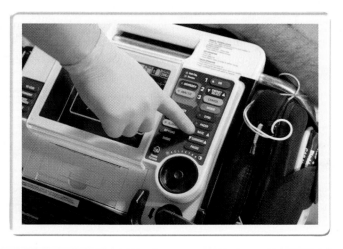

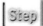 **8** ► **Increase current and observe patient for capture.**

Keeping an eye on the monitor, begin increasing the current to the electrode until capture is achieved. Both electrical and mechanical capture should occur.

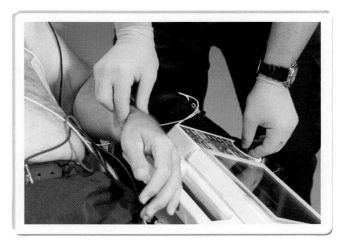

The pacemaker will generate a pacer mark, either a spike or narrow box, when electricity is delivered. Electrical capture occurs when these pacing marks elicit muscular contraction seen as a wide QRS and a tall, broad T wave. In some patients, only a slight change in QRS configuration will occur.

Mechanical capture is evident by a palpable pulse, a rise in blood pressure, an improved level of consciousness, and an improved skin temperature and tissue color. If mechanical capture generates a pulse but there is no improvement of blood pressure, consider increasing the rate up to 100 beats/min. Patients who experience no mechanical capture may not have viable hearts.

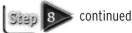 **Step 8** continued

When mechanical capture has been achieved, it is recommended to increase the energy by 2 milliamperes (a unit of current equal to one thousandth (10^{-3}) of an ampere). It is imperative that the pacing energy never be discontinued unless you are sure that underlying rhythm has returned to and can maintain a normal hemodynamic rate. Modern pacemakers have 4:1 ratio features that reduce the pacing pattern to one fourth of the normal pattern. This will allow assessment of the underlying rhythm.

▼

 Step 9 **Obtain rhythm strips for documentation.**

Record the pacing activity for documentation.

12-Lead ECG Acquisition

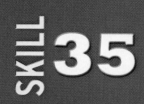
Performance Objective

Given a patient who meets the criteria for a 12-lead electrocardiogram (ECG) tracing, the candidate shall demonstrate the proper placement of electrodes and the procedures for capturing and recording a 12-lead ECG, in 5 minutes or less.

Equipment

The following equipment is required to perform this skill:
- Appropriate body substance isolation/personal protection equipment
- 12-lead ECG monitor
- 12-lead ECG cables
- ECG electrodes

Equipment that may be helpful:
- 4″ × 4″ sponges for drying or abrading skin
- Benzoin spray
- Electric hair clippers/prep razors

Indications

- Patients experiencing chest pain
- Post-arrest patients
- Patients with cardiac or diabetic history complaining of dyspnea or other nondescript complaints, syncope, palpitations, or chest discomfort
- Electrocution
- Poisoning and overdose

Contraindications

- None

Complications

- None

Procedures

Step **1** ▶ **Ensure body substance isolation before beginning procedures.**

Prior to beginning patient care, appropriate body substance isolation procedures should be employed.

▼

Step **2** ▶ **Explain the procedure and prepare the skin for electrode placement.**

Explain the procedure to the patient. Reassure the patient that the machine will not shock him or her.

Prepare the skin by cleaning the chest. Dry the skin with a towel and apply tincture of benzoin, if available. Abrading the skin with a 4″ × 4″ gauze pad or fine grain sandpaper may help to remove dead skin cells, which will interfere with quality tracings. Patients with excessive body hair may need to be shaved for the electrodes to make adequate contact with the skin.

▼

Step **3** ▶ **Position electrodes and attach lead wires.**

Position the electrodes on the patient in the following manner (it may be necessary to attach the lead wire to the electrodes before placing them on the patient).

Limb electrodes need to be placed on the anterior forearm just proximal to the wrists and on the left lower leg just proximal to the ankle. These are labeled:

RA: White
LA: Black
RL: Green
LL: Red

If monitoring electrodes have previously been placed on the chest, additional electrodes will need to

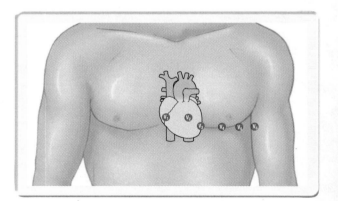

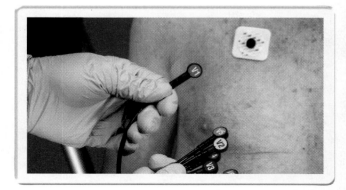

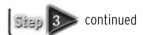

Step 3 continued

be placed on the limbs. The lead wires will then need to be moved to the limb electrodes.

The chest electrodes should be placed in an arching pattern around the left breast.

V_1: Right side of the sternum in the fourth intercostal space
V_2: Left side of the sternum in the fourth intercostal space
V_3: Midway between V_2 and V_4
V_4: Midclavicular line in the fifth intercostal space
V_5: Anterior axillary line at the same level as V_4
V_6: Midaxillary line at the same level as V_4

Attach the cable wires to the appropriate electrodes. Make sure the snap buttons are correctly connected and the monitoring cables have been moved to the limb electrodes as necessary.

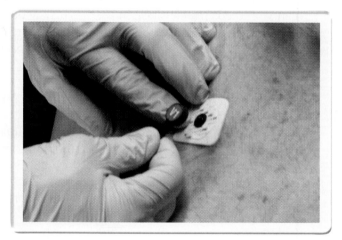

Step 4 Press the Analyze button.

Have the patient remain still throughout the procedure. Press the Analyze button.

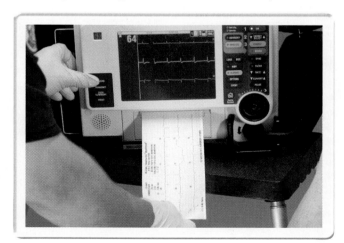

Review tracing.

Review the tracings for indications of ischemia, injury, or infarction. An additional review should be performed to identify possible bundle branch blocks, chamber enlargement, electrolyte imbalance, and axis deviation.

Based on the review of the initial 12-lead tracing, determine if additional views of the right and posterior walls (15- or 18-lead tracings) are needed.

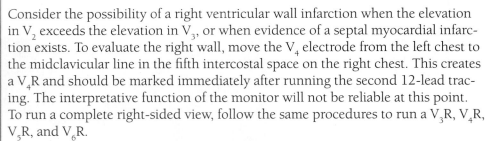 **Evaluate right or posterior walls.**

Consider the possibility of a right ventricular wall infarction when the elevation in V_2 exceeds the elevation in V_3, or when evidence of a septal myocardial infarction exists. To evaluate the right wall, move the V_4 electrode from the left chest to the midclavicular line in the fifth intercostal space on the right chest. This creates a V_4R and should be marked immediately after running the second 12-lead tracing. The interpretative function of the monitor will not be reliable at this point. To run a complete right-sided view, follow the same procedures to run a V_3R, V_4R, V_5R, and V_6R.

Consider the possibility of a posterior wall infarction when the ST depression is seen in V_1 through V_4. To evaluate the posterior wall, move the V_6 electrode from the left chest and place it level with V_4 just to the left of the spinal column (this forms V_9), and move the V_5 electrode level with V_4 just to the base of the scapula (forming V_8). This creates a V_8 and V_9 respectively, and should be marked immediately after running the second 12-lead tracing. The interpretative function of the monitor will not be reliable at this point. To run a complete posterior view, also relocate V_4 to the postaxillary line, level with V_8 and V_9 (in actuality these are now D leads, but that term is seldom, if ever, used).

It is a good practice to always run a V_4R, V_8, and V_9 on the same strip.

 In the Field

12-Lead Interpretation The purpose of the 12-lead tracing in the prehospital setting is to determine the presence of myocardial ischemia, injury, and infarction. In many cases, this is easily identified by looking at the printed interpretation that follows the tracings. However, it is beneficial and more accurate for the interpretation to come from the actual assessment of the tracing by the paramedic, looking for the elevations and inversions that signal myocardial anomalies within the heart. As good as 12-leads are at identifying ischemia, injury, and infarction, they are also an excellent tool for identifying many other problems. With proper training and practice, problems such as ventricular conduction abnormalities, electrical vectors, electrolyte abnormalities, chamber enlargement, and pericarditis can be identified.

ECG Monitoring— Electrode Placement and Lead Selection

Performance Objective

Given a patient in need of cardiac monitoring and the appropriate equipment, the candidate shall demonstrate how to properly attach electrodes to monitor leads I, II, III, MCL_1, and MCL_6, in 5 minutes or less.

Equipment

The following equipment is required to perform this skill:

- Appropriate body substance isolation/personal protection equipment
- Electrocardiogram (ECG) monitor
- ECG cables
- ECG electrodes

Equipment that may be helpful:

- 4" × 4" sponges for drying or abrading skin
- Benzoin spray
- Electric hair clippers/prep razors

Indications

- Any patient with indications of decreased perfusion, trauma, shock, chest pain, dyspnea, altered level of consciousness, burns, electrocution, or chemical exposure (including all poisoning and overdose).

Contraindications

- None

Complications

- None

Procedures

Step 1 ▶ Ensure body substance isolation before beginning procedures.

Prior to beginning patient care, appropriate body substance isolation procedures should be employed.

▼

Step 2 ▶ Explain the procedure and prepare the skin for electrode placement.

Explain the procedure to the patient. Reassure the patient that the machine will not shock him or her. Prepare the skin by cleaning the chest. Dry the skin with a towel and apply tincture of benzoin, if available. Abrading the skin with a 4″ × 4″ sponge or fine grain sandpaper may help to remove dead skin cells, which will interfere with quality tracings. Patients with excessive body hair may need to be shaved for the electrodes to make adequate contact with the skin.

▼

Step 3 ▶ Position electrodes.

Position the electrodes in one of the two following manners:

1. One electrode placed on the soft tissue just inferior to the lateral end of each clavicle and one on the left midaxillary line between the lower rib and the transverse plane of the umbilicus is sufficient for simple ECG monitoring.

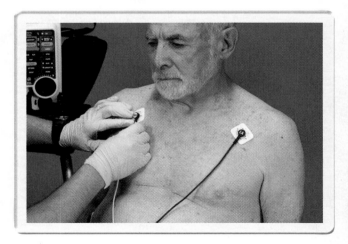

In the Field

Additional Lead Configurations MCL₁ and MCL₆ are used in place of true unipolar precordial leads. With non-12-lead monitors, MCLs can be used to look for or to monitor myocardial ischemia, injury, or infarction. To configure MCLs, set your monitor to run lead II. Place the negative electrode (white) in the left midclavicular line just below the clavicle. The ground electrode (black) should be placed on the right side in the same space. The positive electrode (red) is then positioned for the specific lead to be viewed, starting with MCL₁ on the right side of the sternum in the fourth intercostal space. Move each positive electrode to the position of the appropriate precordial lead.

The Lewis lead is another alternative configuration that can be useful in determining P waves and atrial depolarization. With the monitor set to run lead II, place the negative electrode (white) in the second intercostal space, just to the right of the sternum. The positive electrode (red) is placed just below the negative in the fourth intercostal space. The ground electrode is placed on the left side of the sternum, just across from the negative.

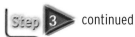 continued

2. For patients who will be getting a 12-lead tracing as well, limb electrodes need to be placed on the anterior forearm just proximal to the wrists and on the left lower leg just proximal to the ankle. Some units require a fourth electrode to be placed on the right lower leg as well. These are labeled:

RA: White
LA: Black
RL: Green
LL: Red

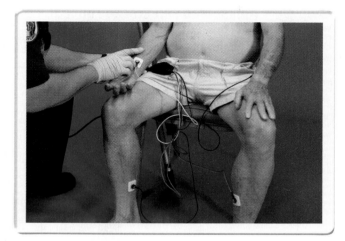

  Attach cables to the appropriate electrode.

Attach the electrodes in the following manner:

RA (white): To the electrode on the right arm or below the right clavicle
LA (black): To the electrode on the left arm or below the left clavicle
LL (red): To the electrode on the left leg or left midaxillary line

In this configuration RA is negative, LA is ground, and LL is positive in lead II.

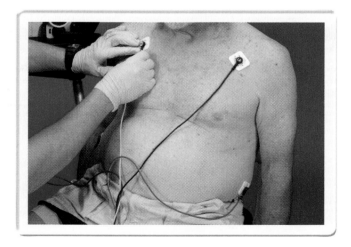

Step 5 ▶ **Turn monitor on and set to lead II.**

Turn the monitor on and set the lead selector to lead II.

▼

 Step 6 ▶ **Adjust lead selector to run lead I and lead III.**

Adjust the monitor's lead selector to view lead I and then lead III.

▼

 Step 7 ▶ **Record tracings.**

Push the Record button to get a paper tracing of each lead. You will have to switch the lead selector as needed.

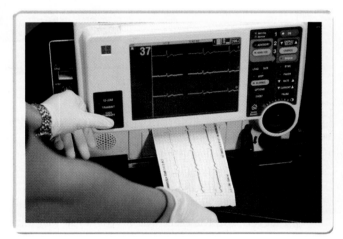

▼

 Step 8 ▶ **Label each strip.**

Label the leads of each strip, and include the patient's name, age, and the time recorded, as appropriate.

Performance Objective

Given a patient with evidence of an imminently life-threatening peri-cardial tamponade, the candidate shall demonstrate the proper proce-dure for pericardiocentesis, in 5 minutes or less.

Equipment

The following equipment is required to perform this skill:
- Appropriate body substance isolation/personal protection equipment
- Sharps container
- 2" 16-gauge or larger catheter (most safety-type catheters will not work because they won't accept a syringe)
- 20-mL syringe
- Cleaning solution
  - Chlorhexidine preps
  - Povidone-iodine preps
  - Alcohol preps

Equipment that may be helpful:
- Prepackaged needle decompression kit
- Ultrasound

Indications

- In the prehospital setting, performing a pericardiocentesis is reserved for traumatic cardiac arrest from a thoracic injury, where other meth-ods of reversing the arrest have failed, or for pericardial effusion with similar deterioration. The patient may be in either a pulseless electri-cal rhythm or in asystole. This is a last-ditch procedure.

Contraindications

- None in asystole or pulseless electrical activity

Complications

- Inadvertent puncture of the myocardial wall, producing a ventricu-lar bleed
- Inadvertent puncture of the pulmonary tissue, producing a tension pneumothorax or hemothorax
- Inadvertent puncture of the liver, producing a hepatic hemorrhage

Procedures

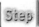 **Step 1** Ensure body substance isolation before beginning procedures.

Prior to beginning patient care, appropriate body substance isolation procedures should be employed.

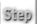 **Step 2** Maintain sterility and safety throughout the procedure.

Ensure that all sterile equipment and the aseptic field are not contaminated. Maintain safety with needles, and use body substance isolation procedures appropriately.

 Step 3 Assess the patient: blood pressure, heart sounds, jugular vein distension, mechanism of injury, and electrocardiogram.

Verify the presence of a pericardial tamponade by assessing the patient's blood pressure, heart sounds, and jugular vein distension. In cases of cardiac arrest from trauma, a mechanism of injury to the chest and pulseless electrical activity or asystole may indicate the presence of a pericardial tamponade.

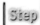 **Step 4** Assemble the equipment.

Gather the necessary equipment to perform the pericardiocentesis. A prepackaged needle decompression kit is preferred because it contains a wire-wrapped catheter. If this is not available, assemble a 2″ 16-gauge or larger catheter, a 20-mL syringe, and chlorhexidine or povidone-iodine swabs and alcohol swabs to cleanse the puncture site.

Remove the cap from the flash chamber and attach the 20-mL syringe. Removal of the catheter from the needle is not necessary and could be detrimental.

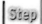

Step 5 ▶ Locate and prepare the site.

Palpate the xiphoid process at the inferior sternum. Prepare the insertion site by cleaning with an antiseptic/antimicrobial agent. A 30-second vigorous scrub using chlorhexidine will kill 99.9% of all colonizing microbes when the solution is dry. If chlorhexidine is not available, povidone-iodine is an acceptable alternative. It is important to allow the povidone-iodine solution to dry completely before injecting the site. Alcohol may be used when the povidone-iodine is dry to clean the dye and improve visualization of the injection site.

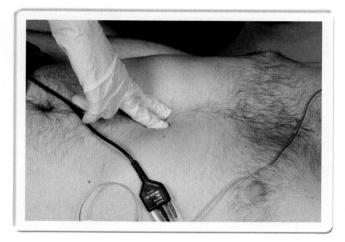

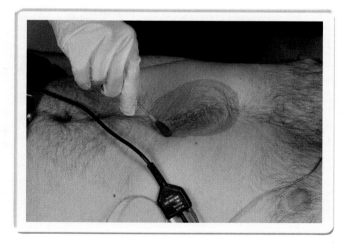

▼

Step 6 ▶ Insert the needle.

Push the IV catheter under the xiphoid process at a 90° angle to the body. Lower the syringe to a 45° angle with the needle pointing toward either midclavicular line. Aiming for the right clavicle reduces the chances of puncturing the heart, while aiming for the left clavicle gives a better chance of reducing a small pericardial tamponade. The right side is safer in the prehospital setting because it decreases the chances of puncturing the heart.

▼

Step **Pull back on the plunger and advance the needle.**

Pull back on the plunger of the syringe to achieve a negative pressure.

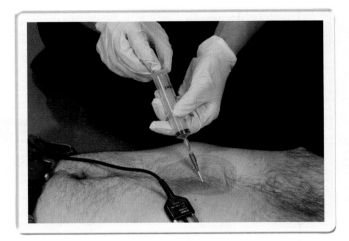

Maintain the negative pressure as you slowly advance the needle into the chest. Watch carefully for blood return into the syringe. As blood begins to fill the syringe, slowly advance the needle to keep the pericardium from pulling off of the needle as it is drained.

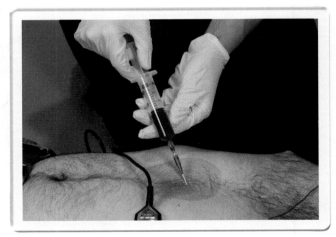

Should you begin to feel pulsations through the syringe before finding a blood return, stop further advancement of the needle. This is an indication that you have reached the heart muscle and that a pericardial tamponade probably does not exist.

▼

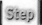 **Evaluate blood return.**

Evaluate the blood that has filled the syringe. In smaller tamponades, blood from the pericardial sac is mixed with pericardial fluid and prevents clotting. Blood that comes from the ventricles of the heart (an inadvertent and undesirable puncture) will clot in a few minutes.

▼

 Properly dispose of the contaminated equipment.

Dispose of needles and all sharp instruments with blood or body fluid contamination in puncture-resistant sharps containers. Other material that has been contaminated by blood or body fluids should be disposed of in biohazard bags. Waste materials that are not contaminated by blood or body fluids can be disposed of in normal trash receptacles.

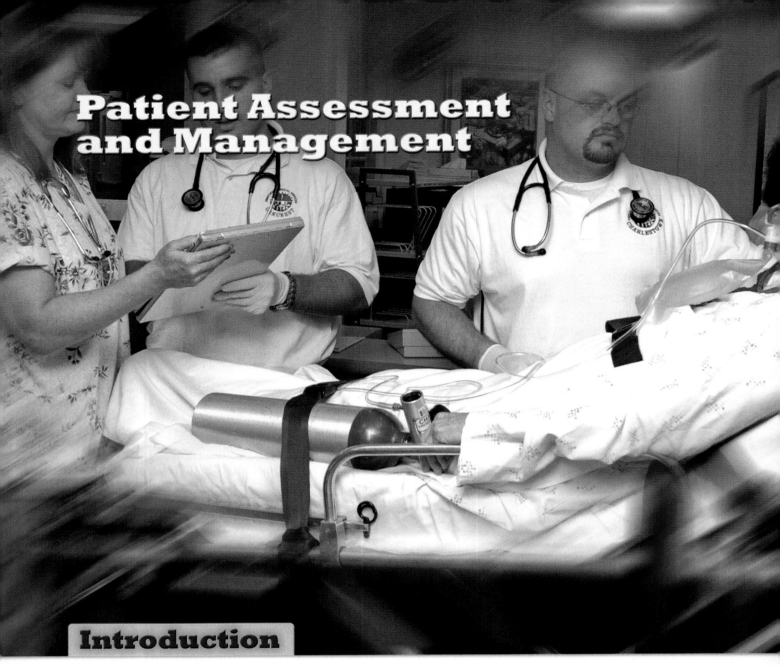

Patient Assessment and Management

Introduction

Proper assessment of a patient is a necessary prerequisite for proper patient management. Thorough assessments, from the first meeting to transfer of care at the receiving facility, lead to appropriate patient care. Accurate oral and written communication skills are vital to this process. For example, the hospital assessment begins with a review of the patient report that is provided by field personnel.

As you practice patient assessment, consider the required documentation that will determine the quality of patient care. Good documentation follows good patient assessment; good patient assessment leads to good documentation. The skills in this section will encourage you to master this important process.

Performance Objective

Given a patient, the proper equipment, and a scenario describing the circumstances of the patient's injury or illness, the candidate shall perform an assessment of the patient, including the scene size-up, initial assessment, and focused history and physical examination or detailed physical examination, and state appropriate interventions for the patient's problems, using the criteria herein prescribed, in 15 minutes or less.

Equipment

The following equipment is required to perform this skill:
- Appropriate body substance isolation/personal protective equipment
- Watch with second hand (or digital equivalent)
- Stethoscope with diaphragm and bell
- Sphygmomanometer, with various-sized cuffs
- Pen and paper (patient care chart)
- Pen light
- Thermometer
- Reflex hammer and/or neurologic (Buck) hammer
- Otoscope
- Familiar object (paper clip, key, coin, pencil, cotton ball)
- Pulse oximeter
- End-tidal carbon dioxide meter

Equipment that may be helpful:
- Ophthalmoscope
- Snellen chart

Indications

- Patient care

Contraindications

- None

Complications

- None

Procedures

 Step 1 Ensure body substance isolation before beginning procedures.

Prior to beginning patient care, appropriate body substance isolation procedures should be employed.

▼

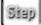 **Step 2** Scene size-up: Determine that the scene or situation is safe.

Prior to initiating patient contact, perform a visual sweep of the scene. Look for any hazards to yourself, other rescuers, and bystanders. Hazards should be identified, and information about hazards should be relayed to other responders. *Do not* enter a scene in which hazards are not stabilized.

▼

 Step 3 Determine mechanism of injury or nature of illness, number of patients, and need for additional help.

Assess the mechanism of injury or the nature of illness. Quickly assess the scene to determine whether other patients are present. Do not assume that no other patients exist in medical emergencies. Situations of stress, poisoning, and environmental problems often produce multiple patients.

Request additional resources if the number of patients or the situation exceeds the capabilities of the initial responding unit. This may include calling for additional ambulances, the fire department, heavy rescue, hazardous materials teams, or utility companies.

▼

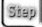 **Step 4** Consider stabilization of the spine (applies when indicated).

Determine whether the patient may have injuries to the spine in association with the chief complaint. If present, apply appropriate stabilization procedures.

▼

Step **5** Initial assessment: Form general impression of patient.

Gather a general impression of the patient upon initial contact. Determine whether the patient looks stable or unstable from her or his initial appearance. Be prepared to change your mind as the survey continues and improvement or deterioration is found. In conscious patients, a simple battery of questions can determine the chief complaint and provide detailed information about the mechanism of injury or nature of illness.

▼

Step **6** Determine responsiveness and level of consciousness.

Quickly determine the patient's level of consciousness through use of the AVPU scale (**A**wake and alert, responds to **V**erbal stimuli, responds to **P**hysical or painful stimuli, **U**nresponsive).

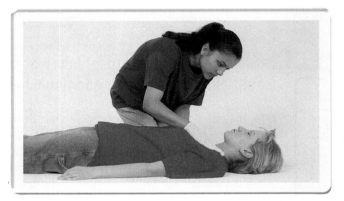

▼

Step **7** Assess airway (with consideration of cervical spine).

Patients who are talking have an open airway. Quickly evaluate the patency to ensure the airway remains open throughout patient care.

In the unresponsive patient, open and assesses the airway. Determine the possibility of cervical injury before opening the airway. If cervical injury is suspected, open the airway using the jaw-thrust maneuver (see Skill 1). Consider inserting an oropharyngeal or nasopharyngeal airway if indicated (see Skill 7 or Skill 9). Quickly inspect the neck for injuries that might interfere with ventilation.

▼

Step 8 ▶ Assess breathing.

Assess breathing and ensure adequate ventilation.

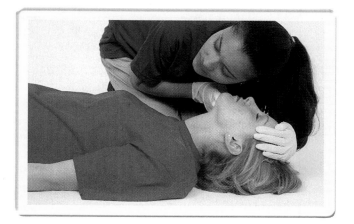

Assess the patient's chest for injuries that might compromise ventilations (tension pneumothorax, flail chest, or sucking chest wound).

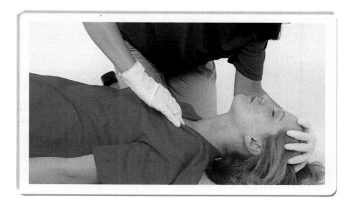

If the ventilations are inadequate, initiate bag-mask ventilations. Apply supplemental oxygen as indicated.

▼

Step 9 ▶ Assess circulation.

Assess for and control major bleeding. Assess the patient's pulse for rate and strength. The patient's skin and tissues should be assessed for tissue color, temperature, and condition. Initiate shock management, including keeping the patient warm and elevating the legs if indicated.

▼

Step  **10** ▶ **Determine chief complaint and apparent life threats.**

From the information gathered, determine the patient's chief complaint and identify apparent threats to life.

▼

Step  **11** ▶ **Identify priority patients and make transport decision.**

In most cases, the goal in patient care is to begin transport as soon as practical—usually within 10 minutes for trauma patients and within 15 minutes for medical patients. Although trauma patients *cannot* be stabilized in the field and require rapid transport, many medical patients can be stabilized in the field. The opportunity to transport should not impede the appropriate delivery of care. Always ask the question, "Will the patient benefit more from rapid transport or from field treatment?"

From the information so far obtained, determine the patient's priority of care and determine the needs for immediate or delayed transport. This can be one of the most difficult decisions associated with patient care. Always go back to the basics: Ensure an airway, maintain breathing, and maintain circulation. If these steps cannot be performed and all available methods available have been employed, transport without delay.

Priority and transport decisions are not one and the same. A patient who is unconscious has, by definition, an unstable airway. Thus, the patient is a high priority. However, the placement of an oropharyngeal airway or endotracheal tube stabilizes the patient, lowering the priority and making transport less urgent. On a similar note, a conscious and alert patient who is developing severe and worsening chest discomfort and dyspnea and has not responded to any therapy you have attempted is a high-priority patient who needs rapid transport. You should note that high priority is always rapid transport, whereas low priority is always delayed transport.

> **High-priority patients.** Altered level of consciousness, airway or ventilatory compromise, poor systemic circulation (low systolic blood pressure), multisystem trauma, etc.
> **Low-priority patients.** Isolated injuries, minor bleeding, minor medical complaint, stable vital signs within normal limits, etc.
> **Rapid transport.** Uncontrolled airway, difficulty ventilating, signs and symptoms of shock, multisystem trauma, compromised medical condition, etc.
> **Delayed transport.** Minor injuries, minor medical complaint, etc.

▼

In the Field
Cardiac Arrest

- **For the EMT.** Cardiac arrest is a rapid, *controlled* transport. The patient needs effective CPR, which cannot be performed during rapid transport.
- **For the paramedic.** Cardiac arrest is *not* a rapid transport situation. The patient will benefit more from proper care delivered *where the patient was found* than from hurried care and rapid transport.

Determine the depth of focused history and physical examination.

- **Trauma patients with no significant mechanism of injury *or* responsive medical patients.** Focus on the body systems involved and the specific injury or illness, guided by the patient's chief complaint (see Steps 13 through 28 and Steps 40 through 43).
- **Trauma patients with serious injuries or mechanisms of injury *or* unresponsive medical patients.** Perform a rapid head-to-toe physical examination (DCAP-BTLS). Assess the size, equality, and reactivity of the pupils; examine the neck for distended jugular veins and tracheal deviation; examine the chest for crepitation, paradoxical motion, and equality of breath sounds; and examine the abdomen for rigidity or distension (see Steps 29 through 43).

▼

Trauma Patients With No Significant Mechanism of Injury or Responsive Medical Patients

 Patient history: Gather history of present illness and/or complete a SAMPLE history.

In conscious medical patients, *always* gather the patient history before conducting a physical examination. In trauma patients, especially trauma involving obvious bleeding, the immediate attention should be the control of bleeding and stabilization of injuries before the gathering of patient information.

Gather the history of present illness from the patient or from family or bystanders if necessary.

- **Cardiac or respiratory patients.** Follow the standard OPQRST approach.
  Onset of symptoms: Was onset sudden or gradual?
  Provocation: What worsens or lessens the condition?
  Quality: Is the pain sharp, throbbing, crushing, or dull?
  Radiation: Does the pain or condition travel to other parts of the body?
  Severity: How badly does it hurt? Determine severity using a scale of 1 to 10, with 10 being the worst pain ever felt by the patient.
  Time: How long ago did the condition begn?
- **Altered mental status patients.** Determine a description of the episode, the onset, the duration, and associated evidence of trauma. Question the patient or family about any interventions already taken and the possibility of seizures or fever.
- **Allergic reaction patients.** Determine history of allergies, what the patient was exposed to and how, the effects and progression of exposure, and any interventions already performed (such as the use of antihistamines or an epinephrine auto-injector).
- **Poisoning/overdose patients.** Determine the toxic substance, the time at which exposure occurred, the type of exposure (ingestion or contact), how much toxin was involved, and over how long a period of time. Also determine what interventions were performed. The patient's weight and the effects of exposure are also important.

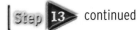 continued

- **Obstetric patients.** First determine the possibility of pregnancy. Determine the length of pregnancy (in weeks, if known), estimated date of confinement, any pain or contractions, bleeding or discharge, and possible crowning. Does the patient feel a need to push? Determine the patient's last menstrual period, previous pregnancies, and the results of each pregnancy (gravida, para, ab, cesarean sections).
- **Behavioral patients.** Start by asking "How do you feel?" Determine if there are thoughts of suicide and whether the patient is a threat to self or others. Ask about any underlying medical problem and any interventions already performed.
- **Environmental emergency patients.** Determine the cause of the problem (heat, cold, water, or altitude), the length of exposure, and any loss of consciousness. Determine what effects have occurred and whether the effects are general or local.

Gather the SAMPLE history from the patient or from family or bystanders if necessary.

Symptoms (history of present illness)
Allergies to medications
Medications currently taken by the patient (prescription and nonprescription)
Past history—pertinent medical information related to current condition
Last oral intake (food, drink), or last menstrual period in obstetric/gynecologic patients
Events leading up to emergency

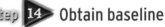 **Obtain baseline vital signs (see Skill 39).**

Determine the patient's level of consciousness (using the patient's orientation to person, place, and time), pulse (rate, strength, and regularity), respirations (rate, depth, and quality), blood pressure, skin temperature and condition, and tissue color.

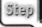 **Apply advanced diagnostic procedures.**

Perform diagnostic procedures as required for the patient. This will involve, based on the level of capabilities, applying a pulse oximeter, an ECG monitor, a 12-lead ECG, testing blood glucose, and assessment of end-tidal carbon dioxide levels.

Using experience and intuition, make a swift and open-minded determination of the patient's general health status. Consider completing a detailed physical examination.

Step 16 Inspect the head.

This area will be one of the most detailed and focused of the system evaluations. Attention to detail is essential to avoid missing important assessments.

- **Head.** Inspect the head for wounds, deformities, or bruising. Inspect the scalp for hair distribution and patterns. Inspect the face and pay attention to the facial expressions, now and at the completion of the examination (evaluates cranial nerve VII). Palpate the temporomandibular joint as the patient moves the jaw. Palpate the scalp for crepitus. Palpate the maxillary sinuses for tenderness. Assess the temporal pulse.

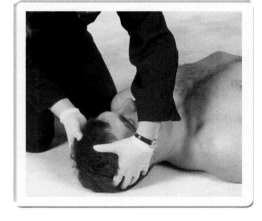

- **Eyes.** Evaluate for signs of obvious trauma, such as corneal abrasions and periorbital ecchymosis. Also look for conjunctivitis, opacities, jaundice, or icterus. Take note of the position of the eyes and look for disconjugate gaze, nystagmus, or other nonpurposeful movements. Evaluate the pupils for shape, size, reaction, and accommodation. Assess the patient's ability to move her or his eyes in all directions using a standard H test (evaluates cranial nerves III, IV, and VI). Determine visual acuity using a Snellen eye chart or by having the patient read standard print (evaluates cranial nerve II). Optionally for EMS evaluation, in a darkened room, use an ophthalmoscope to evaluate the anterior chamber and interior for blood and the condition of blood vessels and the optic nerve.
- **Ears.** Evaluate for signs of trauma, specifically mastoid ecchymosis, symmetry (right to left), lesions, or erythema. Using an otoscope, evaluate the auditory canal and the tympanic membrane. Identify discharge or impacted cerumen. Assess hearing by use of whispered tones or finger clicks (evaluates cranial nerve V).
- **Nose.** Inspect the nose for symmetry, and palpate the nose for crepitus or deformity. Inspect the inner nose for pink mucosa, septal deviations or perforations, bleeding, discharge, or edema. Have the patient breathe in to identify obstructions. Also palpate the sinuses.
- **Mouth/throat.** Inspect the lips, gums, and teeth for abnormalities. Palpate for signs of injury, swelling, erythema, or odors. Note any odors coming from the mouth. Inspect the throat for swelling or enlargement of the tonsils or posterior pharynx. Listen for bruits. Note mobility of the uvula as the patient phonates "ahh," and test gag reflex (evaluates cranial nerves IX and X). Have the patient stick his or her tongue out (evaluates cranial nerve XII).

Step **Inspect the neck.**

Inspect the neck for a midline trachea and jugular vein distension. Auscultate for cannon waves or carotid bruits. Palpate the carotid arteries and lymph nodes, and identify lymphadenitis or enlarged thyroid. Assess the carotid pulse. Assess ability to move without pain or resistance. Assess the shoulder shrug (evaluates cranial nerve XI).

Step **Inspect the chest (posterior and lateral).**

Moving to the back of the patient, inspect the posterior chest and the shape of the thoracic cage. Identify unusual skin characteristics and the symmetry of the shoulders and posterior muscles. Palpate the chest for symmetrical expansion, tactile fremitus, lumps, or tenderness. Run your hand down the spine and assess the length of the spinous processes. Percuss over all lung fields, identifying diaphragmatic excursion, costovertebral angle, and tenderness. Auscultate the equality of breath sounds.

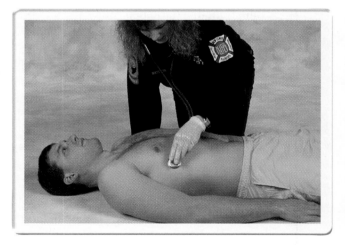

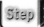 Step **19** ▶ **Inspect the anterior chest.**

- **Pulmonary.** Inspect the quality of respirations and skin characteristics. Palpate for tactile fremitus, lumps, and tenderness. Palpate the axilla and regional nodes. Percuss the lung fields. Auscultate breath sounds with the diaphragm of the stethoscope.
- **Cardiac.** Inspect the precordium for pulsations and heave (lift). Palpate the apical impulse and note location. Palpate the precordium for thrills. With the patient leaning slightly forward, auscultate the heart for murmurs or third heart sounds. Auscultate for apical rate and rhythm, inching from apex to base, first with the diaphragm, then with the bell.
- **Breast examination.** Inspect for symmetry, mobility, and dimpling as the woman lifts her arms over the head, pushes her hands on her hips, and leans forward. Inspect the supraclavicular and infraclavicular areas. Inspect the breast for discharge.

▼

 Step **20** ▶ **Inspect the abdomen.**

With the patient supine, inspect the shape, symmetry, skin characteristics, umbilicus, and pulsation of the abdomen. Auscultate bowel sounds. Palpate all quadrants of the abdomen first using light palpation then using deep palpation. Palpate the liver for aortic pulsations. Assess the abdominal reflexes. Palpate the femoral pulses and inguinal nodes. Assess the femoral pulse. With an assistant's hand placed along the midabdomen, tap the side of the abdomen and assess for fluid waves with the opposite hand.

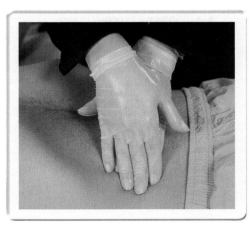

 In the Field

Superficial Reflexes

Abdominal: upper (T7 through T10), lower (T10 through L1)
- Starting with the upper quadrants, lightly stroke the abdomen. The normal reflex is the movement of the umbilicus toward the area being stroked. Repeat the assessment by stroking the lower quadrants.

Plantar: (C6, C7, C8)
- Lightly stroke the plantar surface of the patient's foot, starting at the heel and working up to the ball and across the base of the big toe. The toes should flex slightly (grasping) as the normal response. Dorsiflexion of the big toe with or without fanning of the other toes is an abnormal finding referred to as the Babinski sign.

▼

Step 21 ▶ **Inspect the pelvis.**

Palpate the pelvic area for instability. Verbalize assessment of genitalia/perineum, as needed. Identify sacral edema if present.

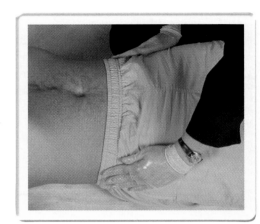

- **Females.** With the patient lying in a lithotomy position, inspect the perineal and perianal areas for injury, lesions, or discharge. If available, save a stool sample for guaiac test.
- **Males.** Sitting in front of the patient as he stands, inspect the penis and scrotum for injury, lesions, or discharge. Palpate the testicles through the scrotal sac. Transluminate if masses are felt. Check for inguinal hernia.

 Step 22 ▶ **Inspect all four extremities.**

Assess distal circulation and motor and sensory function. Assess for the presence of edema and pitting edema.

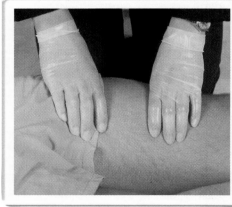

- **Upper extremities.** Assess the patient's ability to move without restriction, and assess muscle strength in the hands, arms, and shoulders.
- **Lower extremities.** Inspect the legs for symmetry, skin characteristics, hair distribution, and varicose veins. Inspect between the toes. Palpate the popliteal, posterior tibial, and dorsalis pedis pulses. Palpate for temperature and pretibial edema. Assess the patient's ability to move without restriction, and assess muscle strength in the hips, knees, ankles, and feet. Evaluate the patient's stride as he/she walks across the room and walks back in a heel-to-toe fashion. Watch as the patient walks a few more steps on his/her toes and then on his/her heels. Have the patient perform shallow knee bends, one for each leg.
- **Spinal column/hips.** As the patient bends over to touch his/her toes, inspect and palpate the spine. Assess the patient's ability to move without resistance as the patient hyperextends, rotates, and laterally bends at the waist.

Step 23 ▸ **Inspect the back.**

If the patient is not immobilized, assess the back for tenderness, deformities, presence of edema in the sacral area, rash, and petechiae.

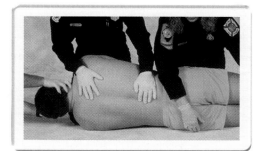

▼

 Step 24 ▸ **Check the neurologic condition of the patient.**

Assess sensory ability to identify superficial pain, light touch, and vibration in selected areas on the face, arms, hands, legs, and feet. Test stereognosis. Assess cerebellar function of the upper extremities using the finger-to-nose test and rapid alternating movements test. Test cerebellar function of the lower extremities by asking the patient to run each heel down the opposite shin. Elicit abdominal and planter superficial reflexes. Elicit the bicep, tricep, brachioradialis, patellar, and Achilles deep tendon reflexes.

▼

 Step 25 ▸ **Perform laboratory/diagnostic procedures.**

Draw blood for blood glucose analysis and cardiac enzymes, using finger stick and point-of-care testing devices. Attach the electrodes to perform 12-lead ECG acquisition.

▼

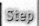 **Step 26** ▸ **Identify and provide interventions.**

From the information gathered, determine the patient's medical problem or extent of injury. Provide interventions appropriate for the patient's condition.

▼

 In the Field

Deep Tendon Reflexes (continued)

Patellar (L2, L3, L4)
- Flex the patient's knee up to 90°, allowing the lower leg to hang loosely. Support the upper leg with your hand, not allowing it to rest against the edge of the examining table. Strike the patellar tendon just below the patella. Contraction of the quadriceps muscle causes extension of the lower leg.

Achilles (S1, S2)
- With the patient sitting, flex the knee to 90° and keep the ankle in neutral position, holding the heel of the foot in your hand. Strike the Achilles tendon at the level of the ankle malleoli. Contraction of the gastrocnemius muscle causes plantar flexion of the foot.

 In the Field

Stereognosis Test

The stereognosis test assesses the patient's ability to recognize objects by feeling their forms, size, and weights.

To perform the test, have the patient close his or her eyes. Place a familiar object (paper clip, key, coin, pencil, cotton ball, etc.) in the patient's hand and ask him or her to identify it. Normally the patient will explore it with his or her fingers and name it correctly.

Step **27** Reevaluate transport decision.

Reevaluate the initial decision to transport. Based on the total picture now available, determine whether to initiate transport or to slow the emergency response.

Step **28** Document abnormal findings.

Document all findings, normal and abnormal, in an appropriate format.

Trauma Patients With Significant Mechanisms of Injury or Unresponsive Medical Patients

Step **29** Obtain or direct assistant to obtain baseline vital signs (see Skill 39).

Determine the patient's level of consciousness (using the patient's orientation to person, place, and time), pulse (rate, strength, and regularity), respirations (rate, depth, and quality), blood pressure, skin temperature and condition, and tissue color. Perform a rapid physical examination as described in Steps 30 through 37.

Step **30** Assess the head.

Inspect/palpate the scalp; inspect/palpate the face; inspect nose, mouth, and ears; inspect eyes and pupils. Look for bleeding, bruising, discoloration, and deformity.

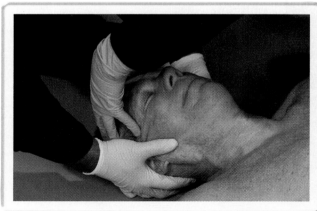

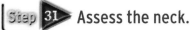 **Assess the neck.**

Inspect/palpate the neck; look for jugular vein distension and tracheal deviation. Apply cervical spine immobilization device on trauma patients. Listen for bruits.

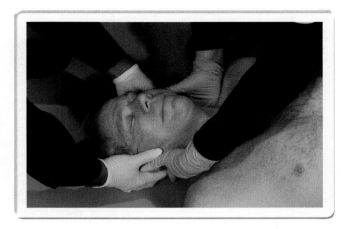

 Assess the chest.

Inspect/palpate the stability of the chest wall; auscultate the equality of breath and heart sounds.

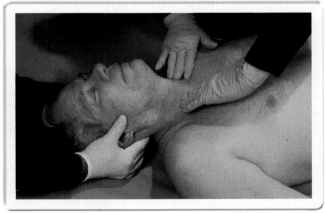

Step 33 ▶ Assess the abdomen and pelvis.

Inspect/palpate all four quadrants. Look for bruising and distension. Palpate for instability in the pelvis. Assessment of genitalia and perineum should be performed if appropriate. Identify sacral edema.

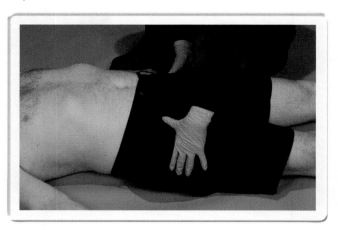

▼

Step 34 ▶ Assess lower extremities.

Inspect/palpate the lower extremities. Look for the quality of circulation and motor and sensory function. Assess the patient's ability to move joints and to move the foot against resistance. Inspect for pitting edema.

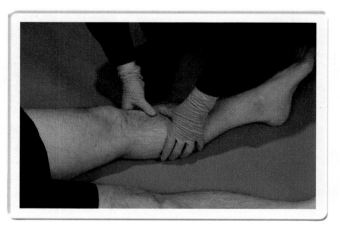

▼

Step 35 **Assess upper extremities.**

Inspect/palpate the upper extremities, looking for the quality of circulation and motor and sensory function. Assess the patient's ability to move joints. Assess grip strength in both hands.

 Step 36 **Assess the back.**

Inspect/palpate thoracic/lumbar spine and the entire back. Make this a thorough inspection. If the patient will be placed on a backboard, this will be the last examination of the back you will be able to perform.

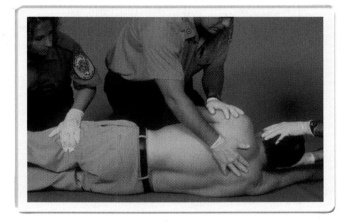

 Step 37 **Manage secondary injuries and wounds appropriately.**

When initial threats to life have been managed, secondary injuries should be managed if the situation allows. This includes stabilizing minor fractures and minor bleeding.

Step **Patient history: Gather the history of present illness.**

In this sequence our patient is either unresponsive or has a significant injury. This means that the following information will likely be gathered from family, friends, or witnesses to the event.

- **Cardiac or respiratory patients.** Follow the standard OPQRST approach.
  Onset of symptoms: Was onset sudden or gradual?
  Provocation: What worsens or lessens the condition?
  Quality: Is the pain sharp, throbbing, crushing, dull?
  Radiation: Does the pain or condition travel to other parts of the body?
  Severity: How badly does it hurt? Determine severity using a scale of 1 to 10, with 10 being the worst pain ever felt by the patient.
  Time: How long ago did the condition begin?
- **Altered mental status patients.** Determine a description of the episode, the onset, the duration, and associated evidence of trauma. Question the family or bystanders about interventions already taken and the possibility of seizures or fever.
- **Allergic reaction patients.** Determine history of allergies, what the patient was exposed to and how, the effects and progression of exposure, and any interventions already performed (such as the use of antihistamines or an epinephrine auto-injector).
- **Poisoning/overdose patients.** Determine the toxic substance, the time at which exposure occurred, the type of exposure (ingestion or contact), how much toxin was involved, and over how long a period of time. Also determine what interventions were performed. The patient's weight and the effects of exposure are also important.
- **Obstetric patients.** First determine the possibility of pregnancy. Determine the length of pregnancy (in weeks if known), estimated date of confinement, any pain or contractions, bleeding or discharge, and possible crowning. Does the patient feel the need to push? Determine the patient's last menstrual period, previous pregnancies, and the results of each pregnancy (gravida, para, ab, cesarean sections).
- **Behavioral patients.** Start by asking "How do you feel?" Determine if there are thoughts of suicide and whether the patient is a threat to self or others. Ask about any underlying medical problem and any interventions already performed.
- **Environmental emergency patients.** Determine the cause of the problem (heat, cold, water, or altitude), the length of exposure, and any loss of consciousness. Determine what effects have occurred and whether the effects are general or local.

▼

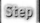 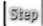

Step 39 ▶ Complete the SAMPLE history.

Gather the SAMPLE history from the patient or from family or bystanders if necessary.

Symptoms (history of present illness)
Allergies to medications
Medications currently taken by the patient (prescription and nonprescription)
Past history—pertinent medical information related to current condition
Last oral intake (food, drink) or last menstrual period in obstetric/gynecologic patients
Events leading up to emergency

▼

Step 40 ▶ Ongoing assessment: Report to hospital after obtaining appropriate information.

The purpose of the hospital radio report is to alert the emergency department of the arrival of a patient. In most cases the information should be as brief as possible. Only in cases where specific treatment orders or physician consultation are desired should a detailed report be given. The information relayed will be used by the emergency department staff to ensure the proper triage of the patient upon arrival.

The report should follow an organized format, giving the following information in order:

- Identification of unit and self
- Age and gender of patient
- Problems found in primary assessment, if any
- Patient's chief complaint
- Estimate of severity of patient's condition
- Brief history of present illness or injury
- Vital signs
- Pertinent treatment provided
- Anticipated time of arrival

> This is Medic 417, paramedic Williams. We are en route to your facility with a 21-year-old female who was involved in a motor vehicle collision. The patient is stable, conscious, and complaining of shoulder and chest pain with dyspnea. Her pulse is 100 beats/min and regular, blood pressure is 114/76 mm Hg, and respirations are 18 breaths/min and regular. We should be in the ED in 15 minutes.

Note: Upon arrival at the receiving facility, a more detailed patient report should be given. This detailed report should be a complete description of the patient's presentation, care delivered, and response to interventions.

▼

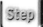 **Step** **Repeat initial assessment and vital signs.**

Repeat the initial assessment. Vital signs should be repeated every 5 minutes for unstable patients (those in the high-priority or rapid-transport categories) and every 15 minutes for stable patients. Reassess the patient's chief complaints and repeat the focused physical examination as necessary. Determine the effects of the interventions performed. A minimum of three sets of recorded vital signs (initial patient contact, just prior to transport, just prior to hospital arrival) should have been performed upon arrival at the emergency department.

▼

 Step **Evaluate patient's response to interventions.**

Following interventions, evaluate the patient to determine if the interventions were effective. Look for improvement in respiratory effort and perfusion, as well as deterioration in condition. Also look for adverse effects from interventions.

▼

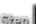 **Step** **Repeat focused assessment regarding patient complaint or injuries.**

If indicated, repeat the focused assessment. This will be essential if responses to interventions are not obvious.

Vital Signs

Performance Objective

Given a patient, the candidate shall assess and interpret the patient's pulse, respirations, palpated and auscultated blood pressure, in 6 minutes or less.

Given the appropriate equipment, the candidate shall also assess the patient's level of consciousness, temperature, red blood cell saturation, end-tidal carbon dioxide, and trauma score, in 5 minutes or less.

Equipment

The following equipment is required to perform this skill:
- Appropriate body substance isolation/personal protective equipment
- Watch with second hand (or digital equivalent)
- Stethoscope with diaphragm and bell
- Sphygmomanometer, with various-sized cuffs
- Pen and paper (patient care chart)
- Thermometer
- Pulse oximeter
- End-tidal carbon dioxide meter

Equipment that may be helpful:
- Reflex hammer
- Pen light

Indications

- General patient assessment
- Determination of patient status

Contraindications

- Blood pressure should not be assessed on the ipsilateral arm of a radical mastectomy patient or on patients with a hemodialysis fistula or an indwelling peripherally inserted central catheter.
- Some patients may have specific reasons why blood pressure should be taken in one arm or another. Those wishes should be honored.

Complications

- None

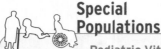

Special Populations

Pediatric Vital Signs

Memorizing normal values for adult vital signs is simple and makes sense. Pediatric vital signs are a completely different issue because of the changes in vital signs as we grow and mature. The normal rates for pulse and respirations will slow, while the normal blood pressure will increase. Even the normal temperature will vary slightly in the early stages of life. Because normal vital signs vary greatly between age groups, it is not necessarily advisable to attempt to memorize all of the varying vital signs for each age group. Instead, get a chart. There are many pediatric vital sign charts on the market, from individual pocket reference cards to a page in a complete pediatric pocket reference guide. Even height-based vital sign tapes are helpful. Use of these reference guides can make determining normal pediatric vital signs simple and convenient.

Procedures

Step 1 Ensure body substance isolation before beginning procedures.

Prior to beginning patient care, appropriate body substance isolation procedures should be employed.

▼

Step 2 Calculate and interpret the radial pulse.

The pulse can be obtained from any palpable artery. For purposes of routine assessment, the radial pulse is most often assessed. The radial pulse can be found by locating the radial prominence just proximal to the thumb. Place your fingers between the radius and the lateral ligament. The radial pulse should be easily felt with minimal pressure.

Using the first two fingers, palpate and count the rate of the radial pulse for 30 seconds, then multiply by two. Describe the quality of the pulse (strong, weak, thready, etc.) and the regularity of the rhythm. Interpret the findings.

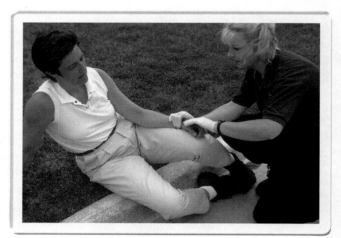

The normal pulse for an adult should be between 60 and 100 beats/min, strong and regular. A pulse rate of less than 60 beats/min is referred to as bradycardia, while a rate of over 100 beats/min is tachycardia.

▼

Step 3 **Calculate and interpret respiratory rate.**

The respiratory rate is the number of times a patient breathes each minute. Usually this rate is based on the patient's own ventilatory effort. Occasionally, as in assisted ventilations or in respiratory arrest, the patient's respiratory rate is, at least in part, a factor of ventilations provided by a bag-mask device.

To accurately determine a patient's ventilatory rate, it is important that the patient not know that their respiratory effort is being counted. This can cause the patient to change how he or she breathes. Often, to measure the respiratory rate, it is best to maintain hold of the patient's wrist as if taking the pulse, just change focus and begin to count the respirations. Respirations can be subtle. Sometimes only slight changes in the rise and fall of the chest will be detected.

Count the rate of the patient's respirations and describe quality (shallow, labored, etc.) and regularity of the respiratory pattern. Interpret the findings.

A normal adult respiratory rate is between 12 and 20 breaths/min; the number varies. Normal respirations are also regular and without effort.

▼

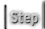 **Step 4** **Palpate and interpret systolic blood pressure.**

A palpated blood pressure is considered to be approximate because it is not exact. It is used to assist in the determination of the blood pressure by identifying a starting point. It is also very helpful if obtaining blood pressure in noisy locations or when the pressure is low and unable to be heard through a stethoscope.

With a cuff properly sized for the patient, apply the cuff snugly to the upper arm, at least 1″ above the antecubital fossa.

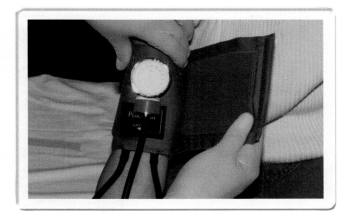

Locate the radial pulse using two fingers. Keep the fingers in place throughout this procedure.

continued

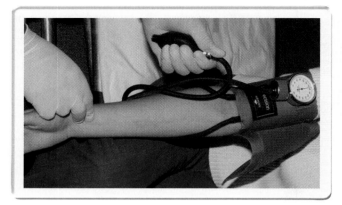

Inflate the cuff gently, feeling for the disappearance of the palpable pulse. After the pulse disappears, give the bulb one or two more squeezes. Carefully and slowly release the air from the blood pressure cuff. Palpate for and note the return of the pulse. The return of the pulse is the palpated systolic blood pressure. Deflate the cuff completely when finished and prior to reinflation (if a second or third attempt is performed). Interpret the findings.

A normal adult systolic blood pressure is between 100 and 120 mm Hg. These numbers will change based on several factors, including: age, gender, physical activity, and weight.

Step 5 Auscultate and interpret blood pressure.

With a cuff properly sized for the patient, apply the cuff snugly to the upper arm, at least 1″ above the antecubital fossa. Place the diaphragm of the stethoscope over the brachial artery.

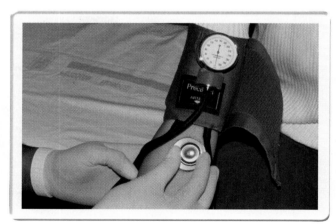

Inflate the cuff gently, listening for Korotkoff sounds to appear as the pressure increases. After the sounds disappear, give the bulb one or two more squeezes. Carefully and slowly release the air from the blood pressure cuff. Listen for the return and disappearance of the Korotkoff sounds. The return of Korotkoff sounds gives the systolic blood pressure, whereas the disappearance gives the diastolic pressure. Deflate the cuff completely when finished and prior to reinflation (if a second or third attempt is performed). Interpret the findings.

A normal adult systolic blood pressure is between 100 and 120 mm Hg. These numbers will change based on several factors, including: age, gender, physical activity, and weight. The normal diastolic pressure is around two thirds of the systolic pressure.

In the Field

Sizing the Blood Pressure Cuff

Choosing the proper blood pressure cuff for the patient is an important part of obtaining an accurate blood pressure.

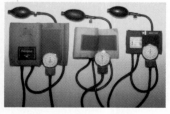

Most blood pressure cuffs have markings to identify the correct size. When the cuff is placed around the patient's arm, the arrow or other markings should fit between the minimum and maximum size indicators.

In the Field

Abnormal Vital Signs

	Low	High
Pulse	• At rest/asleep • Cardiac disease	• Excitement/exercise • Stress • Shock
Respirations	• At rest/asleep • Shock • Respiratory disease	• Exercise • Respiratory disease • Early shock
Blood pressure	• Late shock • Hypoperfusion	• Hypertension • Stress • Neurologic compromise

Advanced Vital Signs

 Step 6 **Assess and interpret level of consciousness.**

The level of consciousness is assessed by three simple means. Used together, and in order, these give a very good picture of the patient's mental status.

The first means of assessing level of consciousness is to determine the level of arousal needed to obtain a response from the patient. This is known as the AVPU scale. Using this scale the patient is either: **A**wake and alert, responsive to **V**erbal stimuli, responsive to **P**hysical or painful stimuli, or is **U**nresponsive (unconscious).

The second means of assessing the level of consciousness is to identify the patient's orientation to person (and others), place, and time. Normally, fully conscious patients are familiar with who they are as well as other people, where they are, and the general time. A patient who knows all parameters is considered to be conscious and alert, oriented to person, place, and time. A patient who has a deficit in one or all is said to be disoriented. Note that because this requires conversations with the patient, it can only be applied to a patient who is awake. Even though it may be possible to obtain some idea of the orientation of a person who is able to be aroused by verbal or physical stimuli, a deficit in level of consciousness has already been determined.

The third means of determining the mental status of a patient is through the use of the Glasgow Coma Scale. The Glasgow Coma Scale measures mental status by assessing three areas: best eye response, best verbal response, and best motor response. The patient is given a score based on the best response in each category, and an overall score is given. A perfect score is 15 points, while the lowest possible score is 3. Because administering the Glasgow Coma Scale is time consuming, it is not expected that it be performed in the initial contact with the patient but rather as a trending scale for ongoing patient assessment.

To assess the mental status of the patient using all three criteria, first make a decision as to whether the patient is awake or if verbal or physical stimuli are needed to stimulate arousal. If the patient does not respond to any stimuli,

Step 6 continued

then he or she is considered to be unresponsive or unconscious. Next, in awake patients, ask the patient if he or she knows his or her name, where he or she is at the present time, and what time it is. Lastly, use the Glasgow Coma Scale to make a final decision about the patient's mental status. When all three assessments are complete, interpret the findings.

Use the Glasgow Coma Scale by assessing the following areas and awarding the assigned points.

Glasgow Coma Scale

Eye Opening		Best Verbal Response		Best Motor Response	
Spontaneous	4	Oriented and converses	5	Follows commands	6
To verbal command	3	Disoriented conversation	4	Localizes pain	5
To pain	2	Speaking but nonsensical	3	Withdraws to pain	4
No response	1	Moans or makes unintelligible sounds	2	Decorticate flexion	3
		No response	1	Decerebrate extension	2
				No response	1

Scores:
14-15: Mild dysfunction
11-13: Moderate to severe dysfunction
10 or less: Severe dysfunction (The lowest possible score is 3.)

Step 7 Assess and interpret temperature.

Temperature is an important vital sign that is all too often overlooked in the prehospital setting. It is an essential part of the complete patient assessment and should be performed on all children, all geriatrics, all patients who present with fever or a potentially infectious disease, and all patients who may be victims of environmental emergencies. Additionally, it is a good practice to obtain a temperature on all patients, if possible.

The best temperature is a core, rectal temperature. However, in the modern world, there are very accurate electronic thermometers that can give a near core temperature by much simpler means. The normal core temperature for children and adults is 98.6°F. Neonates and young infants may have a slightly higher temperature.

With the thermometer used according to the manufacturer's specifications, correctly read the thermometer and interpret the findings.

Step 8 **Assess and interpret red blood cell saturation (pulse oximetry).**

Pulse oximetry is a measure of the saturation of the red blood cells of the body—whether or not the saturation is by oxygen. It is a valuable tool to determine how well the red blood cells carry oxygen, but in some cases, mostly in toxic exposure to gases such as carbon monoxide or cyanide, the reading from the pulse oximeter will be based on nonoxygen saturation. The normal adult patient will have a pulse oximeter reading of 96% to 100%. Pregnant women will have slightly lower numbers, as will patients with emphysema and chronic bronchitis.

It is important to note that a pulse oximeter reading is not equivalent to an arterial oxygen measurement of blood gases. Although these measurements correlate, they are different forms of expressing oxygen in the arteries.

Attach the pulse oximeter sensor to the patient's finger. Correctly read the display and interpret the findings.

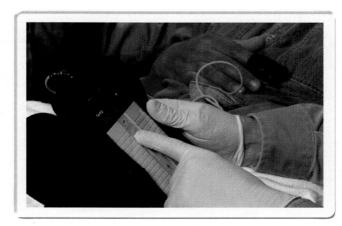

 Step 9 **Assess and interpret end-tidal carbon dioxide level.**

End-tidal carbon dioxide is the amount of carbon dioxide in the expelled air. This is a reflection of how oxygen is utilized in the body and of the workings of the ventilatory activity of the body. End-tidal carbon dioxide is very closely related to the arterial level of carbon dioxide in the blood, and in most cases there is no more than a 5 mm Hg difference. The normal end-tidal carbon dioxide level is between 35 mm Hg and 45 mm Hg.

Attach the end-tidal carbon dioxide cannula to the patient. Correctly read the numeric (capnometry) and wave form (capnography) displays, and interpret the findings.

In the Field

Capnography
Capnometery and capnography are measures of the carbon dioxide in each exhalation. Normally, the carbon dioxide in expired air is 35 mm Hg to 45 mm Hg. By measuring and charting the level of carbon dioxide, it is possible to not only assess the patient but to make improvements in the patient outcome. If the carbon dioxide level is higher than desired, increasing the respiratory rate can bring it down. If the carbon dioxide level is lower than desired, slow the respiratory rate, and the level will rise.

For patients with head injuries, keeping the carbon dioxide level between 35 mm Hg and 40 mm Hg has been shown to maintain lower intracranial pressures. In the intubated patient, constant waveform monitoring is simply the easiest means of ensuring proper tube placement. In short, the use of end-tidal carbon dioxide monitoring is a valuable tool in assessing the ventilatory ability of the patient.

Step 10 **Calculate and interpret the trauma score.**

The revised trauma score is a common trauma score that assigns points for specific ranges of three factors: the Glasgow Coma Scale (GCS), the systolic blood pressure (SPB), and the respiratory rate (RR). After assigning a score to each factor, calculate and interpret the findings (total score 0–12).

Trauma Score

GCS		SBP		RR	
13-15	4	89	4	29	4
9-12	3	76-89	3	10-29	3
6-8	2	50-75	2	6-9	2
4-5	1	1-49	1	1-5	1
3	0	0	0	0	0

Communication

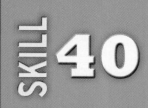

Performance Objective

Given all required information concerning the assessment and management of a patient, the candidate shall relay necessary information to receiving personnel, in 2 minutes or less.

Equipment

The following equipment is required to perform this skill:
- Appropriate body substance isolation/personal protective equipment
- Voice skills
- Radio

Indications

- Radio reports for the purpose of:
  - Notifying the receiving facility of the status of the incoming patient
  - Consulting with the receiving physician concerning further patient care
- Face-to-face report for the transfer of care

Contraindications

- Relaying of patient information to personnel not involved in the continuation of care is prohibited under the Health Insurance Portability and Accountability Act (HIPAA) and may violate other privacy laws as well.

Complications

- None

Procedures

Radio Report for Notification

The purpose of the hospital radio report is to alert the emergency department of the arrival of a patient. In most cases the information should be as brief as possible. The information relayed will be used by the emergency department staff to ensure the proper triage of the patient upon arrival.

 Step 1 ▶ Key microphone.

Key the microphone and wait 1 second before talking.

▼

 Step 2 ▶ Contact receiving facility.

With the microphone approximately 1″ from your lips, make initial contact with the receiving facility. It is best to identify the receiving facility first and then your unit. Stating the hospital name first gains the attention of the receiver and keeps him or her alert as to who is calling.

> Memorial Emergency, this is Medic 16.

▼

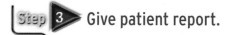

Step 3 ▶ **Give patient report.**

After the receiving facility acknowledges the radio call, key the microphone and wait 1 second. Then, with the microphone held approximately 1″ from your lips, begin the notification report.

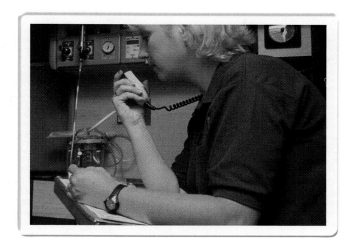

The report should follow an organized format, giving the following information in order:

- Indentification of unit and self
- Age and gender of patient
- Problems found in primary assessment, if any
- Patient's chief complaint
- Estimate of severity of patient's condition
- Brief history of present illness or injury
- Vital signs
- Pertinent treatment provided
- Anticipated time of arrival

This is Medic 16, paramedic Jackson. We are en route to your facility with a 21-year-old female who was involved in a motor vehicle collision. The patient is stable, conscious, and complaining of shoulder and chest pain with dyspnea. Her pulse is 100 beats/min and regular, blood pressure is 114/76 mm Hg, and respirations are 18 breaths/min, regular and nonlabored. We should be in the ED in 15 minutes.

Radio Report for Physician Consultation

The purpose of the physician consultation is to obtain a second opinion on the care of the patient, to determine if the care of the patient needs to follow a path not described in protocol, or to discuss alternative regimens not in the standing orders. Although brief is always better, achieving proper consultation requires that the physician be given enough information to form a complete picture of the patient's situation.

 Key microphone.

Key the microphone and wait 1 second before talking.

 Contact receiving facility.

With the microphone approximately 1″ from your lips, make initial contact with the receiving facility and ask for physician consultation. It is best to identify the receiving facility first and then your unit. Stating the hospital's name first gains the attention of the receiver and keeps him or her alert as to who is calling.

> Memorial Emergency, this is Medic 25. Need to speak with a physician for consultation please.

Step 3 ► Give detailed patient report.

After the physician acknowledges the radio call, key the microphone and wait 1 second. Then, with the microphone approximately 1″ from your lips, begin the consultation report. The report should follow an organized format, giving the following information in order:

- Identification of unit and self
- Age and gender of patient
- Problems found in primary assessment, if any
- Patient's chief complaint, including OPQRST
- History of present illness or injury
- Current findings: vital signs, presentation, electrocardiogram, etc.
- Care rendered
- Description of request (orders needed)

This is Medic 25, paramedic Jackson. We are on the scene with a 58-year-old male who is complaining of retrosternal chest pain radiating into his jaw, left shoulder, and arm. He states that the pain began while watching TV and has been growing steadily worse for the past 2 hours. He denies any previous history of heart problems. At this time he is conscious and alert, denying nausea or shortness of breath. He is showing a sinus rhythm with frequent multiformed premature ventricular contractions on the monitor. Breath sounds are clear and equal bilaterally. Blood pressure is 104/68 mm Hg, pulse 76 beats/min and irregular, respirations 28 breaths/min, skin cool and clammy. We have placed him on 4 L of oxygen and started an IV of normal saline to keep vein open. The patient has shown no improvement. After 2 mg of morphine, the patient is still in considerable pain. There is no change in the respiratory status or blood pressure. I would like to give additional morphine, up to 10 mg.

Face-to-Face Transfer of Care

The purpose of the face-to-face report is to provide the receiving personnel with all of the necessary information about the patient's previous and current condition and the care rendered by EMS.

 Introduce patient to receiving personnel.

Introduce the patient by name to the receiving personnel who will be assuming care. In cases of an unresponsive patient, introduce the receiving personnel to the patient and tell the patient what is happening. Never assume an unresponsive patient is not aware of what is going on around her or him.

> Mr. Smith, this is Sylvia. She is the nurse who will take care of you here in the emergency department.

 Deliver detailed patient report.

Proceeding in an organized fashion, give a detailed description of the patient's condition, giving the following information in order:
- The patient's age and history of chief complaint
- Chief complaint and associated symptoms
- Original assessment findings
- Care given
- Current assessment findings
- Known allergies and medications
- Pertinent past medical history
- Status of continuing interventions (endotracheal tube placement, IV fluid infusion, next required medication doses, drip medications, etc.)

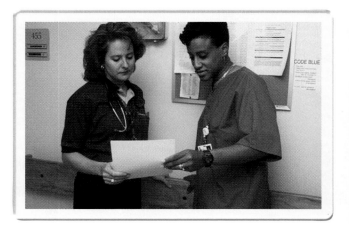

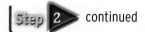 continued

Mr. Smith is 62 years old and woke up this morning complaining of a little nausea. After about 3 hours of taking antacids, he decided he needed to call the ambulance. When we arrived at his house, he was sitting in the living room in moderate distress. He admitted to slight chest pain with the nausea and numbness in his left arm. He rated the pain as a 6. No significant dyspnea reported. We did a 12-lead and found some elevation in the inferior leads but did not see any changes on the right side. His original vitals were all in normal ranges. We placed him on 4 L of oxygen, gave him one 325-mg aspirin, and started the IV, a 16 gauge in the left forearm. He then got one nitro spray and 4 mg of morphine. Currently he still has slight pain rated at a 3, ECG is an ectopy-free normal sinus at 94 beats/min, respirations are 14 breaths/min, and blood pressure is 128/86 mm Hg. The IV is still running with normal saline to keep the vein open; he's had about 50 mL so far, and there are no signs of infiltration or infection.

Documentation

Performance Objective

Following the care of a patient, the candidate shall demonstrate proper documentation of a complete patient report, in 30 minutes or less.

Equipment

The following equipment is required to perform this skill:
- Appropriate body substance isolation/personal protective equipment
- Pen
- Patient care report

Equipment that may be helpful:
- Dictionary
- Thesaurus
- Approved abbreviation list

Indications

- Terminal component of every patient contact, whether patient was transported or not

Contraindications

- None

Complications

- Omitted information can lead to mistakes in the postarrival care of the patient.
- Poorly written reports cast doubt on the quality of patient care.
- Delays in writing reports lead to omitted information and a decline in detail.

Procedures

Writing the SOAP Patient Report

SOAP is an acronym for Subjective, Objective, Assessment, and Patient care, the four components of the patient report. Using this method, specific pieces of information regarding the patient examination and history are divided into two groups: those that cannot be determined, witnessed, or proven by the examiner (subjective) and those that can be determined, witnessed, or proven by the examiner (objective). In other words, this report is a simple division of signs from symptoms.

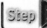 **Step 1 ▶ Subjective.**

Subjective information includes the patient history, whether or not the history comes from the patient directly. Bystander or witness accounts and information supplied by family or neighbors are included in this section, as are the patient's age, past medical condition, allergies, medication taken, chief complaint and associated complaints, and the onset and duration of the problem.

All subjective information is taken at the patient's word rather than being determined by the paramedic. Pain, nausea, dyspnea, and dizziness are also subjective findings because none of them can be proven to exist by the paramedic.

Also included under subjective information are denials from the patient or bystanders, such as loss of consciousness.

▼

  Step 2 ▶ Objective.

Objective information can be determined by the examiner. The location and position of the patient, as well as his or her surroundings, skin temperature, pulse, respiratory rate, and blood pressure are all objective findings. These findings cannot be denied or exaggerated by the patient.

The objective findings should be limited to the *initial* physical examination only and point the assessment toward a specific plan of treatment. All findings from the initial physical examination, vital signs, oxygen saturation as measured by pulse oximetry (S_pO_2), end-tidal carbon dioxide level, and blood glucose level are recorded in this section.

Therapy that was initiated prior to the arrival of EMS should also be documented in this section, such as cardiopulmonary resuscitation performed by a bystander, an IV initiated by a first responder, or bleeding control applied through first aid.

▼

Step 3 ▶ **Assessment.**

The assessment is the patient's problem as seen by the paramedic. It is important to note that although a paramedic cannot make an official medical diagnosis, a paramedic's diagnosis can and must be formed. The patient is treated based on this diagnosis. Without a diagnosis of some kind, treatment of the patient cannot begin.

The paramedic's determination of the patient's condition or problem should match the signs and symptoms noted in the subjective and objective areas of the report and should point toward a specific protocol for treatment. Although the paramedic's diagnosis or opinion of the patient's condition does not need to be as explicit at the physician's official diagnosis, it should reflect the basis for any treatment performed, based on written protocols.

▼

Step 4 ▶ **Patient care (process and procedures, plan).**

The patient care section of the report is a narrative description of the care provided to the patient. The term *plan*, used on physician charts, is not appropriate for a prehospital patient report. When a physician writes a plan, he or she is writing orders to nursing staff and laboratory personnel describing procedures to be carried out in the patient care. Because the "plan" of action on a paramedic's report is actually a retrospective of treatment that has already occurred, a more narrative approach to the actual patient care rendered should be documented.

The patient care section should begin with a description of where the patient encounter initiated and note any additional persons who were important in the assessment of the patient. This should be followed with the assessment of the airway, breathing, and circulation and what determination was made about their status. The report should then proceed to describe each step in the assessment and management of the patient.

The section should also include the response to *all* interventions, any improvement or deterioration in the patient's condition, and what therapeutic adjustments were performed during the course of treatment. The closing of the patient care section and the report should include the transfer of care at the receiving destination. This will include documentation that a report was given to a nurse or physician, as well as the status of continued therapies.

Section	Purpose	Content
Subjective	History and symptoms	What you can't prove, can't see, can't feel
Objective	Physical exam and signs	What you found, saw, heard, felt, smelled
Assessment	Paramedic's diagnosis	Determined and supported by the subjective and objective section findings
Patient care (plan)	Narrative postscript	Detailed explanation of how the assessment, patient interview, therapies, and interventions were carried out; must include responses to all interventions and final disposition of the patient

Patient Report Quality Assurance Checklist

This checklist is to be used to ensure each clinical patient report contains the necessary information.

Subjective Findings

Are all of the following clearly identified as appropriate?

__1   Chief complaint
__2   Associated complaints

SAMPLE History

__3   **S**ymptoms (positive or negative)
__4   **A**llergies: Drug and food
__5   **M**edications: Prescription, over the counter, nonprescription, herbal, compliance
__6   **P**ast medical/surgical history
__7   **L**ast oral intake
__8   **E**vents preceding or leading up to the injury or illness

OPQRST of Chief Complaint

__9   **O**nset
__10 **P**rovocation/palliation
__11 **Q**uality
__12 **R**adiation
__13 **S**everity
__14 **T**ime
__15 Social history: Smoking, alcohol use, drug use, etc.
__16 Caller: Patient, family, bystanders, etc.
__17 Source of information: Patient, family, bystanders, etc.

Special Considerations

Allergies/Anaphylaxis

__18 Allergies
__19 Specifics of previous reactions

Environmental

__20 Exposure
__21 Thermal protection
__22 Fluid/electrolyte intake

Gynecologic/Obstetric

__23 Last menstrual cycle
__24 Possibility of pregnancy
__25 Due date
__26 Gravida, para, ab
__27 Bleeding/discharge

Poisoning/Overdose

__28 Toxin (alone or with alcohol)
__29 How much
__30 Over how long

Trauma: Motor Vehicle

__ 31 Restraints used

__ 32 Patient location in vehicle

Denials

__ 33 Head: Loss of consciousness, headache, dizziness, trauma in last 3 weeks

__ 34 Eyes: Visual difficulty, photophobia, discharge, pain

__ 35 Ears: Change or ringing, discharge

__ 36 Nose: Congestion, pain, discharge

__ 37 Mouth/throat: Pain, trauma or lesions, difficulty speaking/swallowing

__ 38 Chest: Dyspnea, chest pain, palpitations, cough

__ 39 Abdomen: Pain, nausea, emesis, diarrhea

__ 40 GU: Dysuria, hematuria, polyuria, incontinence, discharge

__ 41 Neck/back/extremities: Pain, numbness, tingling

__ 42 Skin: Rashes, lesions, itching

Objective Findings

Are all of the following documented as appropriate for this patient?

Scene Size-Up

__ 43 Scene description (mechanism of injury, environment, vehicle damage, etc.)

__ 44 Patient description and position (weight, supine, prone, driver, back-seat passenger, etc.)

Initial Assessment

__ 45 Level of consciousness (AVPU or estimated Glasgow)

__ 46 Airway

__ 47 Breathing (air movement and effort)

__ 48 Circulation

__ 49 General impression

Physical Examination

Note positive findings for DCAP-BTLS in the following areas. Positive or negative findings should be noted for all other areas as appropriate.

Head

__ 50 Specific examination: Ecchymosis (mastoid, periorbital), drainage (nose, ears), tissue color (conjunctiva, gums), nasal flaring, eye movement, pupil size and response, sclera

Neck

__ 51 Specific examination: Jugular vein distention, carotid bruits, tracheal palpation, spinal palpation, subcutaneous emphysema

Chest

__ 52 Specific examination: Chest rise, paradoxical motion, sucking wounds, breath sounds, respiratory patterns, speech dyspnea, heart sounds, retractions

Abdomen

__ 53 Specific examination: Rigidity, guarding, masses, pulsations, bowel sounds, ecchymosis, rebound, fetal heart tones

Pelvis/Perineum

__ 54 Specific examination: Stability, bleeding, crowning, discharge, incontinence

Posterior (if not included elsewhere)

__ 55 Specific examination

Extremities

__ 56 Specific examination: Motion, sensation, distal circulation, capillary refill, reflexes, strength

Skin

__ 57 Specific examination: Temperature, moisture, tissue color

Trauma Summation

__ 58 "No other deformities, contusions, abrasions, punctures, burns, lacerations, or swelling noted."

Vital Signs and Technology

__ 59 Respiratory rate and quality

__ 60 Pulse rate, strength, and regularity

__ 61 Blood pressure (orthostatic)

__ 62 Electrocardiogram (ECG)

__ 63 12-lead

__ 64 Oxygen saturation as measured by pulse oximetry (S_pO_2); room air and on oxygen

__ 65 End-tidal carbon dioxide level

__ 66 Blood glucose

__ 67 Core temperature

__ 68 I-STAT lab findings

__ 69 Glasgow Coma Scale score

__ 70 Trauma score (on trauma)

Assessment

Is this assessment supported by the signs and symptoms listed in the Subjective and Objective sections?

__ 71 Matches subjective and objective

__ 72 No other problems identified

__ 73 Written as medical diagnosis

Patient Care

Describe in narrative format from patient contact to transfer of care, with times as appropriate.

__ 74 Initial contact

__ 75 Assessment of ABCs

__ 76 History and assessment

__ 77 Initial interventions

__ 78 Response to interventions

__ 79 Reassessment
__ 80 Additional interventions
__ 81 Response to interventions
__ 82 Placement and position on cot
__ 83 Movement to ambulance
__ 84 Loading and securing
__ 85 Movement to final destination
__ 86 Patient report and transfer of care (staff name) and condition of patient
__ 87 Critical status at transfer: IV patient, endotracheal tube placement, fluid volume
        delivered

Procedures

Intravenous Catheterization
__ 88 Size, gauge, and type
__ 89 Location
__ 90 Fluid type and rate
__ 91 Success versus number of attempts—provider

Medication Administration
__ 92 Drug, dose, route, time
__ 93 Intramuscular, subcutaneous: Absence of blood return
__ 94 Intravenous: Positive blood return
__ 95 Provider

Endotracheal Intubation
__ 96 Size and depth
__ 97 Confirmation: Visualization, breath sounds, condensation, end-tidal carbon dioxide,
        esophageal detector (at least three)
__ 98 Secured and collar
__ 99 Reconfirmation with each move: Lifting, defibrillation, loading onto cot, loading into
        ambulance, unloading (constant waveform capnography acceptable)
__ 100 Success versus number of attempts—provider

ET Suctioning
__ 101 Return

Chest Compressions
__ 102 Rate, depth, ratio, pulse generation

Ventilations
__ 103 Rate, volume, compliance

Spinal Motion Restriction
__ 104 Method and procedures (log roll, slide, etc.)
__ 105 Circulation, sensation, and motor function before and after procedure

Orthopaedic Immobilization
__ 106 Method and procedures
__ 107 Circulation, sensation, and motor function before and after procedure
__ 108 Anatomic position
__ 109 Elevated

Defibrillation/Cardioversion
__ 110   Joules and response

Pacing
__ 111   Rate and amperage
__ 112   Capture (electrical/mechanical)

Special Circumstances
Patient Refusal
__ 113   Informed of need for care and/or transportation
__ 114   Informed of consequences of not accepting care or transportation
__ 115   Competency to refuse treatment or transport
__ 116   Advised of critical signs and symptoms

Treat and Release
__ 117   Examination performed
__ 118   Justification of decision why transport is not indicated
__ 119   Accompanied by (mother, spouse, etc.)
__ 120   Advised to seek medical care within ___ hours or days

Deceased
__ 121   Obvious signs of death: Rigor mortis, dependent lividity, decapitation, etc.
__ 122   Time
__ 123   DNR order

Crime Scene
__ 124   Police incident report number
__ 125   Disposition of clothing
__ 126   Preservation of evidence: Bagging of hands, etc.

Family Violence
__ 127   Document location given of nearest family violence center
__ 128   Document injuries that may have resulted from family violence

Child Abuse/Elder Abuse
__ 129   Police incident number (confirming notification)

Termination of Effort
__ 130   Medical control approval
__ 131   Electrocardiogram/end-tidal carbon dioxide at time of termination and no change for 10 minutes

Physician Consultation
__ 132   Physician consultation occurred, including name and time

In the Field

Documentation Methods

In the prehospital setting, several methods of documentation are used and acceptable:

- **Narrative method.** The narrative method is probably the simplest method to write but the most difficult to decipher. This method consists of documenting the patient encounter from start to finish using standard prose. Its strength is that it is simple to learn. Its weakness is that important details are often omitted.

- **CHART or CHARTE method.** CHART stands for **C**hief complaint, **H**istory and physical examination, **A**ssessment, treatment (**R**x), and **T**ransport. To use CHARTE, add **E**xceptions. This method's strength is that it breaks the care and treatment down into smaller sections, which makes it easier to locate specific assessments or care without reading the entire report. Its weakness is that it is difficult to learn.

- **SOAP method.** This is one of the more common forms of documentation, and it is gaining popularity. It is simple to learn, and when it is completed, it provides a simple means for the reader to review the assessment and management.

SOAP Example 1

Subjective

Arrived to find a 55-year-old male complaining of *chest pain (1)*. He admits to *slight dyspnea as well, with mild nausea (2)*. He describes the chest pain as *extreme pressure (11), retrosternal (3), radiating to the left shoulder and jaw (12)*. According to his *wife (17)*, he has had *angina for the past 3 years (6)* and takes *nitroglycerin and nifedipine (5)*. The patient also admits to a history of *hypertension (6)* and *smokes a pack a day (15)*. The *pain is rated as an 8 on a scale of 1 to 10 (13)*. He states the pain began *suddenly (9)* while *sitting watching the news (8)* and has been *present for the past 2 hours (14)*. *Sitting quietly relieves the pain slightly but not to any significant amount (10)*. The patient *denies dizziness, palpitations, or a history of recent cough (38)*. The patient also *denies allergies to drugs or food (4)*. His *last oral intake was dinner just before the pain began, approximately 2 hours ago (7)*.

Objective

The patient was found *sitting on his couch in the living room (43)*. He is *approximately 110 kg (44)*, *diaphoretic (49, 57)*, and *breathes with some distress (47)*. He is *alert; oriented to person, place, and time (45)*; and has a *strong, regular radial pulse (48)*. On physical examination the patient is found to have *ashen oral mucosa (50), equal and reactive pupils approximately 4 mm in diameter (50)*, and *nondistended jugular veins (51)*. His breathing is slightly *labored with equal chest rise (52)*, *breath sounds are clear and equal bilaterally (52)*, and *no heart murmurs or third heart sounds are detected (52)*. *No edema is noted in the sacral area (55) or ankles (56)*. *Distal circulation, sensation, and motor function are found in all extremities (56)*. His *skin is cool to the touch (57)*, his *respirations are 16 breaths/min and slightly labored (59)*, *pulse is 108 beats/min, strong and regular (60)*, and *blood pressure 136/94 mm Hg (61)*. His *ECG is a sinus tachycardia without ectopy (62)*. The *12-lead shows ST elevation in the anterior leads exceeding 2 mm (63)*. His *oxygen saturation is 96% on room air (64)*. The *Glasgow Coma Scale score is 15 (69)* and *blood glucose is 140 mg/dL (66)*.

Assessment

Acute myocardial infarction of the anterior wall (71, 73). Cardiac arrest, postresuscitation coma (71, 73).

Patient Care

Initial examination performed in the *patient's living room, with him remaining in his chair (74)*. The *patient's ABCs were assessed and determined adequate (75)*. The *history was gathered from the patient and his wife (76)* while *vital signs and the ECG were gathered by assisting personnel (76)*. The patient verbally consented to care and transportation. *Oxygen was administered by nasal cannula at 4 L/min (77)*. The *12-lead ECG was gathered as the noninvasive blood pressure was applied (76)*. An *IV was established at 19:01 with an 18-gauge catheter to the right upper forearm on the first attempt by paramedic Tomayo (77, 88, 89, 91)*. The *IV of normal saline was adjusted to run wide open to deliver 500 mL (90)*. One *325-mg aspirin tablet was administered by mouth at 19:04 with 1 ounce of water (92)*. *5-mg morphine sulfate was administered IV push slowly at 19:05 (92)*. The patient was *assisted to the cot and positioned in a semi-Fowler position and secured with straps (82)*. The patient was then *moved to the ambulance, loaded and secured (83, 84)*. Three minutes after giving morphine the patient reported his *pain eased slightly and was now a 6 on a scale of 1 to 10, his pulse oximeter was 99%, and his tissues were beginning to pink (78)*. *Transport was begun to Harris Methodist Fort Worth (85)*. A firefighter accompanied the paramedic in the ambulance. At 19:11, 1 minute into the transport, the *patient looked up and said he felt* "strange" (78). He then lost consciousness and displayed a course ventricular fibrillation on the ECG monitor (79). The head of the cot was lowered to place the patient in a supine position (80). Assessment found the patient without a pulse or respirations (81). Combi-pads were placed and the defibrillator was charged to 200 joules (80). The patient was defibrillated resulting in a conversion to a sinus rhythm with a rate of 74 and no ectopy (110). No immediate return of consciousness occurred, and the patient had a weak radial pulse and breathing remained absent (79). Ventilations were begun at 19:14 with a bag-mask device at 10 breaths/min, creating chest rise (80). Oxygen was attached to the bag in less than 1 minute (80). The noninvasive blood pressure showed a blood pressure of 103/68 mm Hg, and the oxygen saturation was 98% (79, 81). 110 mg of lidocaine was administered via IV push at 19:16 (79, 80, 92) after ensuring IV patency (94), and it was followed by the establishment of a 2 mg/min lidocaine drip at 19:18 by paramedic Tomayo (80, 92, 95). No spontaneous ventilations or gag reflex were present (79). The patient was intubated at 19:22 (80) on one attempt by paramedic Tomayo (100) with a 8.0 endotracheal tube and placed at 24 cm at the lips (96). Placement was ensured by visualization of the tube passing through the cords, breath sounds, and colorimetric capnometry (97). The endotracheal tube was secured with a Thomas tube holder, and a short stiff-neck extrication collar was applied (98). Tube placement was monitored by attaching the side-stream capnograph showing appropriate waveforms (99). Upon arrival at the hospital the patient was taken to trauma room 1 where he was transferred onto the hospital cot (86). The report was given to Ms. Freeman, RN and Dr. Ansohn (86). The ECG monitor, noninvasive blood pressure, and oxygen were changed over to the hospital's systems (86). At the time of transfer the patent remained unresponsive with an ectopy-free sinus rhythm on the ECG. His blood pressure was 112/74 mm Hg, pulse 94 beats/min, and respirations assisted at 12 breaths/min (86). The end-tidal carbon dioxide was 36 mm Hg with appropriate waveforms (87). No spontaneous respirations were present (87). The patient had been given a total of 450 mL of normal saline, 11 mL of lidocaine by IV push, and 5 mL of lidocaine by IV drip (87). Endotracheal tube placement ensured by capnographic waveforms, chest rise, and breath sounds (87, 99).

SOAP Example 2

Subjective

The patient is a 27-year-old male *involved in an industrial accident (8)*. He is *complaining of severe pain to his entire body (1)* following a *flash explosion (9)*. He says his *throat is burning and he is having trouble breathing (1)*. His *coworker (17)* says they were *working on a gas water heater when a spark caused the tank to explode (8)*. The *patient was immediately engulfed in flames, and other workers doused the flames with a garden hose (8)*. The patient says he is very healthy with *no past medical history (6)*, takes no *prescription medications (5)*, and is *allergic to sulfa drugs (4)*. His *last oral intake was 3 hours earlier when he had a full breakfast (7)*. At the time of the explosion the *patient was wearing a polyester/cotton golf shirt, jeans, and boots (9)*. The coworkers state the *shirt was pretty much burned off the patient (17)*. Currently the pain is severe, rated as *a 10 on a scale of 1 to 10 (13)*, and he says *he is very cold (2)*. The incident occurred approximately *10 minutes prior to the arrival of EMS (14)*.

Objective

The *approximately 80 kg patient (44)* was *found lying in a puddle of water with parts of an exploded water tank all around him (43)*. *Coworkers were at his side dousing the patient with cool running water (43)*. The patient is *awake (45)*, shivering, and *moaning in pain (47)*. His *voice is raspy, and he is struggling to breathe (47)*. A *weak radial pulse is present (48)*. He was *obviously in distress from severe burns with respiratory compromise (49)*. On physical examination the patient is found to have *second- and third-degree burns to his face and back of head, circumferential neck and chest, anterior abdomen, and both arms (50, 51, 52, 53, 56, 57)*: an estimated *54% body surface area (57)*. *Soot and charring are present on the patient's teeth, and the oral cavity has mucosal burns (50)*. His *eyelashes and eyebrows are singed and barely perceptible (50)*, and his *pupils are equal and reactive to light at 3 mm (50)*. There is *slight clouding of the right eye (50)*. *Strider is audible without a stethoscope (52)*. *Equal bilateral chest rise is present with clear breath sounds (52)*; *heart sounds reveal no murmurs or third heart sounds (52)*. The *shirt is burned into the chest in several areas (52)*. The patient has *palpable pulses, sensation, and movement in all extremities (56)*. *Abrasions and small lacerations are seen over the face and both arms (50, 56)*. Other than noted, *no other deformities, contusions, abrasions, punctures, lacerations, or swelling are noted (58)*. He has *respirations of 22 breaths/min and labored (59)*, pulse is *102 beats/min, strong and regular (60)*, and *blood pressure 134/84 mm Hg (61)*. He has a *sinus tachycardia without ectopy on the ECG (62)*. His *oxygen saturation is 98% on room air (64)*, his *blood glucose is 140 mg/dL (66)*, and his *core temperature is 96.2°F (67)*. His initial *Glasgow Coma Scale score is 15 (69)*, and his *Trauma score is 12 (70)*.

Assessment

The patient has critical thermal burns with respiratory compromise (71, 73).

Patient Care

An initial assessment and management were conducted at the scene (74). The *airway was assessed and determined to be in danger (75)*; *preparations for facilitated intubation were begun as the history and physical examination were conducted (76)*. *Air transport was called to transport the patient to the burn unit at the hospital (77)*. Consent for treatment and transport was received from the patient. *He was removed from the puddle of water (77)* and placed *on a dry sheet on the cot and covered with a second dry sheet and blanket (82, 77)*. *Oxygen, 12 L/min by nonrebreathing mask, was applied at 09:42 (77)*. The patient immediately *began to relax and said he felt warmer and more comfortable (78)*. His *pain was not eased (78)*. An *IV (77)* of *lactated Ringer's (90)* was established on the *first attempt* by paramedic Crole (91) at 09:45 with a 14-gauge catheter (88) to the right lower forearm (89) and run wide open initially (90). The IV site was secured with sterile roller gauze. After ensuring IV patency (94), 10 mg of morphine was administered at 09:46 IV push over 1 minute (92) followed by 10 mg of midazolam at 09:47 (92). After 2 minutes the patient was still stating the pain was severe with no relief (78). An additional 10 mg of morphine was administered IV push at 09:50 (80). The patient was then informed of the need for intubation and informed of the rapid sequence that intubation involved. He consented to the care and was given 10 mg of vecuronium IV push at 09:52 (80). The patient became flaccid and was intubated as soon as the eyelids did not respond to light pressure (81). Paramedic Jackson attempted to place an 8.0 endotracheal tube through the cords, but laryngeal edema prevented the tube from passing (100). After 1 minute of ventilations, paramedic Crole placed a 7.0 endotracheal tube into the trachea to a depth of 24 cm at the teeth (80, 96). Placement was ensured by visualization of the tube passing the cords, equal breath sounds, and colorimetric capnometry (97). The tube was secured with umbilical cord tape, and a regular Stifneck extrication collar was applied (98). Ventilation was begun at 12 breaths/min with a bag-mask device flowing 15 L/min of oxygen (80). The patient's blood pressure remained steady at 130/80 mm Hg, pulse 108 beats/min, and oxygen saturation 100% (81). Constant monitoring of end-tidal carbon dioxide waveforms confirmed placement of the ET tube (99). An additional 10 mg of morphine was given IV push at 10:01 (80). As air transport landed, a second IV of lactated Ringer's was established in the patient's left mid forearm with a 14-gauge catheter by paramedic Crole on one attempt (80, 88, 89, 91). The IV was adjusted to 200 mL/h (90). The patient was introduced to the flight crew, and a report was given to air transport nurse Moore (86). The patient was transferred to the helicopter stretcher (84). The patient was taken to the helicopter and secured head aft (84). At the time of transport, the patient had been under paralytic control for 6 minutes, had good waveforms on capnography ensuring proper tube placement, and had received 650 mL of lactated Ringer's, slightly over half of the 1,080 mL required for this patient's first hour (87).

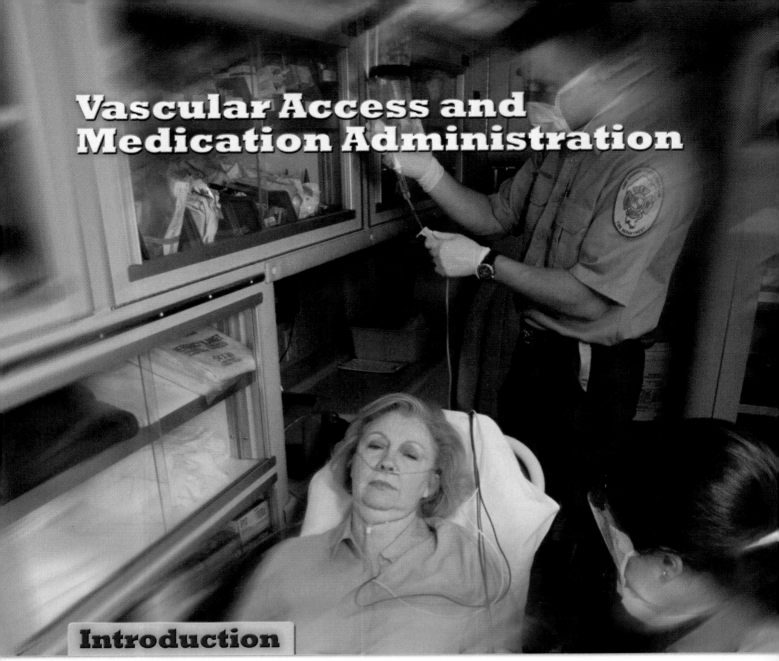

Vascular Access and Medication Administration

Introduction

Administration of medication to any patient carries with it additional responsibilities. Although medications can be lifesaving, they can also be dangerous. Even the simplest medication can have serious side effects if given to a person with an allergy to the drug. Other effects can occur with over dosage or under dosage.

It is essential for all responders to understand the indications, contraindications, complications, side effects, doses, and methods of delivery for every drug carried on their unit. Before providing medication to a patient, after consultation with a physician or according to standing orders, review the *six rights* of medication administration. This ensures the right drug, is given to the right patient, at the right time, by the right route, at the right dose, and with the right documentation in the patient care report. The skills in this section will prepare you to administer medications through a variety of routes.

42 General Rules of Medication Administration

Important Information

Medication administration is both a psychomotor skill, performed by a technician who is capable of performing a task, and an intellectual skill, performed by a practitioner who understands the workings and intricacies of the medication itself. Of these, the most important prerequisite is the intellectual skill. For every medication given, the practitioner needs to know much more than how to jab a needle into a patient's body. It is important that the practitioner have an in-depth knowledge of all aspects of the medication being given.

Components of a Drug Profile

Before administering any medication to the patient, you must ensure that you have a thorough understanding of how the medication will affect the human body, both positively and negatively.

- **Actions (pharmacokinetics).** Actions are actual effects on the body caused by the administration of the drug. Knowing the actions will aid in the understanding of the indications, contraindications, and most importantly, the effects of the drug.
- **Indications for administration.** Indications for administration are therapeutic uses for the medication, usually a very short list.
- **Contraindications to administration.** Contraindications to administration are conditions that outweigh the reason to administer the medication. This may be a simple allergy, a drug interaction, or concomitant medical conditions.
- **Effects of the drug.** The effects of the drug when administered under normal therapeutic conditions and those that are seen when toxic effects occur. There are different categories of effects of the drug, including:
  - **Beneficial effects.** The desired and therapeutic effects of the drug.
  - **Expected side effects.** Tolerable and expected effects of the medication that are not desirable but are not dangerous.
  - **Possible adverse effects.** Intolerable effects of the medication that may indicate overdose, toxicity, or just an anomalous occurrence in some patients. Adverse effects usually require dosage adjustment or stopping of the medication, and frequently additional therapies are required to counteract the adverse effect.
- **Methods of administration.** More than just the route, it is important to know how fast or slow the medication should be given and any special requirements, such as filtered needles, that are needed to safely administer the medication.
- **Related drug and food allergies.** Before giving any medication, it is important to ask the patient not just about their known drug allergies but also about allergies to the specific drug or class of drug that is being given. Also, some patients have allergies to foods that should be considered allergies to drugs.
- **Dosing regimens.** Dosing regimens are the use of repeat doses and administration intervals.
- **Storage requirements.** Storage requirements are a consideration we often miss. Medications are studied and approved for use under controlled situations, which include a temperature range. In EMS, we expose medications to extreme temperature conditions and changes in temperature. There is a process of adulteration caused by heat and cold that has not been adequately studied, but it should be considered given how we store drugs in EMS vehicles.

Cleansing Injection Sites

Prepare insertion sites by cleaning with an antiseptic/antimicrobial agent. A 30-second vigorous scrub using chlorhexidine will kill 99.9% of all colonizing microbes when the solution is dry. Chlorhexidine is safe for adults and children, but because of skin sensitivity, it should not be used on neonates.

If chlorhexidine is not available, povidone-iodine is an acceptable alternative. It is important to allow the povidone-iodine solution to dry completely before injecting the site. Alcohol may be used when the povidone-iodine is dry to clean the dye and improve visualization of the injection site.

For years alcohol has been used as the traditional injecting preparation. Because of its limited ability to kill microbial agents, it should be avoided in all cases unless the patient is allergic to both chlorhexidine and povidone-iodine (persons with shellfish allergies are actually allergic to iodine). Alcohol alone, as a prep for IV or hypodermic injection, should be considered below the standard of care.

Cleanse the site by applying the solution in a circular motion, starting in the center and working out. It is best not to reenter the clean area after it has been cleaned.

The Six Rights of Medication Administration

Before administering any drugs, remember to review the *six rights* of medication administration:

- **Right drug.** Ensure that the drug given to the patient is the correct drug.
- **Right patient.** Ensure that the ordered medication is given to the correct patient.
- **Right dose.** Ensure that the correct amount of drug is given to the patient.
- **Right route.** Ensure that the drug is given through the correct route and method.
- **Right time.** Ensure that the drug is given in a timely manner and that repeat doses are appropriately spaced.
- **Right documentation.** Ensure that all medication administration is properly documented, including drug, dose, route, time, the name of the person who gave the drug, and, very important, responses to the medication.

Pediatric Medication Administration— Length-Based Resuscitation Tapes

When time is crucial, it is usually easier and safer to use a length-based resuscitation tape rather than to estimate a child's weight and calculate a dosage. These tapes provide quick referencing for drug doses as well as for proper sizes of common tubes.

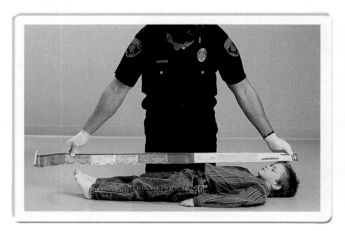

To use the tape, place it on the floor or bed, weight side up, next to the patient, with the head end level with the top of the patient's head. With the tape properly positioned, the weight can be determined by measuring the level at the patient's heel. Length-based tapes are usually divided into color-coded sections. When the initial measurement has been done, all remaining needs can be identified by referencing the color-coded section.

Length-based systems may include complete color-coded kits. The color-coded kit is pre-arranged to contain the proper-sized laryngoscope blades, endotracheal tubes, nasogastric tubes, suction catheters, intravenous catheters, blood pressure cuffs, and other size-specific pieces of equipment.

One final concern is that most resuscitation tapes are based on ideal weights for height. In today's world where childhood obesity is becoming an increasing problem, length-based tapes may be an underestimate when they are used on overweight children. Check with your medical control about the accuracy of these tapes for obese children and the accepted adjustments that should be made.

43 Bronchodilator— Handheld Metered-Dose Inhaler

Performance Objective

Given an adult patient and appropriate equipment and supplies, the candidate shall recognize and select the medication ordered, properly assemble the delivery device, and administer the drug using the criteria herein prescribed, in 5 minutes or less.

Equipment

The following equipment is required to perform this skill:

- Appropriate body substance isolation/personal protective equipment
- Metered-dose inhaler (as prescribed to the patient or carried on the ambulance under approval of medical control)

Equipment that may be helpful:

- Spacer
- Oxygen cylinder, regulator, and key
- Oxygen delivery device (nasal cannula, nonrebreathing mask)
- Stethoscope
- Pulse oximeter
- End-tidal carbon dioxide meter

Indications

- Respiratory distress from upper airway constriction
  - Asthma
  - Bronchiolitis
  - Chronic obstructive pulmonary disease (COPD)
  - Anaphylaxis

Contraindications

- Dependent upon medication used

Complications

- May be ineffective in patients with respiratory failure (maximum effort, minimal air movement)
- Not a "cure-all." Should be used appropriately

Procedures

 Ensure body substance isolation before beginning procedures.

Prior to beginning patient care, appropriate body substance isolation procedures should be employed.

▼

 **Avoid contamination of equipment or replace contaminated equipment prior to use.**

Maintain aseptic technique throughout the skill performance. Keep visual contact with sterile equipment and ensure the sterile field is not compromised.

▼

 Confirm order (medication, dosage, and route).

Repeat order given by physician. Repeat drug, dosage, route, and any additional special considerations. The first step is maintaining the *six rights* of medication administration: right drug, right patient, right dose, right route, right time, right documentation.

▼

 **Inform patient of order for medication and inquire about allergies and recent doses of other bronchodilators.**

Inform the patient of the order received, the need for the therapy, and any concerns about its administration. Ask the patient if he or she has any allergies to the specific drug ordered, as well as to any other drugs, iodine, or pertinent foods.

▼

 **Select correct medication.**

From the medication box, choose the correct medication as ordered by the physician.

▼

Step  6 ▶ **Check medication for contamination and expiration date.**

Inspect the medication label for correct name and appropriate concentration, and the fluid for clarity, discoloration, and obvious contamination or signs of loss of sterility. Check that the expiration date has not passed.

▼

Step  7 ▶ **Shake the inhaler.**

Actively shake the inhaler several times.

▼

Step 8 ▶ **Attach spacer to inhaler, if available.**

If a spacer is available, attach it to the mouthpiece of the inhaler.

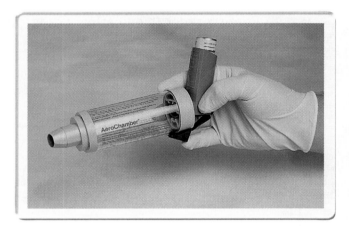

▼

Step 9 ▶ **Recheck the medication label.**

Reinspect the medication label for correct name and appropriate concentration, and the fluid for clarity, discoloration, and obvious contamination or signs of loss of sterility. Check that the expiration date has not passed.

▼

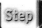 **Remove nonrebreathing mask from patient.**

Remove the oxygen mask from the patient with the oxygen still flowing.

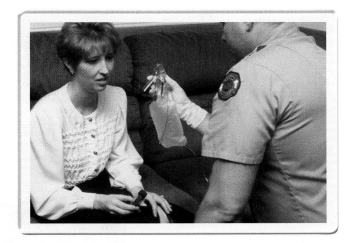

 Instruct patient to exhale deeply.

Explain to the patient how the inhaler works and have the patient take a deep breath and exhale completely.

 Instruct patient to put the mouthpiece in mouth and make a seal with lips.

Have the patient put the mouthpiece in his or her mouth and set the lips tightly.

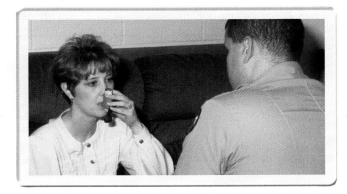

Step **Instruct patient to depress the inhaler canister while inhaling and then hold breath as long as comfortable.**

Instruct the patient to inhale deeply as the canister is depressed. Encourage the patient to hold his or her breath as long as possible.

▼

Step  **Replace nonrebreathing mask on patient.**

Reposition the nonrebreathing mask on the patient and ensure the liter flow is still at 15 L/min.

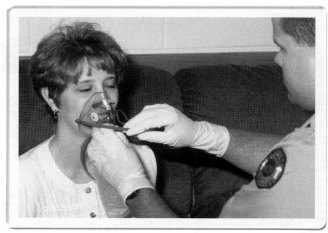

▼

Step **Monitor for effects of medication.**

Monitor the patient for the desired effects of medication administration by reassessing vital signs, tissue color, and difficulty of breathing. Document all changes, beneficial or not, that occur. Adjust management as needed.

Bronchodilator—Small-Volume Nebulizer

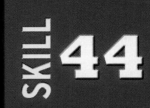

Performance Objective

Given an adult patient and appropriate equipment and supplies, the candidate shall recognize and select the medication ordered, properly assemble the delivery device, and administer the drug using the criteria herein prescribed, in 5 minutes or less.

Equipment

The following equipment is required to perform this skill:
- Appropriate body substance isolation/personal protective equipment
- Oxygen cylinder, regulator, and key
- Oxygen delivery device (nasal cannula, nonrebreathing mask)
- Small-volume nebulizer
- Bronchodilator (as prescribed to the patient or carried on the ambulance under approval of medical control)

Equipment that may be helpful:
- Stethoscope
- Pulse oximeter
- End-tidal carbon dioxide meter

Indications

- Respiratory distress from upper airway constriction
  - Asthma
  - Bronchiolitis
  - Chronic obstructive pulmonary disease (COPD)
  - Anaphylaxis

Contraindications

- Dependent upon medication used

Complications

- May be ineffective in patients with respiratory failure (maximum effort, minimal air movement)
- Not a "cure-all." Should be used appropriately

Procedures

This patient will have a nonrebreathing mask on at the beginning of the scenario.

 Ensure body substance isolation before beginning procedures.

Prior to beginning patient care, appropriate body substance isolation procedures should be employed.

▼

 Avoid contamination of equipment or replace contaminated equipment prior to use.

Maintain aseptic technique throughout the skill performance. Keep visual contact with sterile equipment and ensure the sterile field is not compromised.

▼

 Confirm order (medication, dosage, and route).

Repeat order given by physician. Be sure to repeat the drug, dosage, route, and any special considerations given. The first step is maintaining the *six rights* of medication administration: right drug, right patient, right dose, right route, right time, right documentation.

▼

 Inform patient of order for medication and inquire about allergies and recent doses of other bronchodilators.

Inform the patient of the order received, the need for the therapy, and any concerns about its administration. Ask the patient if he or she has any allergies to the specific drug ordered, as well as to any other drugs, iodine, or pertinent foods.

▼

 **Select correct medication.**

From the medication box, choose the correct medication as ordered by the physician.

▼

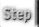 **Step 6** **Visually check medication for contamination and expiration date.**

Visually inspect the medication label for correct name and appropriate concentration, and the fluid for clarity, discoloration, and obvious contamination or signs of loss of sterility. Check that the expiration date has not passed.

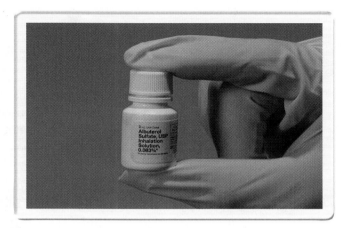

 Step 7 **Add appropriate volume of medication to the nebulizer.**

Open the nebulizer and add the ordered volume. This is normally the entire amount of the container, but mixing the medication with sterile saline or using partial doses may be necessary to achieve the optimal volume of fluid for nebulized function.

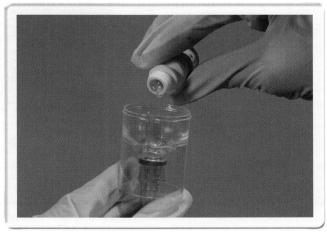

Assemble nebulizer according to the manufacturer's standard (or local protocol) and connect to oxygen regulator.

Reassemble the nebulizer and attach the mouthpiece and exhaust tube. Connect the oxygen tubing to the nebulizer and the oxygen regulator.

▼

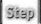 **Recheck the medication label.**

Reinspect the medication label for correct name and appropriate concentration, and the fluid for clarity, discoloration, and obvious contamination or signs of loss of sterility. Check that the expiration date has not passed.

▼

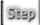 **Adjust oxygen flow as ordered and allow mist to fill breathing tube or mask prior to applying to patient.**

Adjust the oxygen flow to achieve the desired misting effect (usually between 6 to 10 L /min) and wait for a slight mist to come from the end of the tube.

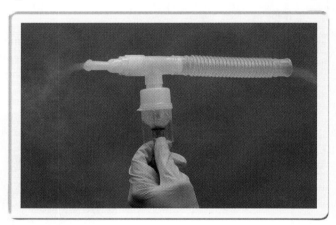

If after several seconds the mist does not form, a slight increase in flow may be necessary.

▼

11 **Remove nonrebreathing mask and position nebulizer device on patient.**

Remove the nonrebreathing mask. Instruct the patient to place the nebulizer to his or her mouth and breathe normally, inhaling the mist. Reassess the patient, recording the respiratory effort, pulse, and breath sounds.

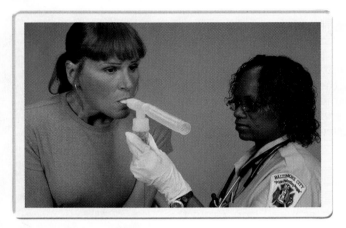

 12 **Monitor for effects of medication.**

Monitor the patient for the desired effects of medication administration by reassessing vital signs, tissue color, and difficulty of breathing. Document all changes, beneficial or not, that occur. Adjust management as needed.

Epinephrine Auto-injectors

Performance Objective

Given an epinephrine auto-injector and appropriate equipment and supplies, the candidate shall be able to recognize and select the medication ordered, properly utilize the auto-injector, and administer the drug using the criteria herein prescribed, in 5 minutes or less.

Equipment

The following equipment is required to perform this skill:

- Appropriate body substance isolation/personal protective equipment
- Epinephrine auto-injector (as prescribed to the patient or carried on the ambulance under approval of medical control)

Equipment that may be helpful:

- Oxygen cylinder, regulator, and key
- Oxygen delivery device (nasal cannula, nonrebreathing mask)
- Stethoscope
- Pulse oximeter
- End-tidal carbon dioxide meter

Indications

- Respiratory distress from severe allergic reactions

Contraindications

- Allergies to epinephrine

Complications

- May cause extreme tachycardia

Procedures

 Ensure body substance isolation before beginning procedures.

Prior to beginning patient care, appropriate body substance isolation procedures should be employed.

 Avoid contamination of equipment or replace contaminated equipment prior to use.

Maintain aseptic technique throughout the skill performance. Keep visual contact with sterile equipment and ensure the sterile field is not compromised.

 **Confirm order (medication, dosage, and route).**

Repeat order given by physician: drug, dosage, route, and any special considerations given. The first step is maintaining the *six rights* of medication administration: right drug, right patient, right dose, right route, right time, right documentation.

 Inform patient of order for medication and inquire about allergies.

Inform the patient of the order received, the need for the therapy, and any concerns about its administration. Ask the patient if he or she has any allergies to the specific drug ordered, as well as to any other drugs, iodine, or pertinent foods.

 In the Field

Use of Epinephrine Auto-injectors

EpiPens deliver 0.3 mg of epinephrine and are appropriate for all adults and for children weighing 30 kg (55 lb) or more. The EpiPen, Jr delivers 0.15 mg and is appropriate for children weighing 15 to 30 kg (33-55 lb).

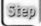 **Select correct medication.**

From the medication box, choose the correct medication as ordered by the physician.

Visually check medication for contamination and expiration date.

Visually inspect the medication label for correct name and appropriate concentration, and the fluid for clarity, discoloration, and obvious contamination or signs of loss of sterility. Check that the expiration date has not passed.

 Select appropriate site.

Locate the correct site for injection, usually the lateral midthigh.

 Recheck the medication label.

Reinspect the medication label for correct name and appropriate concentration, and the fluid for clarity, discoloration, and obvious contamination or signs of loss of sterility. Check that the expiration date has not passed.

 Prepare the injection site.

Choose an injection site in the large muscle of the thigh. If time permits, cleanse the injection site to kill microbial agents that live on the patient's skin. In severe cases of anaphylaxis, it is acceptable to inject the epinephrine through the patient's pants.

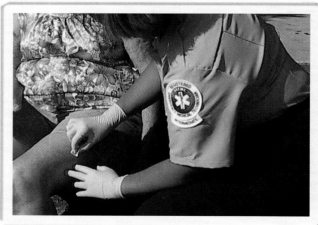

Step 10 Remove safety cap from the auto-injector.

Remove the gray end cap (on the thick end) from the auto-injector.

 Step 11 Place the tip of the auto-injector against the injection site and push the injector firmly against the injection site.

Place the black tip (narrow end) of the auto-injector against the intended injection site. Push firmly and quickly until the needle is released and injects into the patient.

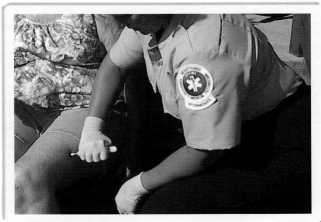

 Step 12 Hold the auto-injector against the site for 10 seconds.

Hold the auto-injector against the injection site for at least 10 seconds.

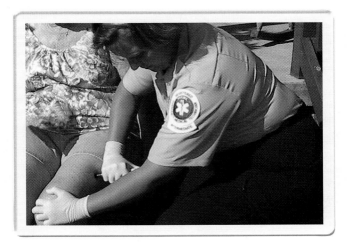

Step 13 ▶ Remove auto-injector and apply pressure.

Quickly remove the auto-injector by pulling it straight out, and apply pressure with a 4″ × 4″ gauze dressing to the injection site. Remember that the auto-injector will have a contaminated needle sticking from the black end.

▼

Step 14 ▶ Dispose of contaminated equipment.

Dispose of the auto-injector by inserting the entire device into a puncture-resistant sharps container, needle first. Use extreme caution with the exposed dirty needle of the auto-injector until it is disposed of.

▼

Step 15 ▶ Monitor for effects of medication.

Monitor the patient for the desired effects of medication administration by reassessing vital signs, tissue color, and difficulty of breathing. Document all changes, beneficial or not, that occur. Adjust management as needed.

Oral Medication Administration

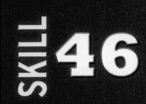

Performance Objective

Given all necessary medications and equipment, the candidate shall be able to recognize and select the medication ordered and administer the drug using the criteria herein prescribed, in 2 minutes or less.

Equipment

The following equipment is required to perform this skill:
- Appropriate body substance isolation/personal protective equipment
- Appropriate medication (as prescribed to the patient or carried on the ambulance under approval of medical control)

Equipment that may be helpful:
- Tongue depressor
- Disposable cup
- Drinking straw
- Stethoscope
- Pulse oximeter
- End-tidal carbon dioxide meter

Indications

- Specific to the medication given

Contraindications

- Patients with altered level of consciousness or who are unresponsive

Complications

- Medication specific

Procedures

Oral medication administration may include giving aspirin, activated charcoal, nitroglycerin, or glucose paste.

 Ensure body substance isolation before beginning procedures.

Prior to beginning patient care, appropriate body substance isolation procedures should be employed.

 Avoid contamination of equipment or replace contaminated equipment prior to use.

Maintain aseptic technique throughout the skill performance. Keep visual contact with sterile equipment and ensure the sterile field is not compromised.

 Confirm order (medication, dosage, and route).

Repeat order given by physician: drug, dosage, route, and any special considerations given. The first step is maintaining the *six rights* of medication administration: right drug, right patient, right dose, right route, right time, right documentation.

 Inform patient of order for medication and inquire about allergies.

Inform the patient of the order received, the need for the therapy, and any concerns about its administration. Ask the patient if he or she has any allergies to the specific drug ordered, as well as to any other drugs, iodine, or pertinent foods.

 Select correct medication.

From the medication box, choose the correct medication as ordered by the physician.

Safety Tips

Inquiring About Drugs and Allergies

It is essential that a complete history be performed before giving a patient any medication. An important question that must be asked before administering nitroglycerin is whether the patient is using medications for erectile dysfunction. Administration of nitroglycerin within 48 hours of a patient taking sildenafil (Viagra) and similar drugs can create serious complications, including death.

Safety Tips

Understanding Medications

Each drug carried on your EMS unit has specific uses. It is *essential* for all EMS personnel who carry drugs on their unit to understand all the indications, contraindications, side effects, precautions, doses, and routes of administration for each drug carried.

6 **Visually check medication for contamination and expiration date.**

Visually inspect the medication label for correct name and appropriate concentration, and the fluid for clarity, discoloration, and obvious contamination or signs of loss of sterility. Check that the expiration date has not passed.

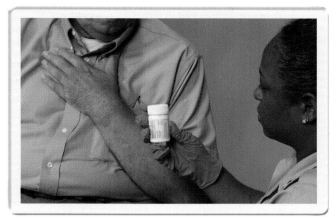

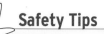 **Safety Tips**

Sublingual Nitroglycerin Spray

Nitroglycerin is a stable compound that will not explode under normal circumstances. However, there are some usage and safety rules that need to be observed. Do not shake the drug container before administration. Ensure that the opening of the spray nozzle is aimed into the patient's mouth, onto or under the tongue. The patient should not swallow or inhale the spray. It is advisable for EMS personnel to wear gloves while administering to avoid nitroglycerin getting on the skin. Even small amounts of nitroglycerin will be absorbed and can result in severe headaches and drops in blood pressure.

 7 **Ensure the patient is conscious and can maintain his or her own airway.**

Before administering oral medications, ensure the patient has the ability to swallow and maintain his or her own airway.

 8 **Place, or instruct patient to place, medication into oral cavity appropriately.**

Place the medication in the oral cavity using the following criteria:

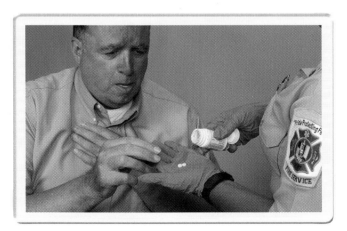

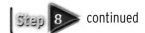
continued

- **Aspirin** should be swallowed. Some EMS systems allow the use of a small amount of water to assist the patient in swallowing the tablet; others require the tablet to either be swallowed dry or to be chewed.
- **Activated charcoal** is administered as a slurry that the patient will drink. Some brands of activated charcoal come as a prepared slurry, whereas others may require you to mix dry activated charcoal with water, magnesium citrate, or another liquid as described in protocols. Place the appropriate amount of the activated charcoal slurry into a cup or other acceptable container. Have the patient drink the activated charcoal either directly or through a straw.
- **Glucose paste** should be given by placing the paste on the end of a tongue depressor and then placing the depressor in the mouth between the cheek and gum. Allow the paste to be absorbed.
- **Nitroglycerin** should be placed under the patient's tongue. Ask the patient to open his or her mouth and lift the tongue. Place the nitroglycerin tablet under the tongue. Have the patient keep the tablet in place until it is dissolved.

▼

 Monitor for effects of medication.

Monitor the patient for the desired effects of medication administration by re-assessing vital signs, tissue color, change in pain, or change in level of consciousness. Document all changes, beneficial or not, that occur. Adjust management as needed.

Performance Objective

Given a patient and all necessary equipment, the candidate shall establish an IV line in an appropriate vein, secure the line and catheter, and establish a drip rate appropriate to the patient's needs, using the criteria herein prescribed, in 6 minutes or less.

Equipment

The following equipment is required to perform this skill:
- Appropriate body substance isolation/personal protection equipment
- Sharps container
- IV pole
- Selection of IV solutions (normal saline, lactated Ringer's)
- Administration sets: macro/micro/extension tubing
- Selection of IV catheters (14, 16, 18, 20, 22 gauge)
- Tape or commercially made IV securing system
- 4" × 4" gauze pads
- Tourniquet
- Cleaning solution
  - Chlorhexidine preps
  - Povidone-iodine preps
  - Alcohol preps
- Bulky dressing
- Adhesive bandages

Equipment that may be helpful:
- Towels
- Vein identification lights

Indications

- Fluid administration
- Medication route

Contraindications

- None in general use

Complications

- Infiltration
- Infection
- Air/catheter embolism

Procedures

 Step 1 Ensure body substance isolation before beginning procedures.

Prior to beginning patient care, appropriate body substance isolation procedures should be employed.

 Step 2 Avoid contamination of equipment.

Maintain sterile/aseptic technique throughout the skill performance. Keep visual contact with sterile equipment and ensure the sterile field is not contaminated or compromised.

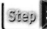 **Step 3** Confirm order (solution and rate).

Repeat the order given by the physician. You must repeat the solution and rate ordered as well as any special considerations given. When following standing orders, it is essential to ensure that the order is followed through with no errors of omission. This is the first step in maintaining the *six rights* of medication administration: right drug, right patient, right dose, right route, right time, right documentation.

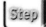 **Step 4** Inform patient of need for fluid therapy.

Inform the patient of the need for starting an IV. Advise the patient of the purpose and the benefits of the procedure, as well as the risks.

Safety Tips

Choosing the Proper Size Solution Bag

Choosing the right IV solution for your patient includes choosing the amount of fluid in the bag. There really is no magic formula for this process.

In trauma patients who will get a lot of fluid over a short period of time, it is best to hang the largest volume available—usually a 1,000-mL bag. However, 500-mL bags or even 250-mL bags will accomplish the same task; they just need to be changed out two to four times as often. With the simple "to keep open" (TKO) IV, the smallest bag available is usually chosen, such as a 250-mL or a 500-mL bag. Again, a 1,000-mL bag will work just fine.

Many people will start a 1,000-mL bag thinking it will last longer. The reality is that most hospitals will change out an IV started in the prehospital setting within 12 hours or so of arrival. That means that a completely new IV bag will be hung anyway.

In short, we generally hang big bags with a lot of fluid if needed and little bags with only a small amount of fluid if needed. Either will work, but pay attention!

Step 5 ▶ Check IV fluid.

Choose the solution ordered by the physician or the most appropriate solution if no specific fluid was ordered. Normal saline is the standard solution for simple to keep open (TKO) IV lines, dehydration, and to accompany blood. Lactated Ringer's solution is used for trauma and burns. Five percent dextrose in water (D_5W) is seldom used for anything other than mixing medications. However, some clinicians still prefer this solution for conditions of overhydration, hypertension, and pulmonary edema. Other solutions, such as blood products, colloids, and electrolyte/glucose mixtures, are seldom used in the prehospital setting.

After choosing the correct solution, inspect the bag for leaks. Ensure the clarity and quality of the solution, looking specifically for signs of discoloration and contamination. Check the expiration date. Discard the solution if it is out of date or if signs of deterioration or contamination exist. Recheck the solution to make sure it is correct (right medication).

▼

  Step 6 ▶ Select appropriate catheter and equipment.

The IV catheter should be chosen based on the patient's condition and relative size. In general, the catheter should be adequate to support the volume intended to be given but (an often overlooked consideration) small enough to fit in the patient's vein. In adults, 14-, 16-, and 18-gauge catheters are used most often. However, in older, smaller, younger, or more fragile patients, catheters as small as 24 gauge may be needed and are perfectly acceptable. Contrary to popular belief, blood can run through *any* size catheter.

You will also need a tourniquet, 4″ × 4″ gauze dressing, adhesive bandage strip, povidone-iodine swab, alcohol swab, and a means of securing the IV catheter. Several commercially made devices exist for the purpose of securing the IV catheter. If these devices are not available, tape should be prepared so the IV can be secured when the tubing is attached. If tape is to be used, tear the tape and have it ready to use before inserting the catheter. Three to four pieces of tape torn into 3″ strips are usually sufficient.

▼

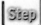 **Step 7** ▶ Select proper administration set and extension set.

From the available equipment, select the administration set and extension appropriate for the patient's condition. In general, a standard infusion and large-bore extension are used when fluid resuscitation will be performed, a microdrip and small-bore extension are used for simple TKO lines, and a volume-controlled set and a small-bore extension is used for children.

▼

In the Field

Saline Locks
The establishment of TKO IVs was a mainstay for patients, but it is rapidly being replaced with saline locks. Saline locks function in much the same way, as a port for medication administration but without the constant infusion of fluid or the burden of the solution bag and tubing.

To establish a saline lock, follow all of the same steps as for the initial IV insertion, but, instead of attaching an administration set:

- Prepare the lock by injecting a small amount of saline to displace the air.
- Attach the saline-filled lock to the end of the IV catheter.
- Flush the catheter with approximately 3 mL of saline.

You now have access for medication administration without a constant flow of fluid. Because there is no fluid to move medications when they are delivered, always remember to flush your lock with at least 3 mL of saline after every drug.

Step 8 ▶ **Connect IV tubing to the IV bag.**

Carefully remove the administration and extension sets from their packaging. Straighten the tubing and untangle any knots. Remove the cap from the extension set first, then remove the cap from the patient end of the administration set. Mate the two ends and give a firm twist. Move the rolling-ball stopcock as close to the drip chamber as possible, and run the ball to the closed position. You are now ready to puncture the IV bag.

Remove the protective cover from the port of the IV bag, and then remove the cap from the needle of the drip chamber. Puncture the IV bag and give a firm twist. Squeeze the drip chamber *one time* and allow the fluid to run into the chamber.

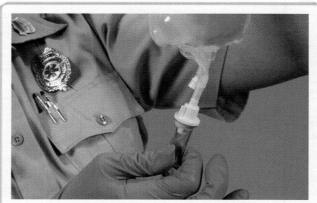

The solution should fill one fourth to one third the volume of the chamber (many solution sets have a mark at this level); additional filling will alter the function of the drip chamber. Open the rolling-ball stopcock and allow the solution to fill the IV line. Before the solution reaches the end, remove the cap until solution runs freely from the line. Shut the clamp and replace the cap of the IV tubing until ready to connect to the IV catheter. This method should produce an air-free IV line; however, inspect the line to ensure that all air bubbles have been run out of the line.

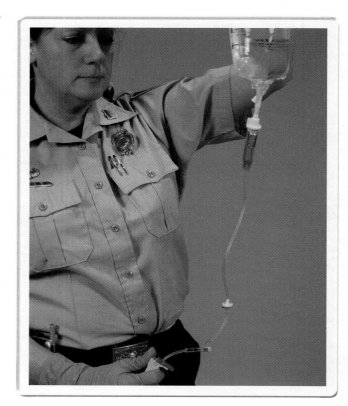

9 **Ensure body substance isolation before beginning invasive procedures and whenever contact with blood or body fluids can be reasonably anticipated.**

Prior to beginning patient care, appropriate body substance isolation procedures should be employed. In most cases, this should include gloves, masks, and eye protection at a minimum. When treating patients with known infectious diseases, especially those spread by respiratory secretions, HEPA filter masks may be required. Occasionally it will be necessary to protect patients from the equipment. Patients with latex allergies and elderly patients with thin skin may need special care when applying tourniquets and tape.

▼

 10 **Apply tourniquet.**

Place the tourniquet 4″ to 6″ above the intended puncture site. Check the distal pulse to ensure that an arterial tourniquet has not been applied.

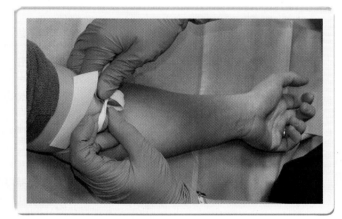

For scalp veins in infants, use a rubber band applied around the circumference of the head.

▼

 Special Populations

Important Considerations

Trauma patients with thoracic injuries above the nipple line should have the IV started on the opposite arm, if possible. This will prevent fluid leakage out of injured vessels.

An IV should not be started in the arm with an associated dialysis shunt, and the shunt itself should not be used for IV access except in *extreme* cases.

Mastectomy patients have a surgically altered lymphatic system in the affected arm. To avoid problems with infiltration and drainage, avoid starting an IV in the affected arm. However, in the case of bilateral mastectomies, you will have no choice but to start an IV in one of the arms. The use of leg veins poses risks of phlebitis and other complications and should not be considered.

Palpate suitable vein.

Palpate the veins in the intended site to choose the most appropriate vessel. A firm, rubbery, relatively large surface vein is usually a good choice.

The IV should be started in the lowest possible location on the chosen extremity. This will allow for additional IVs to be placed later in the care of the patient, moving up the extremity as the care continues. Additional considerations for the site of the IV are determined by the patient's needs. Obviously, in the most dire of circumstances, you take what you can get. In the prehospital setting, IVs should be started in the forearm away from joints. The back of the hand is acceptable on calm, cooperative patients who pose little concern for pulling the IV out of the vein. Critical heart patients and cardiac arrest patients should have an IV started in the antecubital fossa or higher. This is the only patient group that requires an antecubital IV, and with the exception of this site being the only vein available, it is a poor practice for the management of *all* other conditions.

▼

 Prepare injection site.

Prepare the insertion site by cleaning with an antiseptic/antimicrobial agent. A 30-second vigorous scrub using chlorhexidine will kill 99.9% of all colonizing microbes when the solution is dry. Chlorhexidine is safe for adults and children, but because of skin sensitivity, it should not be used on neonates.

If chlorhexidine is not available, povidone iodine is an acceptable alternative. It is important to allow the povidone-iodine solution to dry completely before injecting the site. Alcohol may be used when the povidone iodine is dry to clean the dye and improve visualization of the injection site.

For years alcohol has been used as the traditional injecting preparation. Because of its limited ability to kill microbial agents, it should be avoided in all cases unless the patient is allergic to both chlorhexidine and povidone iodine (persons with shellfish allergies are allergic to iodine). Alcohol alone, as a prep for IV or hypodermic injection, should be considered below the standard of care.

Cleanse the site by applying the solution in a circular motion, starting in the center and working out. It is best not to reenter the clean area after it is cleaned.

▼

Step 13 ▶ Perform venipuncture.

Remove the chosen catheter from the package, and remove the plastic needle guard. Inspect the catheter for defects. It is helpful to loosen the catheter from the needle stylet by giving a slight lift and twist, making sure the end of the catheter does not go past the end of the needle. Reseat the catheter on the flash chamber of the needle.

With your nondominant hand, stabilize the intended vein by pulling the skin tight. Make sure that all your fingers are kept out of the sterile field and that the IV catheter will not have to pass directly over a finger to puncture the skin.

With the bevel of the needle facing up, approach the vein at a 15° to 45° angle. Puncture the vein with a quick, controlled stab.

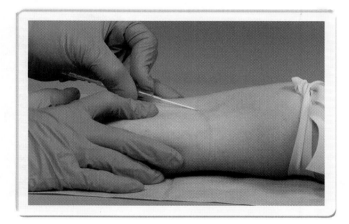

As blood begins to enter the flash chamber, slowly advance the entire catheter-needle unit into the vein between one eighth and one fourth of an inch.

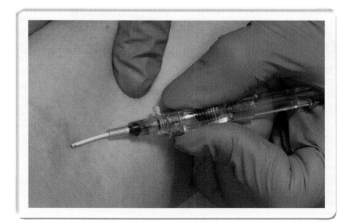

Stabilizing the needle, slowly advance the catheter off of the needle stylet and into the vein. Do not completely remove the needle from the catheter.

Resistance usually means that the catheter is not traveling into a vein. If evaluation finds this to be the case, remove the tourniquet and the needle and apply pressure to the puncture site. Reattempt the IV with a new catheter.

▼

In the Field

Drawing Blood From the IV Site

If time permits, a syringe can be attached to the catheter hub for the purpose of drawing blood samples. When the syringe is filled, the blood should be placed in appropriate collecting tubes, labeled, and taken with the patient to the hospital. This will prevent unnecessary needle sticks to draw additional blood in the hospital.

Using venous blood as the source for glucometers will serve a basic purpose of identifying high or low levels of blood glucose, but keep in mind that most glucometers are calibrated to measure capillary blood, not venous blood. For an accurate reading, always use blood collected from a finger stick process in a glucometer.

Safety Tips

The Missed IV
It is not uncommon for an IV to be missed. Should an IV attempt fail, it is important to ensure that the puncture site be properly cared for. Hematomas can be reduced by applying pressure over the areas where the bleeding is occurring, which may be slightly upstream from the actual puncture site.

Whether to attempt a second IV will depend on policy and patient need. In severe cases, if the IV has failed, it may be time to start an intraosseous line. If a second attempt at the IV is deemed necessary, always pick a site away or upstream from the first site.

Step 14 Remove constricting band.

Always and without exception, remove the tourniquet before removing the needle stylet from the catheter. Failure to do this will cause excessive and often impressive bleeding through the catheter.

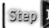
Step 15 Attach tubing to the catheter hub.

With the catheter held securely, pull the needle stylet from the catheter.

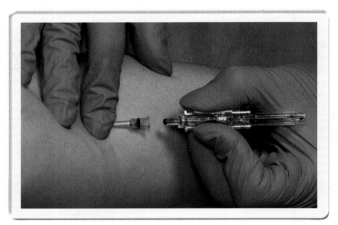

Remove the cap from the IV tubing, connect the IV tubing to the catheter hub, and give a twist to lock it in place.

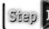
Step 16 Dispose of needle in proper container.

Dispose of needles and all sharp instruments with blood or body fluid contamination in puncture-resistant sharps containers.

Step **17**▶ **Run IV for a brief period to ensure a patent line.**

Open the flow control and begin running fluid. In patients with fragile veins, it is best to begin slowly rather than to widely open the control. Verify if the flow of fluid is running into the vein. A large edematous area at the end of the catheter, or a line that will not run, indicates improper IV placement; it may be necessary to restart the IV.

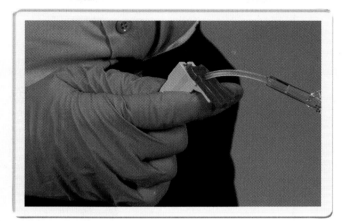

 18▶ **Secure the catheter and dress the site.**

There are several appropriate methods of securing an IV. The most common today are commercially made devices intended specifically for the purpose of securing an IV. These devices usually include a transparent dressing that allows the injection site to remain visible to the caregiver as well as act as a barrier to infectious agents.

The traditional approach, and first backup to commercially made devices, is to use simple adhesive tape. Generally, three 3″ strips of 1″ tape and two 3″ strips of ½″ tape are used. Place these strips within easy reach of the intended IV site. Place the two ½″ strips of tape over the hub of the catheter by placing the tape under the hub, and fold it over the top to form a chevron. It is imperative that the tape does not cover the actual puncture site. When the hub is secured, apply the remaining three pieces of tape to the IV line approximately 1″ from the hub and, working backwards, along the IV line. The tubing should be looped, with the last two pieces of tape holding the loop in place. Transparent dressings should be placed over the injection site if available. This will allow the inspection of the injection site for inflammation, hematomas, or other complications. If no transparent dressing is available, apply a 1″ adhesive bandage over the puncture site.

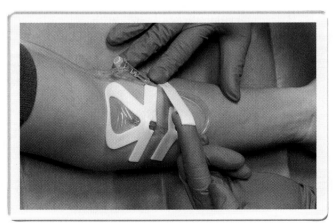

19 Adjust flow rate as appropriate.

Adjust the drip rate as appropriate for the patient's needs. Count the number of drops in a 15-second period and multiply by four until you are close. Then count the drops for a full minute to make the final adjustment.

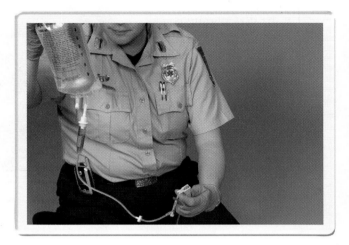

 20 Dispose of contaminated equipment.

Dispose of needles and all sharp instruments with blood or body fluid contamination in puncture-resistant sharps containers. Other materials that have been contaminated by blood or body fluids should be disposed of in biohazard bags. Waste materials that are not contaminated by blood or body fluids can be disposed of in normal trash receptacles.

 21 Label site.

Using a small piece of tape, write the catheter size, the date the IV was started, and your initials. Place this piece of tape across the hub of the IV catheter.

Step 22 ▶ **Double check patency.**

The final step in beginning an IV is to ensure that the line is patent. This should also be performed before administering IV medications through either bolus or drip and when transferring care of the patient. Always document checks of patency.

Patency can be checked by:

- Lowering the IV bag below the level of insertion. Blood entering the IV tubing ensures patency.
- Inserting a syringe into the medication port and pulling back on the plunger. Blood entering the IV tubing ensures patency.
- Injecting saline into the medication port. An unrestricted injection and no signs of infiltration ensures patency.

Special Populations

Scalp Vein Access in Infants

There is little reason to start a scalp vein in most EMS systems today. In severe cases, intraosseous infusion has become the mainstay of emergent venous access. In the newborn, the umbilical cord is readily available. The use of scalp vein access is limited and reserved for those rare times when an IV must be established in the moderately sick infant.

A rubber band placed around the infant's brow serves well as a tourniquet. As the veins begin to fill, choose any suitable site that will hold the intravenous catheter. Note that arteries and veins often run close together in the infant's scalp. To ensure the vessel is a vein and not an artery, always palpate for the presence of a pulse. Scalp veins run from the crown to the feet, so always insert the catheter toward the tourniquet.

Intraosseous Infusion

Performance Objective

Given a patient who meets the criteria for intraosseous infusion and all necessary equipment, the candidate shall demonstrate the procedure for establishing an intraosseous line, within 6 minutes or less.

Equipment

The following equipment is required to perform this skill:
- Appropriate body substance isolation/personal protection equipment
- Sharps container
- IV pole
- Selection of IV solutions (normal saline, lactated Ringer's)
- Administration sets: macro/micro/extension tubing
- Intraosseous needles
- Syringes (various sizes)
- Tape or commercially made IV securing system
- 4" × 4" gauze pads
- Cleaning solution
  - Chlorhexidine preps
  - Povidone-iodine preps
  - Alcohol preps
- Bulky dressing

Equipment that may be helpful:
- Towels
- Pressure infusion bag
- Commercially made insertion system (EZ-IO, Bone Injection Gun, FAST1 device)

Indications

- Cardiac arrest
  - This procedure can be performed on patients of any age, although many prehospital protocols limit its use to children younger than 3 to 6 years of age.
- When standard IV attempts have failed and vascular access is essential

Contraindications

- Fractures of the bone being used
- Previous intraosseous infusion in the same bone
- Osteomyelitis or cellulitis
- History of chronic bone disease

Complications

- Osteomyelitis
- Pain

Special Considerations

Intraosseous (IO) infusion is a painful procedure and is usually limited to unconscious patients. However, if it is imperative to obtain an intraosseous line in the conscious patient, sedation and/or local anesthesia can be used if time and the patient's condition permits.

When an intraosseous line has been established, it should remain for only a few hours, with removal as soon as other IV access has been established.

When established, the intraosseous line can be used like any other vascular access line. Be sure to follow the instructions of your medical director concerning which drugs are acceptable through the IO route.

Procedures

 Ensure body substance isolation before beginning procedures.

Prior to beginning patient care, appropriate body substance isolation procedures should be employed.

▼

 Avoid contamination of equipment.

Maintain sterile/aseptic technique throughout the skill performance. Keep visual contact with sterile equipment, and ensure that the sterile field is not contaminated or compromised.

▼

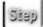 **Confirm order (solution and rate).**

Repeat the order given by the physician. You must repeat the solution and rate ordered as well as any special considerations given. When following standing orders, it is essential to ensure that the order is followed through with no errors of omission. This is the first step in maintaining the *six rights* of medication administration: right drug, right patient, right dose, right route, right time, right documentation.

▼

4 ▶ **Inform patient or family of need for fluid therapy.**

Inform the patient of the need for starting an IV. Advise the patient of the purpose and the benefits of the procedure, as well as the risks.

When it becomes necessary to perform intraosseous injection in a conscious patient, local anesthesia through lidocaine infiltration should be performed. See Skill 49, *Local Anesthesia for Intraosseous Infusion*.

▼

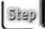 **5** ▶ **Check IV fluid.**

Choose the solution ordered by the physician or the most appropriate solution if no specific fluid was ordered. Normal saline is the standard solution for simple to keep open (TKO) IV lines, dehydration, and to accompany blood. Lactated Ringer's solution is used for trauma and burns. Five percent dextrose in water (D_5W) is seldom used for anything other than mixing medications. However, some clinicians still prefer this solution for overhydration conditions, hypertension, and pulmonary edema. Other solutions, such as blood products, colloids, and electrolyte/glucose mixtures, are seldom used in the prehospital setting.

After choosing the correct solution, inspect the bag for leaks. Ensure the clarity and quality of the solution, looking specifically for signs of discoloration and contamination, and check the expiration date. Discard the solution if it is out of date or if signs of deterioration or contamination exist. Recheck the solution to make sure it is correct (right medication).

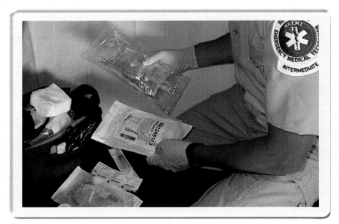

▼

Step 6 ▶ Select appropriate equipment.

Gather the necessary equipment for starting an IV line. You will need the fluid, administration set, tape, povidone-iodine swabs and alcohol swabs. In addition, you will need to choose either a sternal or iliac aspiration needle or a power driver, such as the EZ-IO. Attach a 5-mL syringe to an extension set, and fill the extension set with the IV fluid. Do not fill the 5-mL syringe because it may be used later to aspirate the bone marrow from the needle.

The sternal or iliac aspiration needles are preferred over standard hypodermic needles because they are stouter, with an obturating trocar placed in the lumen. This prevents coring of the bone tissue and adds strength to the needle. The wings on the iliac needle also act as a handle and aid in the twisting motion required in this procedure. In the event that neither of these needles are available, a standard hypodermic needle can be used by attaching a 5-mL syringe as a handle.

Modern innovations have brought us power-driven intraosseous needles, such as the EZ-IO, *FAST1*® intraosseous infusion system, and Bone Injection Gun (BIG; adult and pediatric).

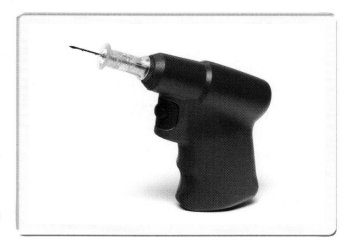

EZ-IO

Safety Tips

Powered IO Placement Devices

There are several devices on the market that use springs and batteries to power the IO needle into the injection site, such as the Bone Injection Gun and the EZ-IO. These devices are simply another way to accomplish the IO process, and for the most part all the rules for insertion apply. Because of government regulations, which are constantly changing, there may be limitations of where the needle can be placed. When using these devices be sure to read the manufacturers' recommendations for placement and for use in adults, children, and infants.

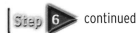 continued

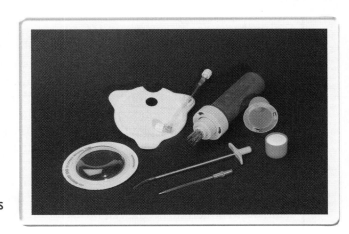

FAST1® intraosseous infusion system

These devices are quickly becoming the standard of care and should be considered over the hand-driven devices, such as the Jamshedi needle, for safety and speed. Other than the device, no other alterations in the intraosseous procedure exist.

Prepare the IV fluid and administration set. Adjust the maximum depth of the aspiration needle by turning the base. It is advisable to adjust slightly deep, approximately one third to one half the diameter of the patient's palpable tibia.

▼

 Select proper administration set and extension set.

From the available equipment, select a macrodrip administration set and extension set. Other types of administration sets are inappropriate for intraosseous infusion. Use of a macrodrip administration set will allow the use of pressure infusion.

▼

8 ▶ **Connect administration set to bag.**

Carefully remove the administration and extension sets from their packaging. Straighten the tubing and untangle any knots. Remove the cap from the extension set first, then remove the cap from the patient end of the administration set. Mate the two ends and give a firm twist. Move the rolling-ball stopcock as close to the drip chamber as possible, and run the ball to the closed position. You are now ready to puncture the IV bag.

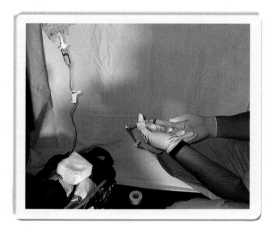

Remove the protective cover from the port of the IV bag, and then remove the cap from the needle of the drip chamber. Puncture the IV bag, and give a firm twist. Squeeze the drip chamber *one time* and allow the fluid to run into the chamber. The solution should fill one fourth to one third the volume of the chamber (many solution sets have a mark at this level); additional filling will alter the function of the drip chamber. Open the rolling-ball stopcock and allow the solution to fill the IV line. Before the solution reaches the end, remove the cap until solution runs freely from the line. Shut the clamp and replace the cap of the IV tubing until ready to connect to the IV catheter. This method should produce an air-free IV line; however, inspect the line to ensure that all air bubbles have been run out of the line.

▼

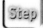 **9** ▶ **Cut or tear tape.**

Prepare for the securing of the infusion needle by tearing three to four 3″ pieces of tape. Place these in an area that can be easily reached when the needle is in place. *Do not* stick tape to your clothing because blood on your gloves may contaminate your clothing.

▼

10 Ensure body substance isolation before beginning invasive procedures and whenever contact with blood or body fluids can be reasonably anticipated.

Prior to beginning patient care, appropriate body substance isolation procedures should be employed. In most cases, this should include gloves, masks, and eye protection at a minimum. When treating patients with known infectious diseases, especially those spread by respiratory secretions, HEPA filter masks may be required.

▼

 11 Identify proper anatomic site for IO puncture.

- **Tibial tuberosity (proximal tibia).** With the knee supported on a 1″ to 2″ pad and the foot externally rotated, position the proximal tibia so the flat, medial surface is level. Choose a site approximately two fingerbreadths below the top of the palpable tibia (one fingerbreadth in infants).

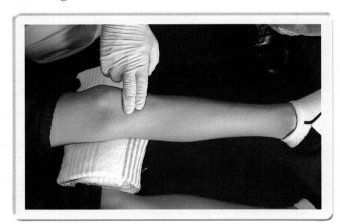

- **Medial malleolus (distal tibia).** With the leg rotated so the foot is parallel to the floor, locate the medial malleolus at the ankle. Make the puncture approximately one fingerbreadth to two fingerbreadths above the peak of the malleolus.
- **Distal femur.** With the knee supported on a 1″ to 2″ pad, position the knee so it is straight, with the patella facing up. Choose a site approximately two fingerbreadths above the top of the patella (one fingerbreadth in infants).
- **Proximal humerus.** With the arm against the side and the hand placed over the abdomen, palpate the midshaft of the humerus. Continue to palpate up the humerus to locate the humeral head. Insert the needle into the center of the humeral head into the greater tubercle.

▼

Prepare injection site.

Prepare the insertion site by cleaning with an antiseptic/antimicrobial agent. A 30-second vigorous scrub using chlorhexidine will kill 99.9% of all colonizing microbes when the solution is dry. Chlorhexidine is safe for adults and children, but because of skin sensitivity, it should not be used on neonates.

If chlorhexidine is not available, povidone-iodine is an acceptable alternative. It is important to allow the povidone-iodine solution to dry completely before injecting the site. Alcohol may be used when the povidone-iodine is dry to clean the dye and improve visualization of the injection site.

For years alcohol has been used as the traditional injecting preparation. Because of its limited ability to kill microbial agents, it should be avoided in all cases unless the patient is allergic to both chlorhexidine and povidone-iodine (persons with shellfish allergies are actually allergic to iodine). Alcohol alone, as a prep for IV or hypodermic injection, should be considered below the standard of care.

Cleanse the site by applying the solution in a circular motion, starting in the center and working out. It is best not to reenter the clean area after it is cleaned.

▼

  Perform IO puncture.

Stabilize the injection site with your nondominant hand by grasping from the front. Do not place your hand behind the needle insertion site. Insert the needle into the tibia, perpendicular (90°) to the bone.

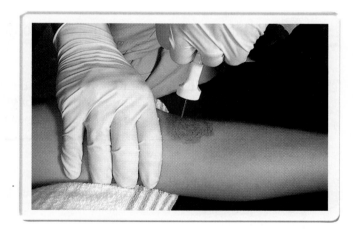

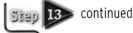 **13** continued

Inserting the needle at an angle increases the possibility of bending the needle or splitting the bone. A slowly advancing, twisting motion will prevent damage to the end of the needle and make the process less damaging to the patient. When resistance is suddenly lost, the bone marrow has been reached. Carefully release the trocar and pull it from the needle.

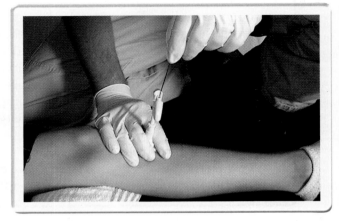

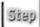 **Dispose of needle in proper container.**

Discard the trocar in a puncture-resistant sharps container.

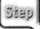 **Attach syringe and extension set to IO and aspirate (*optional, not recommended*).**

Attach the partially filled 5-mL syringe and extension set to the IO needle and aspirate for return of blood and marrow. Although this is acceptable, it can clog the needle and greatly reduce the effectiveness of venous flow.

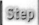 **Slowly inject saline to ensure proper placement of needle.**

Palpate and visualize, looking and feeling for any signs of infiltration.

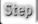 **Connect administration set and adjust flow rate as appropriate.**

Attach the administration set and begin the flow of fluid. A steady drip to a wide-open rate should be possible. Adjust the flow to the desired rate. The application of a pressure infuser may be necessary to keep a steady flow.

In the Field

Sternal Intraosseous Infusion and the FAST1

The FAST1 Intraosseous Infusion System is a means of establishing intravenous access through the marrow in the patient's sternum. Because the exact position of the needle in sternal infusion is crucial, it is important that the proper steps for insertion be followed.

Insertion

1. **Expose sternum and cleanse site.**
2. **Locate landmarks and attach target guide.** Remove the top part of the *patch* backing (labeled "Remove 1"). Locate the sternal notch with your index finger held perpendicular to the manubrium. Using your index finger, align the notch in the *patch* with the patient's sternal notch. Verify that the *target zone* (circular hole in the *patch*) is over the patient's midline. Secure the top half of the *patch* to the patient. Remove the bottom half of the *patch* backing. Press firmly to secure the *patch* to the patient. Verify the location; the notch in the *patch* should match the sternal notch, and the *target zone* should be over the patient's midline. Take corrective action if there is an error greater than about 1 cm.
3. **Place device into target guide.** Remove the protective cover from the bone probe cluster and place it in the *target zone*. Ensure that the introducer axis is perpendicular (90°) to the skin at the insertion site. Ensure the entire bone probe cluster is within the *target zone*.
4. **Apply steady pressure and insert.** Pressing straight along the introducer axis, with your hand and elbow inline, push with firm and constant force until a distinct release is heard and felt. The introducer must remain perpendicular to the skin during insertion. After release, lift straight back to remove the introducer, exposing the *infusion tube*. Push the used bone probe cluster into the foam-filled sharps plug.
5. **Attach short tubing and check placement.** Attach the right-angle female connector on the *patch* to the infusion tube. Increase the fluid flow rate by flushing the system with 10 mL of normal saline.
6. **Attach fluids and adjust flow.** Attach the straight connector on the *patch* to the purged source of fluid or drugs. Fluid can now flow to the site.
7. **Place sterile cover.** Place the *dome* over the *patch* and press down firmly to engage the Velcro fastening.
8. **Secure the removal tool to chest.** Attach the *unopened* sterile *remover* package to the patient (the manufacturer recommends placing the *remover* on the arm or leg, or attach it to the chart; however, taping the *remover* to the chest next to the dome focuses attention on its importance). The *remover* is needed to remove the infusion tube from the patient's bone when intraosseous access is no longer required.

Although removal usually will be performed at the hospital, it may be the responsibility of the EMS system to perform the procedure.

Removal

9. **Shut off fluid flow and remove dome.** Clamp the administration set to stop the flow of fluids. Remove the dome from the *patch*.
10. **Disconnect tubing.** Disconnect the infusion tube from the male connector.
11. **Insert removal tool.** Maintaining aseptic technique, open the *remover* package and take out the *remover*. Remove the protection from the *remover*'s threaded tip, and insert the *remover* into the infusion tube. Hold the infusion tube straight out from the patient (90° to the *patch*) as the *remover* is being placed. Advance the *remover*, and turn it clockwise until it stops turning to engage the threads in the proximal tip of the infusion tube.
12. **Pull out catheter.** Pull the *remover* straight out to remove the infusion tube. Dispose of the *remover* in a sharps container.
13. **Remove *patch*.** Remove the *patch* and apply steady pressure over the injection site to control bleeding. Dress the wound.

18 Secure the needle with tape and support with bulky dressing.

Adjust the base of the needle to the level of the patient's skin. Do not turn the base tight because it will physically remove the needle from the bone. In most cases, the needle will be secure as it is, much like a nail in a board. However, to ensure the stability of the needle, tape and a bulky bandage can be applied to hold it in place. Monitor the position of the needle and the flow of fluid throughout transport.

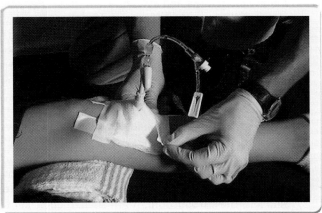

Local Anesthesia for Intraosseous Infusion

Performance Objective

Given a conscious patient who meets the criteria for intraosseous infusion and all necessary equipment, the candidate shall demonstrate the procedure for performing local anesthesia in conjunction with the placement of the intraosseous line, within 8 minutes or less.

Equipment

The following equipment is required to perform this skill:
- Appropriate body substance isolation/personal protection equipment
- Sharps container
- Lidocaine 1% or 2%
- Syringes (various sizes)
- Hypodermic needles (various sizes)
- Cleaning solution
  - Chlorhexidine preps
  - Povidone-iodine preps
  - Alcohol preps

Indications

- Pain reduction in the initiation and maintenance of an intraosseous line in conscious patients

Contraindications

- Allergies to lidocaine

Complications

- None

Procedures

 Step 1 ▶ **Ensure body substance isolation before beginning procedures.**

Prior to beginning patient care, appropriate body substance isolation procedures should be employed.

▼

 Step 2 ▶ **Prepare the intraosseous site.**

Prepare the insertion site by cleaning with an antiseptic/antimicrobial agent. A 30-second vigorous scrub using chlorhexidine will kill 99.9% of all colonizing microbes when the solution is dry. Chlorhexidine is safe for adults and children, but because of skin sensitivity, it should not be used on neonates.

If chlorhexidine is not available, povidone-iodine is an acceptable alternative. It is important to allow the povidone-iodine solution to dry completely before injecting the site. Alcohol may be used when the povidone-iodine is dry to clean the dye and improve visualization of the injection site.

For years alcohol has been used as the traditional injecting preparation. Because of its limited ability to kill microbial agents, it should be avoided in all cases unless the patient is allergic to both chlorhexidine and povidone-iodine (persons with shellfish allergies are allergic to iodine). Alcohol alone, as a prep for IV or hypodermic injection, should be considered below the standard of care.

Cleanse the site by applying the solution in a circular motion, starting in the center and working out. It is best not to reenter the clean area after it is cleaned.

▼

 In the Field

Using Lidocaine
Infiltration of the injection site with 1% lidocaine (the standard 100 mg/10 mL lidocaine used for cardiac arrhythmias) will remove the pain response from the skin and periosteum, but it will not totally remove the pain from the bone itself. In comparison, the injection of the needle is not as painful as it may seem, but the infusion of drugs or fluids can be excruciating.

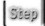 **Step 3** ▶ **Anesthetize the skin.**

Inject approximately 0.5 mL of lidocaine 1% or 0.25 mL of lidocaine 2% intradermal (wheal infiltration).

▼

Step 4 ▶ Anesthetize the bone.

Remove the needle from the skin and reinsert at a 90° angle to the bone until the resistance of the bone is felt. Inject 1 to 2 mL of lidocaine 1% or 0.5 to 1 mL of lidocaine 2% to infiltrate the periosteum (if resistance is felt, pull back slightly on the needle until you are able to inject—"periosteal occlusion").

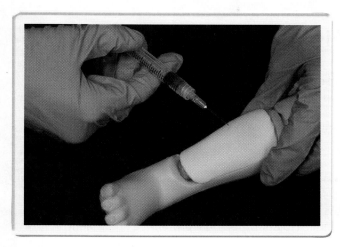

▼

Step 5 ▶ Compress the infiltrated tissue.

Compress the infiltrated area with your thumb. This will disperse the excess lidocaine into the tissues for greater anesthesia and will decrease the resistance for the intraosseous (IO) needle.

▼

Step 6 ▶ Insert the IO needle.

After a short period of time to allow the lidocaine to take effect, perform the IO technique of choice as usual.

▼

Step 7 ▶ Anesthetize the marrow channels.

Inject 4 mL of the lidocaine 1% or 2 mL of lidocaine 2% into the IO apparatus to anesthetize the marrow channels. After a short period of time to allow the lidocaine to take effect, use the IO as usual.

Implanted Venous Port Access

Performance Objective

Given a training model and other appropriate equipment, the candidate shall establish an IV line in an implanted venous port, secure the line and needle, and establish a drip rate of 30 drops/min using the criteria herein prescribed, in 8 minutes or less.

Equipment

The following equipment is required to perform this skill:
- Appropriate body substance isolation/personal protective equipment
- Appropriately sized sterile gloves
- Sharps container
- IV pole
- Selection of IV solutions (normal saline, lactated Ringer's)
- Administration sets: macro/micro/extension tubing
- Noncoring needle (Huber, Gripper)
- Tape or commercially made IV securing system
- 4" × 4" gauze pads
- Cleaning solution
  - Chlorhexidine preps   • Povidone-iodine preps
  - Alcohol preps
- Transparent dressing
- 4- and 10-mL syringes
- Selection of sterile needles
- Blood collection tubes

Equipment that may be helpful:
- Towels   ■ Topical lidocaine cream

Indications

- Immediate need for intravenous access in a patient with an implanted port

Contraindications

- None in emergency situations

Complications

- Thromboembolism or air embolism
- Infection   ■ Septicemia–septic shock

Procedures

 Ensure body substance isolation before beginning procedures.

Prior to beginning patient care, appropriate body substance isolation procedures should be employed.

▼

 **Avoid contamination of equipment.**

Maintain sterile/aseptic technique throughout the skill performance. Keep visual contact with sterile equipment and ensure the sterile field is not contaminated or compromised.

▼

 **Confirm order (solution and rate).**

Repeat the order given by the physician. You must repeat the solution and rate ordered as well as any special considerations given. When following standing orders, it is essential to ensure that the order is followed through with no errors of omission. This is the first step in maintaining the *six rights* of medication administration: right drug, right patient, right dose, right route, right time, right documentation.

▼

 Inform patient of need for fluid therapy.

Inform the patient of the need for accessing the indwelling port. Advise the patient of the purpose and the benefits of the procedure, as well as the risks. Many patients will ask about the use of lidocaine cream to provide local anesthesia. The use of lidocaine cream will depend on the ability to wait 15 to 20 minutes for the cream to take effect.

▼

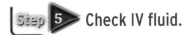 **Check IV fluid.**

Choose the solution ordered by the physician or the most appropriate solution if no specific fluid was ordered. Normal saline is the standard solution for simple to keep open (TKO) IV lines, dehydration, and to accompany blood. Lactated Ringer's solution is used for trauma and burns. Five percent dextrose in water (D_5W) is seldom used for anything other than mixing medications. However, some clinicians still prefer this solution for overhydration conditions, hypertension, and pulmonary edema. Other solutions, such as blood products, colloids, and electrolyte/glucose mixtures, are seldom used in the prehospital setting.

After choosing the correct solution, inspect the bag for leaks. Ensure the clarity and quality of the solution, looking specifically for signs of discoloration and contamination, and check the expiration date. Discard the solution if it is out of date or if signs of deterioration or contamination exist. Recheck the solution to make sure it is correct (right medication).

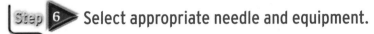 **Select appropriate needle and equipment.**

The needle should be chosen based on the patient's relative size. In general, the patient or family will know the length of needle that is typically used. The needle should be noncoring (Huber, Gripper).

You will also need an adhesive transparent dressing (if this is not available, use 4″ × 4″ gauze), povidone-iodine swabs and alcohol swabs (or chlorhexidine), and adhesive tape torn into appropriately sized strips for securing the tubing. Place these strips within easy reach of the intended site.

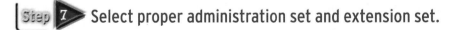 **Select proper administration set and extension set.**

From the available equipment, select the administration set and extension appropriate for the patient's condition. In general, a standard infusion and large-bore extension are used when fluid resuscitation will be performed; a microdrip and smaller-bore extension are used for simple TKO lines.

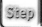 **Connect IV tubing to the IV bag.**

Carefully remove the administration and extension sets from their packaging. Straighten the tubing and untangle any knots. Remove the cap from the extension set first, and then remove the cap from the patient end of the administration set. Mate the two ends and give a firm twist. Move the rolling-ball stopcock as close to the drip chamber as possible, and run the ball to the closed position. You are now ready to puncture the IV bag.

Remove the protective cover from the port of the IV bag, and then remove the cap from the needle of the drip chamber. Puncture the IV bag, and give a firm twist. Squeeze the drip chamber *one time* and allow the fluid to run into the chamber. The solution should fill one fourth to one third the volume of the chamber (many solution sets have a mark at this level); additional filling will alter the function of the drip chamber. Open the rolling-ball stopcock and allow the solution to fill the IV line. Before the solution reaches the end, remove the cap until solution runs freely from the line. Shut the clamp and replace the cap of the IV tubing until ready to connect to the IV catheter. This method should produce an air-free IV line; however, inspect the line to ensure that all air bubbles have been run out of the line.

 Ensure body substance isolation before beginning invasive procedures and whenever contact with blood or body fluids can be reasonably anticipated.

Prior to beginning patient care, appropriate body substance isolation procedures should be employed. In most cases, this should include gloves, masks, and eye protection at a minimum. When treating patients with known infectious diseases, especially those spread by respiratory secretions, HEPA filter masks may be required.

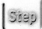 **Set up sterile field.**

Open the package of the sterile gloves, removing and opening the inner package on a steady surface. *Do not* don the gloves. Use the inner packaging of the gloves as a sterile field. Place the necessary items on the fingertip portion of the sterile field while maintaining the sterility of the items and the field. These items are four 10-mL syringes, a noncoring needle (Huber or Gripper), a transparent dressing, an attachable injection site (better known as a hep lock or saline lock), and a needle for drawing up saline (18 or 21 gauge).

Step **Locate the port.**

Palpate to find the flat face, contour, edges, and mobility of the port.

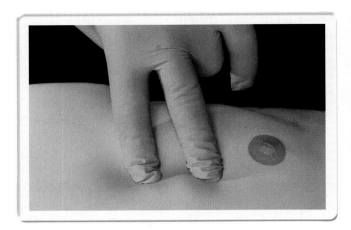

Step **Prepare the site.**

Prepare the insertion site by cleaning with an antiseptic/antimicrobial agent. A 30-second vigorous scrub using chlorhexidine will kill 99.9% of all colonizing microbes when the solution is dry. Chlorhexidine is safe for adults and children, but because of skin sensitivity, it should not be used on neonates.

If chlorhexidine is not available, povidone-iodine is an acceptable alternative. It is important to allow the povidone-iodine solution to dry completely before injecting the site. Alcohol may be used when the povidone-iodine is dry to clean the dye and improve visualization of the injection site. Cleanse the site by applying the solution in a circular motion, starting in the center and working out. It is best not to reenter the clean area after it is cleaned.

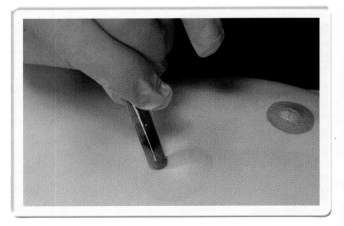

Step 13 ▶ Don sterile gloves.

Open the wrapper to expose both gloves. Note that both gloves have a cuff, exposing the inner part of the glove. The inner exposed part will eventually come in contact with your skin and is considered to be nonsterile. This part is safe to touch without compromising the sterile field. The remainder of the glove and the package remain sterile and must be kept sterile by using appropriate aseptic technique.

To don the gloves, grasp the first glove by the inner cuff without touching any of the sterile portion. Holding the glove by the cuff with the fingers pointing down, slip the opposite hand as deep inside as possible. *Do not* attempt to make the glove fit tight. Final adjustments will be made when both gloves are in place.

Now, with the gloved hand, slide your fingertips under the cuff of the second glove, and lift it off of the sterile wrapper. Slide the ungloved hand into the second glove, working the fingers into place. Adjust each glove to fit, reaching under the cuff to pull up and then unroll the cuff up your wrist. When you have donned the sterile gloves, keep your hands in front of you and above your waist. Do not touch anything outside the sterile field.

▼

Step 14 ▶ Prepare the noncoring needle.

First, remove all end caps from all syringes, if present.

Attach a needle to a 10-mL syringe, and draw up approximately 5 mL of air. Have an assistant hold up a vial of normal saline. The assistant should hold the vial upside down in one hand and brace the wrist with the other hand. Insert the needle into the vial, inject the air, and draw up approximately 5 mL of solution. When it is filled, remove the needle from the vial and safely recap. Return the filled syringe to the sterile field. Repeat this procedure with a second syringe filled to a full 10 mL.

Attach a saline lock injection site to the tubing of the noncoring needle. Insert the needle of the syringe that contains 5 mL of saline, and flush the fluid through to the end of the needle. This should leave at least 3 mL in the syringe.

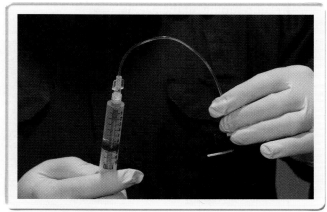

Note: If a vial of normal saline is not available, the syringes can be filled using the injection port of the chosen IV solution. Ensure that this is performed in a sterile manner.

Note: If an injection site is not available, you can attach flushed IV tubing directly to the flushed tubing of the noncoring needle prior to dressing the site.

▼

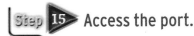

Step 15 ▶ **Access the port.**

Pick up the noncoring needle and remove the plastic needle guard. Inspect the needle for defects. With your nondominant hand, stabilize the port by holding it tight between your thumb and index finger (when this hand has touched the patient, only the thumb and forefinger remain sterile). The remainder of the hand should not reenter the sterile field. Hold the needle with the dominant hand at a 90° angle to the face of the port and slowly insert. Advance the needle until resistance is felt as it makes contact with the port's metal back. Verify placement by aspirating the syringe for blood return. If no blood is returned, discontinue the procedure by removing the needle.

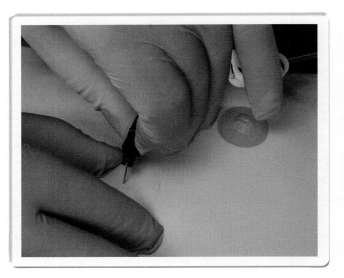

If blood is obtained, continue to withdraw blood until the syringe is full, then clamp tubing on the needle.

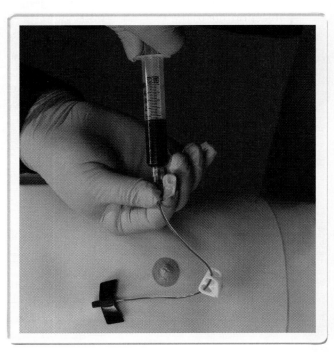

Step 15 continued

This syringe is waste and should be handled appropriately. Attach a second 10-mL syringe, unclamp the needle tubing, withdraw 5 to 10 mL of blood, and reclamp the tubing. This syringe is also waste. Attach a third 10-mL syringe, unclamp the needle tubing, withdraw 10 mL of blood, and reclamp the tubing. This syringe should be handed to your assistant, who will place the blood into appropriate and available lab tubes.

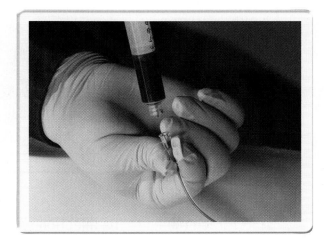

Attach the syringe with 10 mL of saline, unclamp the tubing, and flush with the full 10 mL of saline.

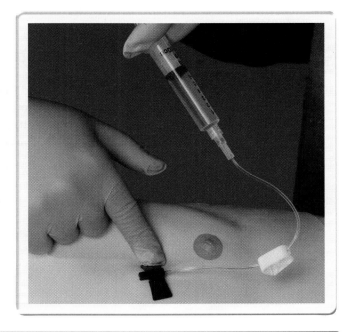

Step  16 Stabilize and dress the site.

If the appropriate size needle was used, there should be little space between the 90° bend in the needle and the skin. If, however, there is a space, fill the gap with a sterile 2″ × 2″ gauze or a folded 4″ × 4″ gauze. Cover it with the transparent dressing.

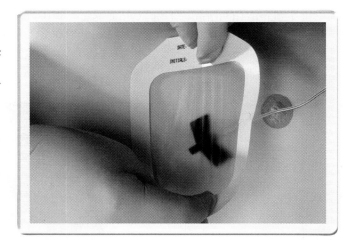

Step  17 Attach tubing to the injection site if not already done.

Connect the IV tubing to the injection site. Twist the connections to form a proper seat.

Step  18 Run IV for a brief period to ensure patent line.

Open the flow control and begin running fluid to verify that the port access is patent. An IV line that will not run indicates improper needle placement. It may be necessary to restart the port access procedure.

Step  19 Adjust flow rate as appropriate.

Adjust the drip rate as appropriate for the patient's needs. Count the number of drops in a 15-second period and multiply by four until you have achieved the desired rate. Count the drops for a full minute to make the final adjustment and ensure accuracy.

Dispose of contaminated equipment.

Dispose of needles and all sharp instruments with blood or body fluid contamination in puncture-resistant sharps containers. Other materials that have been contaminated by blood or body fluids should be disposed of in biohazard bags. Waste materials that are not contaminated by blood or body fluids can be disposed of in normal trash receptacles.

▼

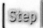 **Verify patency again.**

The final step in beginning any venous access is to ensure that the line is patent. This should also be performed before administering IV medications through either bolus or drip and when transferring care of the patient. Always document all checks of patency.
   Patency can be checked by:

- Lowering the IV bag below the level of insertion. Blood entering the IV tubing ensures patency.
- Inserting a syringe into the medication port and pulling back on the plunger. Blood entering the IV tubing ensures patency.
- Injecting saline into the medication port. An unrestricted injection and no signs of infiltration ensure patency.

Performance Objective

Given a supply of medications in vials and ampules and an assortment of syringes and hypodermic needles, the candidate shall be able to identify the prescribed or ordered medication and draw the appropriate volume into a syringe using the criteria herein prescribed, in 2 minutes or less.

Equipment

The following equipment is required to perform this skill:
- Appropriate body substance isolation/personal protection equipment
- Sharps container
- Selection of syringes
- Selection of hypodermic needles (filtered and nonfiltered)
- Medications in ampules and vials

Equipment that may be helpful:
- 2" × 2" or 4" × 4" gauze pads

Indications

- Preparing medications for injection

Contraindications

- None

Complications

- Aspiration and eventual injection of glass or rubber emboli
- Sterile abscess

Procedures

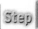 **Step 1** Ensure body substance isolation before beginning procedures.

Prior to beginning patient care, appropriate body substance isolation procedures should be employed.

▼

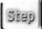 **Step 2** Maintain sterility throughout procedure.

Maintain the sterility of the medication at all times. Use extreme caution that the needle, inside of the syringe, and the medication itself do not come in contact with a nonsterile object or surface.

▼

 Step 3 Identify appropriate medication as prescribed or ordered.

From the available drugs, select the prescribed or ordered medication.

▼

 Step 4 Inspect medication label for proper concentration and expiration date.

Confirm that the medication is the correct concentration. Check that the expiration date has not passed. This is the first step in maintaining the *six rights* of medication administration: right drug, right patient, right dose, right route, right time, right documentation. From the medication box, choose the correct medication based on protocol or as ordered by the physician.

▼

 Step 5 Choose appropriate syringe.

From the available supply, choose the smallest syringe that will contain the desired amount of medication.

▼

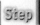 **Step 6** Choose and attach appropriate needle using aseptic technique.

From the available supply, choose a needle that will allow for the most appropriate removal of the medication from the vial or ampule. To draw medication from a vial, complete Steps 7–15. To draw medication from an ampule, complete Steps 16–22.

▼

Drawing Medications From a Vial

 7 Check to be sure you have the correct medication.

Before drawing up the medication, ensure that the right medication and concentration have been chosen and the expiration date has not passed. Choose the smallest available needle to insert into the rubber stopper of the vial. This will reduce the possibility of coring a small piece of rubber into the syringe.

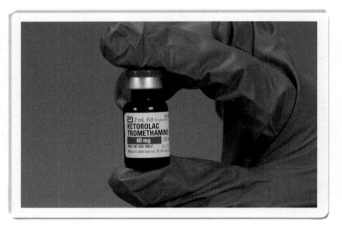

  8 Remove the cap from the vial (if present).

Remove the cap from the vial and wipe with an alcohol prep.

 9 Determine the amount of medication you will need and draw that amount of air into the syringe.

Draw the appropriate amount of air into the syringe.

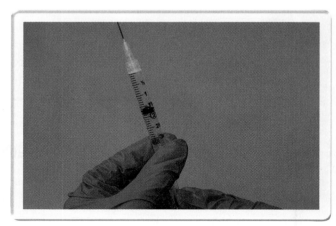

Step **10** ▶ Inject the vial with air.

With the vial placed on a firm surface, insert the needle through the rubber stopper and inject the air into the vial from the syringe.

▼

Step **11** ▶ Invert the vial.

Invert the vial and pull the needle to the lower neck of the vial.

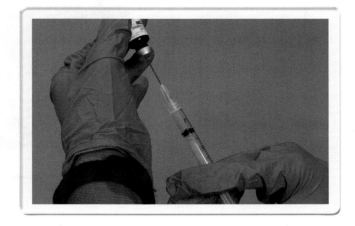

▼

Step **12** ▶ Draw the medication into the syringe.

Draw slightly more than the desired amount of medication into the syringe.

▼

Step **13** ▶ Remove the needle from the vial.

Withdraw the needle from the vial and expel any air from the syringe.

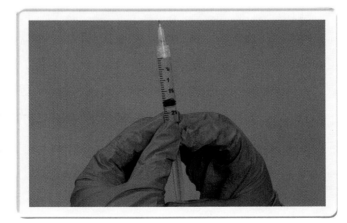

▼

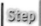

Safety Tips

Recapping Needles
There is a widespread and correct rule that you should never recap a needle. This is a correct statement *after* the needle has been used on the patient. Before administration to the patient, recapping the needle helps prevent compromise to the needle's sterility. It is also important to recap the needle if you are going to remove it to attach a different needle.

Step **14** **Recap the needle.**

Recap the needle using the one-handed method. Because this needle has never been used in a patient, and because the one-handed method runs a risk of contamination of the needle, it is also considered appropriate to recap the needle by simply placing the cover back on the needle. Do not use this method when the needle is contaminated.

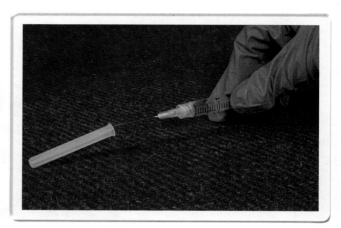

Step **15** **Change needle for injection.**

Remove the needle from the syringe and dispose of it in an appropriate puncture-resistant container. Attach a second needle to the syringe that is appropriate for the method of injection. Volume, order, or medication will determine the site and method of medication administration.

Medication Administration Sites						
	Deltoid Muscle	Dorsogluteal Muscle	Ventrogluteal Muscle	Vastus Lateralis Muscle	Arm, Abdomen, Thigh	Forearm
Type	Intramuscular (IM)	Intramuscular (IM)	Intramuscular (IM)	Intramuscular (IM)	Subcutaneous (SC)	Intradermal (ID)
Size	23 to 25 gauge, $5/8$" to 1"	20 to 23 gauge, $1 1/2$" to 3"	20 to 23 gauge, $1 1/2$" to 3"	23 to 25 gauge, $5/8$" to $1 1/2$"	25 to 27 gauge, $1/2$" to $5/8$"	26 to 27 gauge, $3/8$"
Range	0.5-2 mL	1-5 mL	1-5 mL	1-5 mL	0.5-1.5 mL	0.001-1 mL

Drawing Medications From an Ampule

Step 16 Check to be sure you have the correct medication.

Before drawing up the medication, ensure that the right medication and concentration has been chosen and the expiration date has not passed. Choose a filtered needle to prevent the aspiration of small pieces of glass that may enter the ampule when the top is broken.

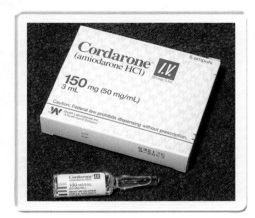

Step 17 Ensure that all medication is in the bottom of the ampule.

Any medication in the top of the ampule can be moved to the bottom by holding the base and tapping the top of the ampule to shake the medication to the base.

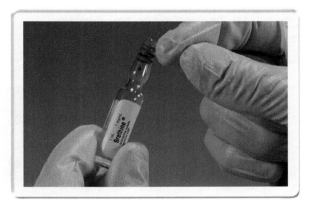

Step 18 Break the ampule along the scored neck, taking precautions against injury.

Wrapping the neck of the ampule with a 4″ × 4″ gauze pad or an alcohol prep can prevent you from being cut by the neck of the ampule should it not break clean.

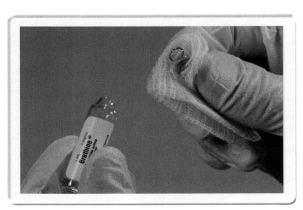

Step 19 Insert the needle into the neck of the ampule and draw the medication into the syringe.

Insert the needle into the ampule without touching the outside of the ampule. Draw the medication into the syringe. For ampules containing 5 mL or less, carefully invert the ampule to draw the medication; larger ampules should be tilted to bring the mediation in reach of the needle, but it should not be completely inverted.

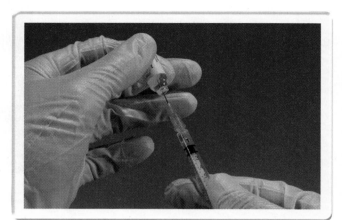

 Step 20 Loosen air trapped inside.

Hold the syringe with the needle pointing up, and gently tap the barrel to loosen air trapped inside.

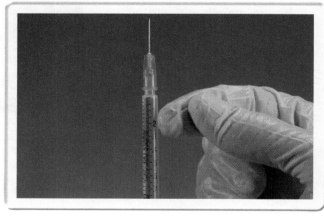

Step 21 Dispel any air bubbles and recap the needle.

Press gently on the plunger to dispel any air bubbles. Recap the needle using the one-handed method.

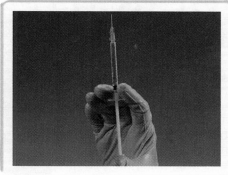

Step 22 Change needle for injection.

Remove the needle from the syringe and dispose of it in an appropriate puncture-resistant container. Attach a second needle to the syringe that is appropriate for the method of injection.

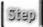

In the Field

Reconstituting Dry Powdered Medications

An increasing number of medications are not stable in a liquid state for reasonable periods of time and are instead placed into vials as a dry powder. These medications must be reconstituted with sterile water or saline before being administered to the patient. Pharmaceutical companies often package these medications with a vial that contains the appropriate amount of fluid for reconstituting the powder. To reconstitute the powder, draw up the appropriate amount of fluid into a syringe and inject the fluid into the vial that contains the powder. With the syringe still in the vial, carefully shake the vial to thoroughly mix the powder. Draw up the reconstituted medication, and prepare for injection. It is normal for the medication to be somewhat milky in most cases.

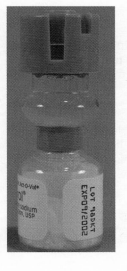

Some powdered drugs, such as methylprednisolone sodium succinate, are stored in an hourglass-shaped vial with a rubber disk that separates the liquid diluent from the powder (shown at right). To reconstitute the drug you simply push on the top of the stopper. The pressure will force the center stopper down into the bottom part that contains the powder. Shake the vial thoroughly to mix, and draw up as you would any normal vial.

Hypodermic Medication Administration

Performance Objective

Given a patient and appropriate equipment, the candidate shall be able to recognize and select appropriate medication as ordered, identify an appropriate administration site, and administer a drug using the criteria herein prescribed, in 3 minutes or less per component.

Equipment

The following equipment is required to perform this skill:

- Appropriate body substance isolation/personal protection equipment
- Sharps container
- Appropriate medications in prefilled syringes, ampules, and vials
- Selection of syringes
- Selection of hypodermic needles (filtered and nonfiltered)
- Cleaning solution
  - Chlorhexidine preps
  - Povidone-iodine preps
  - Alcohol preps
- Adhesive bandages

Equipment that may be helpful:
- 2" × 2" or 4" × 4" gauze pads

Indications

- Medical necessity of medication
- Medication capable of being appropriately absorbed
- Medication compatible with chosen route

Contraindications

- None

Complications

- Inadvertent puncture of artery or vein
- Sterile abscess

Procedures

 Ensure body substance isolation before beginning procedures.

Prior to beginning patient care, appropriate body substance isolation procedures should be employed.

▼

 **Inform patient of need for therapy and ask about known allergies to drugs and foods.**

Inform the patient of the order received, the need for the therapy, and any concerns about its administration. Ask the patient if he or she has had any allergies to the specific drug ordered, as well as any other drugs, iodine, or pertinent foods. It may be necessary to check the patient for allergy bands, medical ID tags, or hospital records, if available.

▼

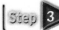 **Confirm order and select correct medication.**

Confirm the medication as ordered or as listed in the protocol. Check that the expiration date has not passed. This is the first step in maintaining the *six rights* of medication administration: right drug, right patient, right dose, right route, right time, right documentation. From the medication box, choose the correct medication, based on protocol or as ordered by the physician.

▼

 Ensure correct concentration of drug.

Inspect the medication for correct name, appropriate concentration, fluid clarity, discoloration, and obvious contamination or signs of loss of sterility.

▼

Prepare correct amount of medication for administration.

In the appropriate syringe, draw up the desired amount of medication. Remove the needle and replace with the appropriate needle for the type and location of injection. Hold the syringe needle up, and tap the syringe to force air bubbles to the top. Depress the plunger of the syringe to force the air out through the needle. For hypodermic administration, expel excess medication until you have only the desired amount to be delivered to the patient.

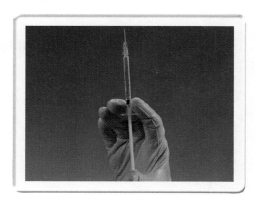

 Select appropriate administration site.

Select the appropriate administration site for the volume of the medication to be given. See the table below for examples. Volume, order, or medication will determine the site and method of medication administration.

Medication Administration Sites						
	Deltoid Muscle	Dorsogluteal Muscle	Ventrogluteal Muscle	Vastus Lateralis Muscle	Arm, Abdomen, Thigh	Forearm
Type	Intramuscular (IM)	Intramuscular (IM)	Intramuscular (IM)	Intramuscular (IM)	Subcutaneous (SC)	Intradermal (ID)
Size	23 to 25 gauge, $5/8$" to 1"	20 to 23 gauge, $1\frac{1}{2}$" to 3"	20 to 23 gauge, $1\frac{1}{2}$" to 3"	23 to 25 gauge, $5/8$" to $1\frac{1}{2}$"	25 to 27 gauge, $1/2$" to $5/8$"	26 to 27 gauge, $3/8$"
Range	0.5-2 mL	1-5 mL	1-5 mL	1-5 mL	0.5-1.5 mL	0.001-1 mL

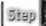 **7** ▶ Prepare injection site.

Prepare the injection site by cleaning with an antiseptic/antimicrobial agent. A 30-second vigorous scrub using chlorhexidine will kill 99.9% of all colonizing microbes when the solution is dry. Chlorhexidine is safe for adults and children, but because of skin sensitivity, it should not be used on neonates.

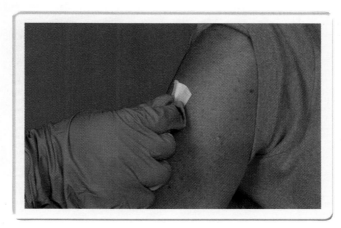

If chlorhexidine is not available, povidone-iodine is an acceptable alternative. It is important to allow the povidone-iodine solution to dry completely before injecting the site. Alcohol may be used when the povidone-iodine is dry to clean the dye and improve visualization of the injection site.

For years alcohol has been used as the traditional injecting preparation. Because of its limited ability to kill microbial agents, it should be avoided in all cases unless the patient is allergic to both chlorhexidine and povidone-iodine (persons with shellfish allergies are actually allergic to iodine). Alcohol alone, as a prep for IV or hypodermic injection, should be considered below the standard of care.

Cleanse the site by applying the solution in a circular motion, starting in the center and working out. It is best not to reenter the clean area after it is cleaned.

▼

8 ▶ Reconfirm medication.

Inspect the medication for correct name, appropriate concentration, fluid clarity, discoloration, and obvious contamination or signs of loss of sterility. Check that the expiration date has not passed.

▼

Step 9 Perform needle insertion.

Prepare for the injection by informing the patient of the procedure and that he or she may feel slight discomfort.

Intramuscular Injection

Stretch skin and hold tight. Hold the syringe at a 90° angle to the skin. With a steady, sharp, and controlled motion, insert the needle into the muscle tissue. Release tension on the skin.

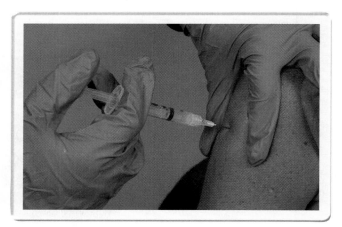

Subcutaneous Injection

Pinch the skin between two fingers. Hold the syringe at a 45° angle, and insert the needle below the skin using a sharp and controlled motion.

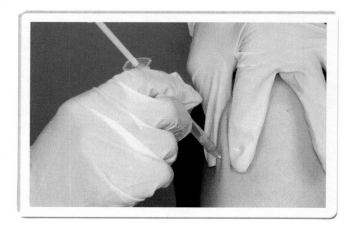

 In the Field

Subcutaneous and Intramuscular Injections

Subcutaneous (SC) and intramuscular (IM) injections should not be given to patients with inadequate perfusion.

Intradermal Injection

Pull the skin tight. Hold the syringe at a 10° to 15° angle, and insert the needle into the skin using a sharp and controlled motion. Insert the needle just deep enough to put the lumen into the skin.

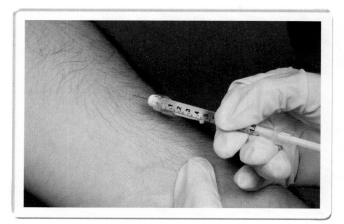

Aspirate for absence of blood return.

Holding the syringe steady, pull back on the syringe. Absence of a blood return indicates that the needle is not in a vessel.

  Administer correct dose at the proper push rate with aseptic technique maintained throughout.

Inject the contents of the syringe.

  Withdraw needle.

Remove the needle at the angle at which it was inserted. Apply direct pressure over the injection site with a sterile wipe and hold for a few seconds. *Do not recap needle.* Do not apply pressure after intradermal injection.

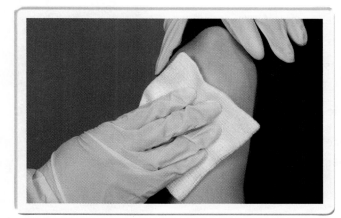

  Dispose of syringe and needle in proper container.

Dispose of all contaminated equipment using puncture-resistant sharps containers and biohazard equipment as appropriate. Remember that not all equipment used is a biological hazard. Any used equipment or supplies that do not pose a threat of injury or biohazard exposure should be disposed of in normal trash receptacles.

Monitor for desired or adverse effects of medication.

Watch the patient for the desired effects and for any adverse effects of the delivered medication. Be sure to document the response that has occurred.

Safety Tips

Minimizing Risk of Needlestick

- Immediately dispose of all sharps in a puncture-proof sharps container. Do not drop the sharps on the floor for later disposal, and do not attempt to recap a needle and syringe before placing it in the sharps container.
- When possible, perform all invasive procedures at the scene. If your patient's condition warrants starting an IV or administering a medication en route to the hospital, use extreme caution. Although most paramedics become proficient at starting IVs in the back of a moving ambulance, it may be necessary to have your partner briefly stop the ambulance, especially if you are traveling over rough terrain.
- Recap needles only as an absolute last resort. If you must recap a needle, use the one-handed technique. Place the needle cover on a stationary surface, then slide the needle—with one hand—into the needle cap.

Mucosal Atomizer Medication Administration

Performance Objective

Given a patient and appropriate equipment, the candidate shall be able to recognize and select appropriate medication as ordered, identify an appropriate administration site, and administer the drug using the criteria herein prescribed, in 3 minutes or less per component.

Equipment

The following equipment is required to perform this skill:
- Appropriate body substance isolation/personal protection equipment
- Sharps container
- Appropriate medications in prefilled syringes, ampules, and vials
- Selection of syringes
- Selection of hypodermic needles (filtered and nonfiltered)
- Mucosal atomizer device

Equipment that may be helpful:
- Facial tissue

Indications

- Medical necessity of medication
- Medication capable of being appropriately absorbed
- Medication compatible with chosen route

Contraindications

- None

Complications

- Nasal irritation

Procedures

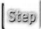 **Ensure body substance isolation before beginning procedures.**

Prior to beginning patient care, appropriate body substance isolation procedures should be employed.

▼

  Inform patient of need for therapy and ask about known allergies to drugs or foods.

Inform the patient of the order received, the need for the therapy, and any concerns about its administration. Ask the patient if he or she has had any allergies to the specific drug ordered, as well as any other drugs, iodine, or pertinent foods. It may be necessary to check the patient for allergy bands, medical ID tags, or hospital records, if available.

▼

 **Confirm order and select correct medication.**

Confirm the medication as ordered or as listed in the protocol. Check that the expiration date has not passed. This is the first step in maintaining the *six rights* of medication administration: right drug, right patient, right dose, right route, right time, right documentation. From the medication box, choose the correct medication, based on protocol or as ordered by the physician.

▼

  Ensure correct concentration of drug.

Inspect the medication for correct name, appropriate concentration, fluid clarity, discoloration, and obvious contamination or signs of loss of sterility.

▼

5 Prepare correct amount of medication for administration.

In an appropriate syringe, draw up the desired amount of medication. Remove the needle and replace with the mucosal atomizer device.

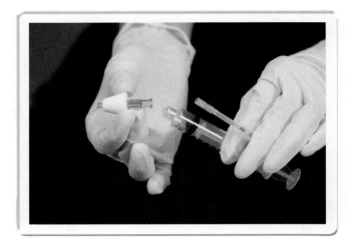

Hold the syringe tip up; tap the syringe to force air bubbles to the top. Depress the plunger of the syringe to force the air out through the atomizer. Expel excess medication until you have only the desired amount to be delivered to the patient. Each naris will be able to absorb 0.5 to 1 mL of medication.

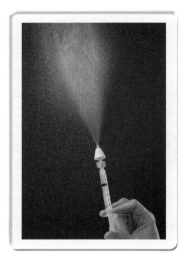

 In the Field

The Intranasal Route

Intranasal medications are rapidly absorbed, providing a more rapid onset of drug action than via the intramuscular route. Administration of emergency medications via the intranasal route is performed using a mucosal atomizer device.

 6 Reconfirm medication.

Inspect the medication for correct name, appropriate concentration, fluid clarity, discoloration, and obvious contamination or signs of loss of sterility. Check that the expiration date has not passed.

Step 7 ▶ Place atomizer into naris and atomize the medication.

Place the mucosal atomizer into the desired naris. Using a steady pressure, depress the plunger to atomize the medication into the naris. If the amount of medication needed exceeds the 1 mL maximum for the naris, a second dose can be administered into the other naris.

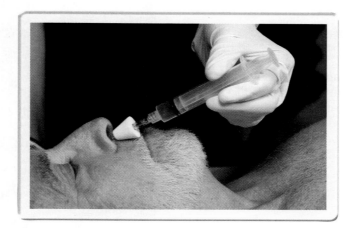

▼

Step 8 ▶ Dispose of syringe and needle in proper container.

Dispose of all contaminated equipment using puncture-resistant sharps containers and biohazard equipment as appropriate. Remember that not all equipment used is a biological hazard. Any used equipment or supplies that do not pose a threat of injury or biohazard exposure should be disposed of in normal trash receptacles.

▼

Step 9 ▶ Monitor for desired or adverse effects of medication.

Watch the patient for the desired effects and for any adverse effects of the delivered medication. Be sure to document the response that has occurred.

Intravenous Bolus Medication Administration

Performance Objective

Given a patient and all appropriate equipment, the candidate shall be able to recognize and select appropriate medication as ordered, identify an appropriate administration site, and administer the drug using the criteria herein prescribed, in 3 minutes or less per component.

Equipment

The following equipment is required to perform this skill:
- Appropriate body substance isolation/personal protection equipment
- Patient intravenous access line (previously established)
- Sharps container
- Appropriate medication in prefilled syringes, ampules, or vials
- Syringes and needles (various sizes)
- Cleaning solution
  - Chlorhexidine preps
  - Povidone-iodine preps
  - Alcohol preps

Indications

- Medical necessity of medication
- Medication capable of being appropriately absorbed

Contraindications

- Usually drug dependent, not procedure dependent

Complications

- Air embolism

Procedures

 Ensure body substance isolation before beginning procedures.

Prior to beginning patient care, appropriate body substance isolation procedures should be employed.

▼

 **Inform patient of need for therapy and ask about known allergies to drugs and foods.**

Inform the patient of the order received, the need for the therapy, and any concerns about its administration. Ask the patient if he or she has had any allergies to the specific drug ordered, as well as any other drugs, iodine, or pertinent foods. It may be necessary to check the patient for allergy bands, medical ID tags, or hospital records, if available.

▼

 Confirm order and select correct medication.

Confirm the medication as ordered or as listed in the protocol. Check that the expiration date has not passed. This is the first step in maintaining the *six rights* of medication administration: right drug, right patient, right dose, right route, right time, right documentation.

▼

 **Ensure correct concentration of drug.**

Inspect the medication for correct name, appropriate concentration, fluid clarity, discoloration, and obvious contamination or signs of loss of sterility.

▼

 Draw up medication.

In an appropriate syringe, draw up the desired amount of medication. Hold the syringe needle up, and tap the syringe to force the air bubbles to the top. Remove the needle and replace with the appropriate needle for the type and location of injection. Depress the plunger of the syringe to force all remaining air out through the needle. Many IV drugs come supplied in prefilled syringes. Follow the instructions on the package to see how to assemble the syringe.

▼

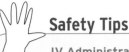
Step **6** ▶ **Cleanse injection site.**

Clean the injection port with chlorhexidine or a povidone-iodine or alcohol wipe. If using a needleless system, remove the protective cap.

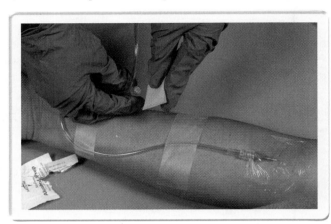

Step **7** ▶ **Reconfirm medication.**

Inspect the medication for correct name, appropriate concentration, fluid clarity, discoloration, and obvious contamination or signs of loss of sterility. Check that the expiration date has not passed.

Step **8** ▶ **Stop IV flow by pinching tubing or occluding flow.**

Holding the injection port carefully, insert the needle through the rubber stopper. Pinch the infusion tubing above the injection port, as close to the port as possible.

Step **9** ▶ **Ensure patency of IV.**

Patency can be checked by:

- Lowering the IV bag below the level of insertion. Blood entering the IV tubing ensures patency.
- Inserting a syringe into the medication port and pulling back on the plunger. Blood entering the IV tubing ensures patency.
- Injecting saline into the medication port. An unrestricted injection and no signs of infiltration ensures patency.

Administer correct dose at proper push rate with aseptic technique maintained throughout.

Inject the medication into the IV port at a rate appropriate for the medication being administered. When in doubt, administer the medication slowly. Ensure that the sterile fields are not contaminated.

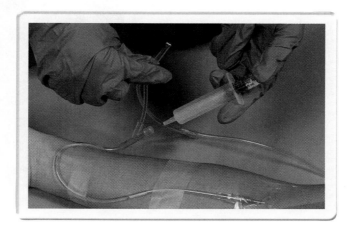

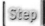 **Dispose of the syringe and needle in proper container.**

Dispose of all contaminated equipment using puncture-resistant sharps containers and biohazard equipment as appropriate. Remember that not all equipment used is a biological hazard. Any used equipment or supplies that do not pose a threat of injury or biohazard exposure should be disposed of in normal trash receptacles.

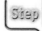 **Flush tubing.**

Remove the needle from the injection port and flush the IV line with fluid. It is helpful to give a bolus of at least 20 mL of IV fluid to help push the drug into the system. In cardiac arrest, shock, or other serious conditions it may be necessary to elevate the arm and "milk" the medication into the thorax. This will ensure that the medication reaches the central circulation and does not remain dormant in the arm.

13 Adjust drip rate to keep open (TKO).

Adjust the IV drip to a to keep open (TKO) rate, or to the original setting as appropriate.

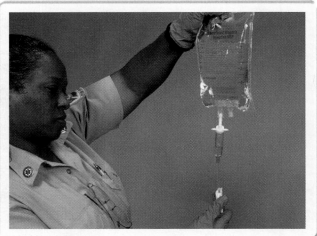

 14 Monitor for desired or adverse effects of medication.

Watch the patient for the desired effects and for any adverse effects of the delivered medication. Be sure to document the response that has occurred.

Endotracheal Medication Administration

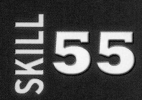

Performance Objective

Given a patient and all appropriate equipment, the candidate shall be able to recognize and select appropriate medication as per order, identify an appropriate administration site, and administer the drug using the criteria herein prescribed, in 3 minutes or less per component.

Equipment

The following equipment is required to perform this skill:
- Appropriate body substance isolation/personal protection equipment
- Sharps container
- Appropriate medication in prefilled syringes, ampules, or vials
- Syringes and needles (various sizes)
- Bag-valve device
- Endotracheal tube

Indications

- Administration of atropine, lidocaine, or epinephrine in cardiac arrest when no IV access can be established.

Contraindications

- Vascular access by any other means, such as intraosseous

Complications

- None

Procedures

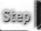 **Step 1** Ensure body substance isolation before beginning procedures.

Prior to beginning patient care, appropriate body substance isolation procedures should be employed.

▼

 Step 2 Ask family or caregiver about any known allergies to drugs or foods.

Ask the patient's family or caregiver if he or she has had any allergies to the specific drug ordered, as well as to any other drugs, iodine, or pertinent foods. It may be necessary to check the patient for allergy bands, medical ID tags, or hospital records, if available.

▼

 Step 3 Confirm order and select correct medication.

Confirm the medication as ordered or as listed in the protocol. Check that the expiration date has not passed. This is the first step in maintaining the *six rights* of medication administration: right drug, right patient, right dose, right route, right time, right documentation.

▼

 Step 4 Ensure correct concentration of drug.

Inspect the medication for correct name, appropriate concentration, fluid clarity, discoloration, and obvious contamination or signs of loss of sterility.

▼

 Step 5 Prepare correct amount of medication for administration.

In an appropriate syringe, draw up the desired amount of medication. According to proper protocol or physician order, prepare the medication to a minimum of 10 mL. Dosages that are carried in less than 10 mL will need to be diluted to this minimum volume. Many protocols allow for medications given via an endotracheal tube to be doubled or tripled from an IV order. Before automatically doubling or tripling the order, ensure that the physician has approved this action.

▼

Step **Instruct partner to hyperventilate patient.**

Instruct your partner to hyperventilate the patient at a rate of 20 to 30 breaths/min. After 2 to 3 minutes, you will be able to remove the bag-valve device and administer the medication. You will have only 20 seconds to begin the next breath.

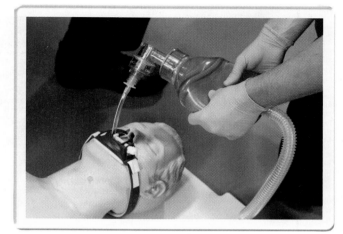

Step **Recheck the medication label.**

Inspect the medication for correct name, appropriate concentration, fluid clarity, discoloration, and obvious contamination or signs of loss of sterility. Check that the expiration date has not passed.

Step **Administer the medication.**

After 2 to 3 minutes of hyperventilation, disconnect the bag-valve device from the endotracheal tube. If a needle is attached to the syringe, it should be removed if possible. Rapidly instill the medication into the endotracheal tube. The application of a flexible catheter to the syringe may be used to assist the delivery of the medication to the bronchial tree.

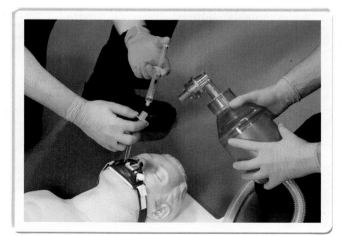

Step 9 Instruct partner to hyperventilate patient.

Have your partner attach the bag-valve device back onto the endotracheal tube and begin hyperventilation of the patient for another 2 to 3 minutes.

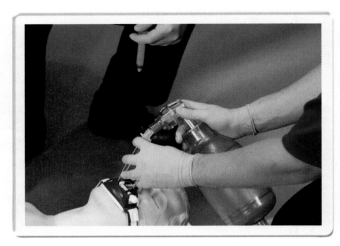

Step 10 Dispose of syringe and needle in proper container.

Dispose of all contaminated equipment using puncture-resistant sharps containers and biohazard equipment as appropriate. Remember that not all equipment used is a biological hazard. Any used equipment or supplies that do not pose a threat of injury or biohazard exposure should be disposed of in normal trash receptacles.

Step 11 Monitor for desired or adverse effects of medication.

Watch the patient for the desired effects and for any adverse effects of the delivered medication. Be sure to document the response that has occurred.

In the Field

Effectiveness of Endotracheal Medication Administration

Most studies have found little evidence to support the continued use of the endotracheal route for the administration of medications. Over the years, several recommendations have been made regarding how much medication must be given via the endotracheal route to be equivalent to an IV dose. Little evidence exists to support any of these recommendations. With the advances and innovations in intraosseous access, there seems to be little need for the endotracheal route as a routine method of medication administration.

Continuous Medication Infusion

Performance Objective

Given a patient and all appropriate equipment, the candidate shall be able to recognize and select appropriate medication as per order, identify an appropriate administration site, and administer the drug using the criteria herein prescribed, in 8 minutes or less per component.

Equipment

The following equipment is required to perform this skill:
- Appropriate body substance isolation/personal protection equipment
- Sharps container
- Selection of IV solutions (normal saline, 5% dextrose in water)
- Administration sets: Macro/micro/extension tubing
- Appropriate medication in prefilled syringes, ampules, or vials
- Syringes and needles (various sizes)
- Tape
- Cleaning solution
  - Chlorhexidine preps
  - Alcohol preps
  - Povidone-iodine preps

Equipment that may be helpful:
- Medication pump
- Pump tubing

Indications

- Medical necessity of medication
- Continuous delivery of medication, maintenance of therapeutic level

Contraindications

- None

Complications

- Air embolism
- Overdose

Procedures

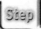 **Ensure body substance isolation before beginning procedures.**

Prior to beginning patient care, appropriate body substance isolation procedures should be employed.

  Inform patient of need for therapy and ask about known allergies to drugs or foods.

Inform the patient of the order received, the need for the therapy, and any concerns about its administration. Ask the patient if he or she has had any allergies to the specific drug ordered, as well as any other drugs, iodine, or pertinent foods. It may be necessary to check the patient for allergy bands, medical ID tags, or hospital records, if available.

 **Confirm order and select correct medication.**

Confirm the medication as ordered or as listed in the protocol. Check that the expiration date has not passed. This is the first step in maintaining the *six rights* of medication administration: right drug, right patient, right dose, right route, right time, right documentation.

  Ensure correct concentration of drug.

Inspect the medication for correct name, appropriate concentration, fluid clarity, discoloration, and obvious contamination or signs of loss of sterility.

  Prepare the correct amount of medication for administration.

In an appropriate syringe, draw up the desired amount of medication. Draw up only the amount intended to be placed in the IV bag.

Many drugs that are intended for continuous infusion come supplied in pre-mixed bags. Prefilled bags need no additional preparation.

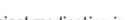 ## Step 6 ▶ Recheck the medication label.

Inspect the medication for correct name, appropriate concentration, fluid clarity, discoloration, and obvious contamination or signs of loss of sterility. Check that the expiration date has not passed.

▼

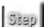 ## Step 7 ▶ Inject medication into secondary IV bag and mix solution.

Using chlorhexidine or a povidone-iodine or an alcohol swab, clean the injection port of the IV bag. Inject the appropriate amount of medication through the injection port, and gently mix the solution.

   If the amount of medication added to the bag exceeds 10% of the volume of the bag, you will need to remove fluid from the bag before injecting the medication.

   Skip this step if you are using a premixed bag.

▼

Step 8 ▶ Label medicated IV bag with name of drug and amount added.

Write the name of the drug, the amount added, and the time and date the solution was mixed on an adhesive label or to a large piece of adhesive tape. Attach the label to the IV bag. *Do not* write directly on the solution bag.

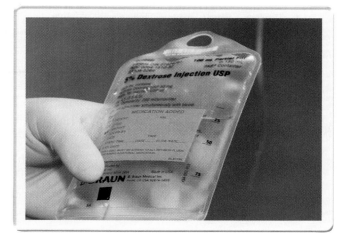

   It is a good idea to apply a tape label to the IV line just below the rolling ball stopcock when it is positioned. This provides a "flag" to identify which IV line controls the medication infusion. When multiple infusions are used, the name of the drug should be written on the label to ensure the proper medication is being adjusted.

▼

9 Connect the IV tubing and needle to the solution and expel air.

Prepare the administration set by unwrapping it from the packaging and running the rolling ball stopcock to the top of the set next to the drip chamber. Attach an 18- to 22-gauge needle to the end of the administration set.

Using sterile/aseptic technique, remove the covers from the injection port of the IV bag and then from the needle of the drip chamber. Puncture the IV bag and twist the needle of the drip chamber into place. With the rolling ball stopcock closed, squeeze the drip chamber one time.

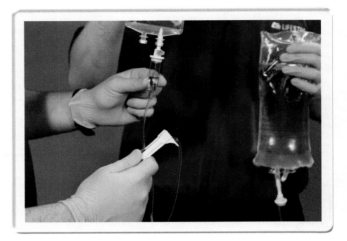

After the drip chamber has filled to one fourth to one third the volume of the chamber (usually to a mark on the chamber), open the stopcock chamber and allow the medication to fill the IV tubing. It is best to uncap the needle on the administration end until the medication runs out. Shut off the rolling ball stopcock and carefully recap the needle.

▼

 10 Ensure patency of original IV line.

Lower the primary IV bag below the level of the patient's arm and check for a blood return. A patent IV line should give a blood return. If no blood return occurs, a new IV should be started before starting the piggyback medication.

▼

 11 Cleanse injection port.

Clean the injection port with chlorhexidine, povidone-iodine, or an alcohol wipe.

▼

Step **Connect piggyback solution by inserting the needle into the injection port.**

Uncap the needle from the piggyback line and insert it into the injection port.

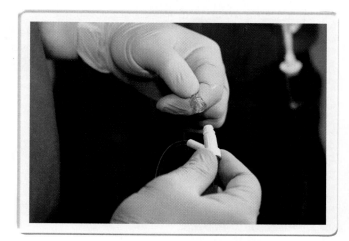

In most cases, it is best to use the injection port closest to the IV catheter. In the event a previous medication is already in the closest site, or when push medications are anticipated, a second IV may be necessary depending on medication compatibility.

Step  **Dispose of syringe and needle in proper container.**

Dispose of all contaminated equipment using puncture-resistant sharps containers and biohazard equipment as appropriate. Remember that not all equipment used is a biological hazard. Any used equipment or supplies that do not pose a threat of injury or biohazard exposure should be disposed of in normal trash receptacles.

Step  **Monitor for desired or adverse effects of medication.**

Watch the patient for the desired effects and for any adverse effects of the delivered medication. Be sure to document the response that has occurred.

 In the Field

Medication Infusion Pumps

Medication infusion pumps are the mainstay of hospital infusion therapy. Unfortunately, prehospital medicine has been very slow to utilize this safe and convenient piece of equipment. There are many different manufacturers of infusion pumps, each with slight differences in operation and, of course, each with a different type of infusion tubing, which means that the odds are low that your IV pump tubing is compatible with the pump tubing of the receiving hospital.

Modern infusion pumps are near miracles, especially for people who are mathematically challenged. You set up the infusion by programming in the amount of fluid in the bag, the amount of drug in or added to the bag, and the desired dosage. The pump calculates the drip rate.

There are some problems that will come up from time to time in the use of pumps. Most often these are line occlusions or air in the tubing. If they can be cleared, then the pump continues to work normally. If they can't be cleared, or if the battery fails, a standard drip infusion will have to be used as a backup system.

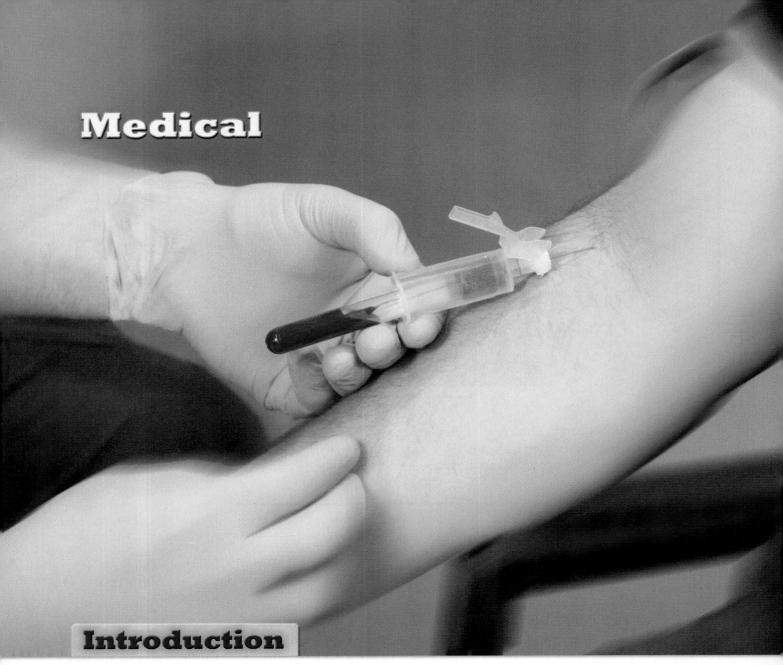

Medical

Introduction

General medical skills are used in all aspects of patient care. Although many of the skills in this section may be considered hospital skills, the reality is that there are also benefits to performing these skills in the prehospital setting.

The skills in this section include skills necessary for performing laboratory studies, as well as for the long-term management of patients.

Blood Collection

Performance Objective

Given a patient from which a sample of blood must be drawn and all the necessary equipment, the candidate shall demonstrate the procedure for performing multi-draw blood collection using vacuum tubes, in 10 minutes or less.

Equipment

The following equipment is required to perform this skill:

- Appropriate body substance isolation/personal protection equipment
- Sharps container
- Multidraw needle
- Multidraw vacuum tube barrel
- Blood collection vacuum tubes (appropriate for sample and desired tests)
- 4" × 4" gauze pads
- Tourniquet
- Cleaning solution
  - Chlorhexidine preps
  - Povidone-iodine preps
  - Alcohol preps
- Adhesive bandages

Equipment that may be helpful:

- Towels
- Vein identification lights
- Patient identification labels

Indications

- Collection of blood for laboratory studies

Contraindications

- None

Complications

- Infection
- Sterile abscess

Procedures

  Assemble equipment.

Gather the necessary equipment for performing multidraw blood collection: a multidraw needle, puncture-resistant sharps container, multidraw vacuum tube barrel, blood collection vacuum tubes for the lab tests ordered, a tourniquet, gloves, eye protection, a sterile 4″ × 4″ gauze pad, tape, an adhesive bandage, povidone-iodine swabs, and alcohol swabs.

   Assemble the needle barrel combination by breaking the paper seal. Screw the needle onto the barrel. Do not remove the second needle cover.

▼

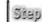 **Ensure body substance isolation before beginning invasive procedures and whenever contact with blood or body fluids can be reasonably anticipated.**

Prior to beginning patient care, appropriate body substance isolation procedures should be employed. In most cases, this should include gloves, masks, and eye protection, at a minimum. When treating patients with known infectious diseases, especially those spread by respiratory secretions, HEPA filter masks may be required.

▼

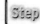 **Apply tourniquet and check pulse.**

Place the tourniquet 4″ to 6″ above the intended puncture site. Check the distal pulse to ensure that an arterial tourniquet has not been applied.

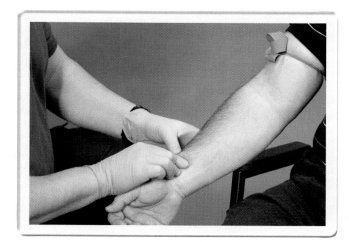

▼

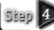 **Locate intended puncture site.**

Palpate the veins in the intended site to choose the most appropriate vessel. A firm, rubbery, relatively large surface vein is usually a good choice. This procedure is usually performed in the antecubital fossa, which offers three veins on most patients. Generally, the medial and lateral veins will stand up well, while a more centralized vein may be deeper. This central vein is used more often than the other veins.

▼

 Prepare injection site.

Prepare the insertion site by cleaning with an antiseptic/antimicrobial agent. A 30-second vigorous scrub using chlorhexidine will kill 99.9% of all colonizing microbes when the solution is dry. Chlorhexidine is safe for adults and children, but because of skin sensitivity, it should not be used on neonates.

If chlorhexidine is not available, povidone-iodine is an acceptable alternative. It is important to allow the povidone-iodine solution to dry completely before injecting the site. Alcohol may be used when the povidone-iodine is dry to clean the dye and improve visualization of the injection site.

Alcohol alone, as a prep for IV or hypodermic injection, should be considered below the standard of care. When assessing the patient's blood alcohol level, the use of alcohol to clean the site can place doubt on the accuracy of the test.

Cleanse the site by applying the solution in a circular motion, starting in the center and working out. It is best not to reenter the clean area after it is cleaned.

▼

Step 6 Insert needle and stabilize.

With the needle held at a 45° angle to the skin and the bevel up, make a quick, short stab into the vein. Be sure to push the entire lumen of the needle into the vein, or leaking around the puncture wound will occur. Stabilize the barrel, keeping the needle at a 45° angle.

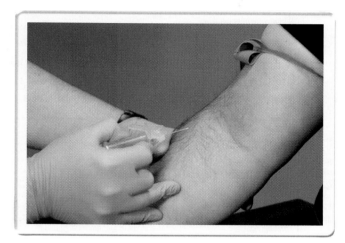

The method of holding the barrel as you make the puncture is a matter of personal preference. The best methods allow the needle to be held in your dominant hand until the puncture is made, then your nondominant hand will take control of the barrel and stabilize it in the vein. It is important that when the needle enters the vein, its position should not change, either by degree or depth.

Step 7 Advance blood collection tubes and ensure proper filling.

Place a vacuum tube into the barrel and gently push it onto the rubber-covered needle. Blood should begin to shoot into the collection tube. Adjust the vacuum tube to draw in the correct amount of volume into the tube. Be sure to allow the tube to finish filling.

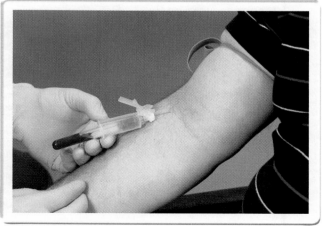

In the Field

How Much Blood is Needed?

For blood tubes to be viable for testing, they must be at least three fourths full. Follow local protocols for the types of blood tubes to fill.

Step 8 ▶ **Remove tube and invert.**

Keeping the needle in the current position, carefully remove the vacuum tube from the barrel and invert the tube several times.

▼

Step 9 ▶ **Repeat Steps 7 and 8 until last tube begins to fill.**

Continue the process of pushing a tube onto the needle, filling the tube, removing, and inverting until you are filling the last tube. Throughout this procedure, ensure the needle holds its position in the vein.

▼

Step 10 ▶ **Remove tourniquet.**

With the last tube filling in the barrel, remove the tourniquet from the patient. Be careful not to allow the tails of the tourniquet to enter the puncture site area and contaminate the sterile field.

▼

Step 11 ▶ **Remove last tube and invert.**

Remove the final tube, and invert it several times.

▼

Step 12 ▶ **Remove needle and discard.**

Place a 4″ × 4″ gauze pad over the puncture site, and carefully remove the needle from the vein. *Do not* hold pressure at the site while the needle is being withdrawn. Keep your attention focused on the needle, and immediately place it in a puncture-resistant sharps container. The barrel is not always considered to be disposable unless it is contaminated with blood.

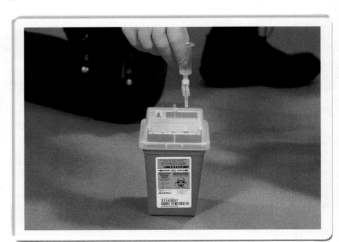

▼

Step 13 **Apply pressure to puncture site.**

Apply pressure to the puncture site. If the antecubital fossa was used to draw the blood, the patient can be instructed to bend the elbow to help hold pressure at the site. However, keeping the arm straight is preferred.

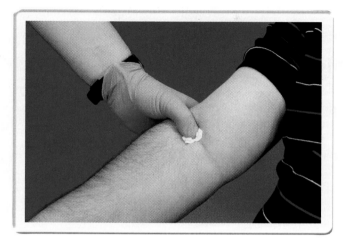

Step 14 **Invert tubes.**

Invert the tubes several more times to ensure a good mix of any chemicals that the tubes contain. *Do not* shake the tubes because this may injure the blood cells.

Step 15 **Label tubes.**

All tubes should be labeled with the patient's name, the time, the date the blood was drawn, and the initials of the person who collected the sample.

Step 16 **Apply ointment and dress puncture site.**

Place an antibiotic ointment on the pad of an adhesive bandage and place it on the puncture site.

Step 17 **Properly dispose of contaminated equipment.**

Dispose of contaminated equipment. Material that has been contaminated by blood or body fluids should be disposed of in biohazard bags. Waste materials that are not contaminated by blood or body fluids can be disposed of in normal trash receptacles.

Blood Glucose Measurement

Performance Objective

Given a patient with the need for blood glucose measurement, the candidate shall demonstrate the ability to perform a finger stick blood glucose assessment and perform the required interventions, in 5 minutes or less.

Equipment

The following equipment is required to perform this skill:
- Appropriate body substance isolation/personal protection equipment
- Sharps container
- Lancet
- Glucometer (with test strips or cassette)
- 4″ × 4″ gauze pads
- Cleaning solution
  - Chlorhexidine preps
  - Povidone-iodine preps
  - Alcohol preps
- Adhesive bandages

Equipment that may be helpful:
- Spring-loaded lancet device

Indications

- Altered mental status of possible diabetic or hypoglycemic origin
- Rule out hypoglycemia as cause of altered mental status

Contraindications

- None in emergency situations

Complications

- None in emergency situations

Procedures

 Ensure body substance isolation before beginning procedures.

Prior to beginning patient care, appropriate body substance isolation procedures should be employed.

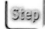 **Assemble equipment.**

Gather the necessary equipment for performing finger stick blood glucose measurement using a glucometer. At a minimum, this should include gloves, eye protection, a glucometer with matching test strips or cassettes, povidone-iodine swabs and alcohol swabs, sterile 4″ × 4″ gauze pads, adhesive bandages, and lancets or a spring-loaded puncture device.

 Prepare glucometer.

Turn the glucometer on and perform initial self-test of start-up procedures. With many glucometers on the market, be sure to follow the procedures specified by the individual manufacturer. This may include initial calibration using check strip tests or high/low calibration tests.

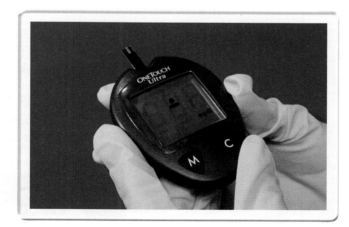

 In the Field

Calibrating and Preparing the Glucometer

Preparing the glucometer is an important step for accurately measuring the blood glucose level. This is done by following the manufacturer's recommendations and should be performed prior to being needed by the patient. Each glucometer will have specific schedules outlining how often and to what level calibration should be performed. At the very least, be sure to perform calibration and tests during the daily check of the ambulance equipment.

Step **4** ▶ **Select and prepare puncture site.**

Begin by washing the patient's hands with soap and water (if available). Wet wipes may be used if soap and water are not immediately available. Dry the hands thoroughly when finished.

Examine the end of the patient's fingers to find a fingertip free of calluses or scar tissue. The most preferable sites are the tip of the middle or ring fingers;

however, any fingertip will work. Prepare the finger for puncture by allowing it to dangle for 10 to 15 seconds. Clean the finger with povidone-iodine swabs and/or alcohol swabs. Allow the finger to dry thoroughly before performing the stick with the lancet.

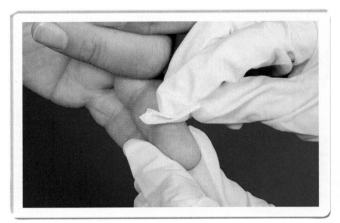

Step **5** ▶ **Perform finger stick.**

Target the lancet or spring-loaded device to make a puncture slightly off center on the fleshy part of the fingertip. Perform the puncture using one of the following procedures:

- Using a simple lancet, twist off the cover of the needle. With your nondominant hand, hold the target finger firmly. Make a quick and deep jab with the lancet into the target area of the fingertip.
- If using a spring-loaded device, load the needle according to the manufacturer's recommendations. With your nondominant hand, hold the target finger firmly. Hold the tip of the device against the target area, and release the trigger.

Gently squeeze the finger to obtain a large drop of blood. Wipe the first drop of blood with a 4″ × 4″ gauze pad, and squeeze a second drop of blood.

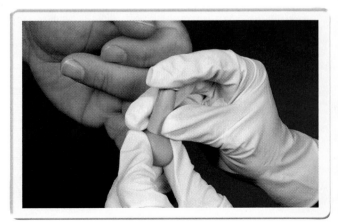

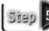

Safety Tips

Normal Blood Glucose Values
Adult: 70 to 110 mg/dL
Neonatal: 30 to 60 mg/dL

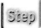 **Step 6 > Dispose of sharps.**

Dispose of the used lancet or sharp from the spring-loaded device into a sharps container.

▼

 Step 7 > Apply an adequate drop of blood to the test strip/cassette.

Following the manufacturer's recommendation, apply the drop of blood to the test strip or cassette. Allow the blood to enter the strip or cassette completely. If the test strip or cassette has difficulty collecting the blood, use a second strip or cassette to obtain the sample. Never reuse a strip or cassette, even on the same patient.

▼

Step 8 > Obtain blood glucose concentration measurement.

Insert the test strip or cassette into the glucometer as recommended by the manufacturer. Follow the recommended steps to obtain the concentration measurement. It may take between 10 to 60 seconds for the machine to read the concentration.

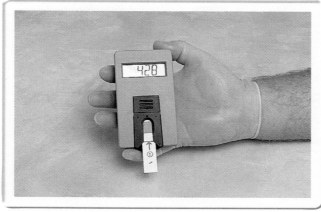

▼

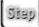 **Step 9 > Place an adhesive bandage on the finger stick site if desired by patient.**

If desired by the patient, complete the procedure by applying an adhesive bandage over the puncture site.

▼

In the Field

Finger Stick or Venous Blood Sample?

Glucometers are calibrated to measure capillary blood collected from the fingertip. The use of plasma or serum samples collected through an IV or from a multidraw tube sample will be inaccurate and are usually off by as much as 10% or higher. To achieve accurate readings from venous blood, it is necessary to reoxygenate the sample. Because this is nearly impossible to perform outside of the laboratory, it is best to always use a fingertip sample when measuring blood glucose.

 Step 10 **Perform appropriate management of patient.**

Management of the patient should be guided by the overall assessment and presentation. Blood glucose levels are simply one tool in this assessment. Although blood glucose measurements are usually accurate, be prepared to manage the patient based on the total findings and not the results of one test. In simple terms, always treat the patient and not the glucometer.

For low blood glucose levels, or for other indications of hypoglycemia, the administration of glucose is an essential element of patient care. Base the method of administration on established protocols as written and approved by your medical director. This may include, but is not limited to, the administration of oral glucose or an intramuscular injection of glucagon.

Foley Catheterization

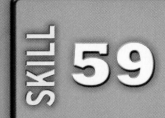

Performance Objective

Given a patient who meets the criteria for urinary catheterization and all necessary equipment, the candidate shall demonstrate the proper procedures for placing a Foley catheter, in both male and female patients, in 5 minutes or less per patient.

Equipment

The following equipment is required to perform this skill:
- Appropriate body substance isolation/personal protection equipment
- Prepackaged urinary catheterization tray (highly recommended), containing:
  - Urinary catheter
  - Urine collection bag
  - Sterile gloves
  - Sterile water-soluble jelly
  - Cotton balls
  - Povidone-iodine solution
  - Tweezers
  - Saline-filled syringe (appropriate for catheter)
- Tape

Indications

- Management of urinary incontinence
- Monitoring of urinary output in the critically ill or injured

Contraindications

- Bleeding meatus
- Scrotal hematoma

Complications

- Urinary tract/kidney infection
- Septicemia
- Urethral injury
- Bladder stones
- Hematuria

Procedures

 Assemble equipment.

Open the urinary catheterization set with proper sterile procedure. Remove the set from the plastic wrap and place on flat surface. Remove the glove package and put aside.

 Ensure body substance isolation before beginning invasive procedures and whenever contact with blood or bodily fluids can be reasonably anticipated.

Prior to beginning patient care, appropriate body substance isolation procedures should be employed. In most cases, this should include gloves, masks, and eye protection, at a minimum. When treating patients with known infectious diseases, especially those spread by respiratory secretions, HEPA filter masks may be required.

 Prepare sterile field.

Open the paper flaps: top flap away from you first, both side flaps, then the bottom flap toward you. This is now a sterile field and should not be touched without sterile gloves.

Don the sterile gloves. Position the draping over the perineal area. Ensure the urethral opening is accessible through the opening in the drape. Open the povidone-iodine and pour it over the swabs.

Prepare the lubrication for the catheter by squirting the jelly onto the sterile tray.

Test the patency of the cuff by inflating with the saline-filled syringe provided, then deflate, leaving the syringe attached to the port.

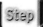 **Step 4 ▶ Clean urethral opening.**

Females

With your nondominant hand, open the labia. With your sterile dominant hand, wipe the povidone-iodine swabs over the urethral opening from top to bottom. Ensure that the immediate surroundings of the labia are cleansed. *Do not* wipe through the vagina or anus into the urethral field. Be sure to use each swab, and use each swab only once. This should give a minimum of four cleansing wipes. A final wipe with a clean swab will reduce burning as the catheter is inserted.

Males

Grasp the penis in your nondominant hand. With the sterile dominant hand, wipe the glans penis with the povidone-iodine swabs using circular motions. Be sure to use each swab, and use each swab only once. This should give a minimum of four cleansing wipes. Active scrubbing is not necessary. A final wipe with a clean swab will reduce burning as the catheter is inserted.

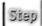 **Step 5 ▶ Lubricate catheter.**

With the sterile hand, pick up the urinary catheter and lubricate the end with sterile jelly from the tray. Wrapping the catheter in the hand will prevent dragging it through a nonsterile area. Ensure the insertion area remains sterile throughout the application procedure. An unclean labia or foreskin can contaminate the sterile field.

 In the Field

Inserting a Catheter
Catheters may remain in place (indwelling catheters, such as Foley catheters) or may be used intermittently (straight catheters). The principles for catheterization remain the same for both genders, but anatomy differences change the process.

Step 6 ▶ Insert catheter.

Females

Locate the urinary meatus anterior to the vagina and insert the catheter.

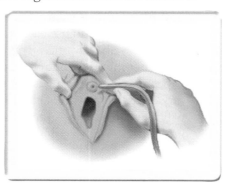

Insert the catheter until urine appears in the collection tube. Insert a few centimeters more and stop.

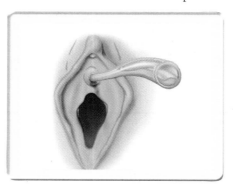

Males

Hold the catheter at a 90° angle to the body and insert the catheter.

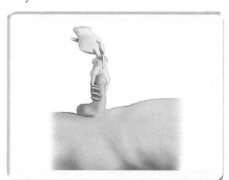

Insert the catheter as far as it will go. The balloon port should be in contact with the glans penis.

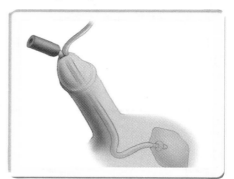

Step 7 ▶ Inflate cuff.

Inflate the cuff to the amount specified on the collar of the port, and remove the syringe.

8 ▶ **Pull the catheter into position.**

Pull the catheter back carefully until resistance is felt.

▼

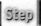 ▶ **Lower the urine collection bag.**

The sterile procedure is now complete. Lower the catheter bag and evaluate the urine return. Tear the drape from around the catheter and discard.

Females

Males

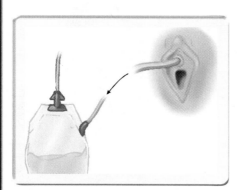 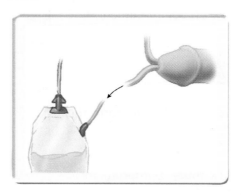

▼

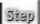 ▶ **Secure the catheter.**

Secure the catheter to the patient's thigh or abdomen with a piece of adhesive tape.

Nasogastric Tube Insertion

Performance Objective

Given a patient who meets the criteria for placement of a nasogastric tube and all necessary equipment, the candidate shall demonstrate proper placement, in 5 minutes or less.

Equipment

The following equipment is required to perform this skill:

- Appropriate body substance isolation/personal protection equipment
- A Salem sump (nasogastric tube) appropriate for patient (usually 14F to 18F for adults)
- 60-mL syringe with catheter tip
- Stethoscope
- Water-soluble lubricating jelly
- Suction device
- Tape

Equipment that may be helpful:

- Towel

Indications

- All intubated patients
- Toxic substance ingestion (as appropriate for toxin)

Contraindications

- Facial fracture
- Caustic substance ingestion
- Use caution in patients with esophageal varices

Complications

- Stimulation of gag reflex and vomiting
- Nasal bleeding/pharyngeal bleeding
- Tracheal intubation
- Gastric ulcers from constant suctioning

Procedures

 Step 1 ▶ Ensure body substance isolation before beginning procedures.

Prior to beginning patient care, appropriate body substance isolation procedures should be employed.

 Step 2 ▶ Assemble equipment.

Gather the necessary equipment for nasogastric tube insertion. You will need a Salem sump (nasogastric tube) 14F to 18F, 60-mL syringe with catheter tip, stethoscope, lubricating jelly, suction device, and tape. Towels and other draping material are helpful.

In the Field
Anesthetic Spray
Occasionally, patients with sensitive gag reflexes will benefit from the application of an anesthetic to the uvula and back of the tongue. Topical sprays are available for this purpose.

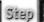 **Step 3 ▶ Measure tube.**

Measure the tube by positioning the tip at the patient's sternum and pulling up to the ear, bending the tube to the tip of the nose. Tubes are marked in 10-cm increments. Note the location of the closest mark.

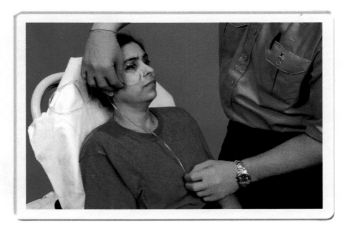

In the Field
Orogastric Tubes
Orogastric tubes may also be inserted in a similar manner. Simply measure from the navel to the jaw and bend to the mouth. Orogastric tubes can be placed easily in intubated patients where no gag reflex exists.

Step **4** Lubricate tube.

Apply lubricating jelly to the tip of the tube.

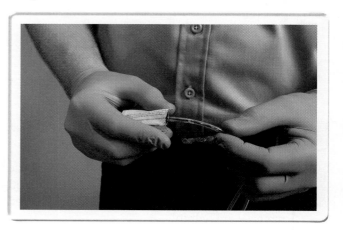

In the Field

Controlling Nasal Bleeding
To reduce the risk of nosebleed during the introduction of the nasogastric tube, alpha-adrenergic agents can be administered nasally. This will constrict nasal blood vessels and limit bleeding from mucosal injury.

 Step **5** Insert through naris.

Gently guide the tube straight back, perpendicular to the face, instead of following the bridge of the nose.

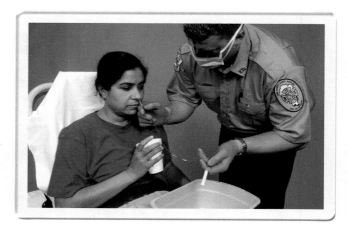

Slight resistance will be felt at the back of the nasal cavity. Twist the tube through this point and have the patient begin to swallow. Lifting the patient's head will flex the neck and help prevent tracheal aspiration of the nasogastric tube. Continue to insert the tube until it has reached the desired depth, without stopping and while continuing to coach the patient to swallow.

Step 6 ▷ **Assess position.**

Attach a 60-mL syringe filled with air to the end of the tube. With a stethoscope positioned over the epigastrium, rapidly push the air into the tube. A rapid burping sound should be heard through the stethoscope if the tube is in the correct position. Gastric contents in the tube can help confirm placement but are not absolutes. Conscious patients should be able to talk with the tube properly placed.

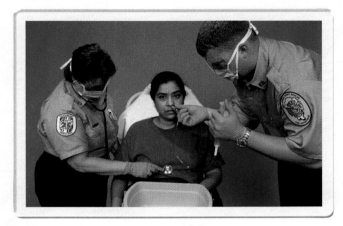

Step 7 ▷ **Secure the tube.**

Secure the nasogastric tube to the patient's nose with a short piece of tape. The tube should be closed off if it is not attached to suction or used for lavage.

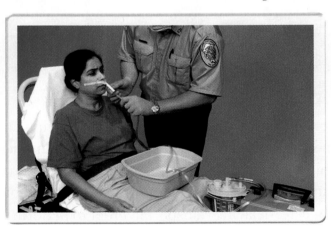

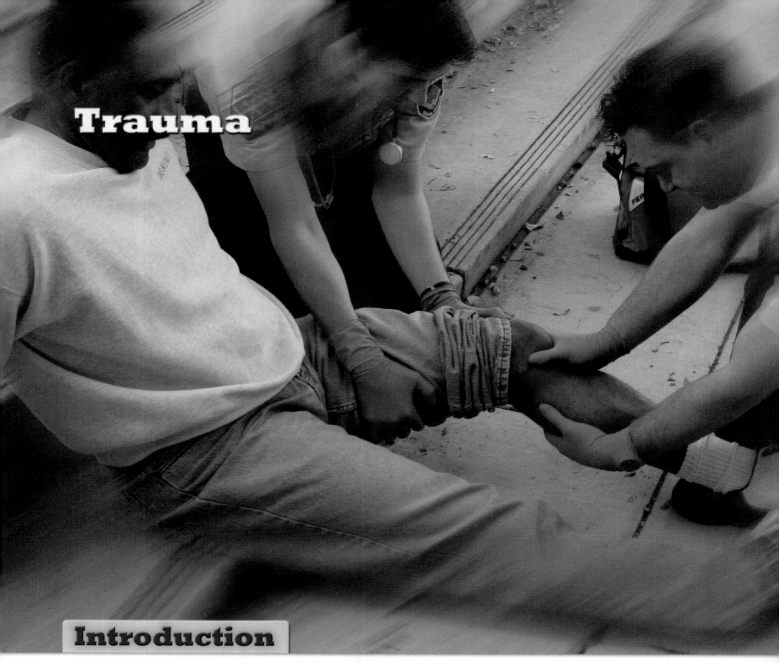

Trauma

Introduction

Trauma is the number one killer of children and young adults. Trauma management skills are important in the control of bleeding and in the stabilization of spinal injuries, fractures, and dislocations.

The most important trauma skill in the management of a trauma patient is often rapid transport. Although the management of bleeding and the stabilization of spinal injuries and fractures are a part of total patient care, delaying transport in order to perform such skills can be a fatal error. Always weigh the importance of patient care against the immediate needs of the patient. In general, trauma care for a patient with serious injuries should involve assurance of an airway, management of serious hemorrhage, stabilization of the cervical and thoracic spine, and rapid transport. Bleeding control and splinting can be deferred or performed en route to the hospital.

It is important to learn how to perform each of the skills in this section and to learn when they should be used. Proper management of trauma patients is essential in reducing death and disability.

General Bandaging Techniques

Performance Objective

Given a patient and a description of the patient's injuries, the candidate shall apply a dressing and bandage according to the principles of hemorrhage control and aseptic technique, in 10 minutes or less.

Equipment

The following equipment is required to perform this skill:

- Appropriate body substance isolation/personal protective equipment
- 4" × 4" gauze dressings
- 5" × 9" dressings
- 3" roller bandages
- 6" roller bandages
- Triangular bandages
- 1" tape (cloth or silk)

Equipment that may be helpful:

- Multitrauma dressings
- Elastic roller bandages
- Sterile saline (500 mL and 1,000 mL bottles)

Indications

- Control of external hemorrhage

Contraindications

- None

Complications

- Tight bandages may lead to constriction of distal circulation.

Procedures

 Ensure body substance isolation before beginning procedures.

Prior to beginning patient care, appropriate body substance isolation procedures should be employed.

 Check circulation (capillary refill or pulse) distal to injury before bandaging.

A check of the distal circulation through capillary refill or pulse check must be performed when appropriate and possible.

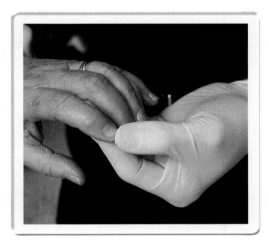

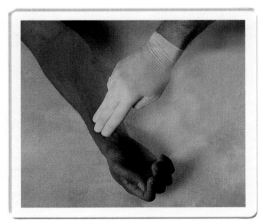

Step 3 ▶ Check sensation distal to injury before bandaging.

Assessment of sensation must be performed on all extremities. This step is not possible for wounds to the head, eye, or neck or in situations of amputation.

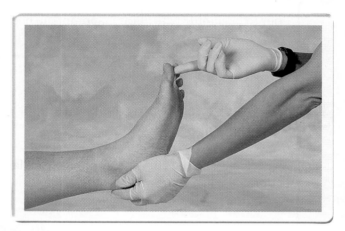

Step 4 ▶ Check motor function distal to injury before bandaging.

Assessment of motor function must be performed on all extremities. This step is not possible for wounds to the head, eye, or neck or in situations of amputation.

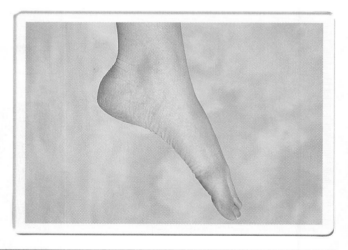

Step 5 Cover injury completely with clean dressing(s) demonstrating aseptic technique.

A clean (preferably sterile) dressing must cover the entire wound. The technique used to apply the dressing must not contaminate the surface of the dressing that will be placed next to the wound.

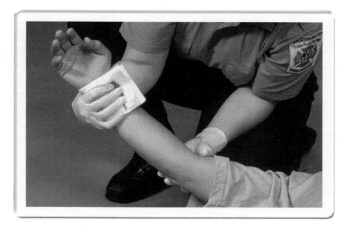

Step 6 Secure dressing using appropriate pressure with no excessive movement.

Apply pressure sufficient to control hemorrhage without compromising circulation, unless pressure is contraindicated. Adequate bulk must be applied when pressure is contraindicated.

Bandages must completely cover all dressing materials and be secure enough to hold both the dressing and bandage in place without slippage. The entire process of dressing and bandaging must not cause excessive movement. Excessive movement is defined as any movement that would lead to the aggravation of the injury and cause harm to the patient.

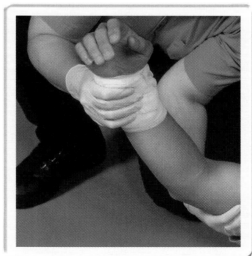

Use bandaging technique appropriate to injury.

Technique must control hemorrhage without aggravation of the injury.
See suggested procedures in Skill 63 for techniques appropriate for specific types of injuries.

▼

 Reassess circulation (capillary refill or pulse), sensation, and motor function distal to injury after bandaging.

A check of the distal circulation through capillary refill or pulse check must be performed when appropriate and possible. Reassessment of motor function and sensation must be performed on all extremities. This step is not possible for wounds to the head, eye, or neck or in situations of amputation.

Bleeding Control and Shock Management

Performance Objective

Given a patient and a description of the patient's injuries, the candidate shall apply the principles of hemorrhage control and shock management, in 10 minutes or less.

Equipment

The following equipment is required to perform this skill:
- Appropriate body substance isolation/personal protection equipment
- 4" × 4" gauze dressings
- 5" × 9" dressings
- 3" roller bandages
- 6" roller bandages
- Triangular bandages
- 1" tape (cloth or silk)
- Blanket

Equipment that may be helpful:
- Multitrauma dressings
- Elastic roller bandages
- Sterile saline (500 mL and 1,000 mL bottles)

Indications

- Control of external hemorrhage and shock

Contraindications

- None

Complications

- None

Procedures

This is a sequential procedure. The actual care of the patient will dictate which of the following steps are included. Assessment of circulation, sensation, and motor function distal to the injury should be performed at some point in this sequence (as described in Skill 61). The actual point at which this assessment takes place will depend on the severity of the situation. Less severe bleeding will allow more opportunities for distal assessment than life-threatening hemorrhage.

 Ensure body substance isolation before beginning procedures.

Prior to beginning patient care, appropriate body substance isolation procedures should be employed.

 Identify wound and apply dressing and direct pressure.

Upon identification of a bleeding wound, immediately apply a dressing and direct pressure.

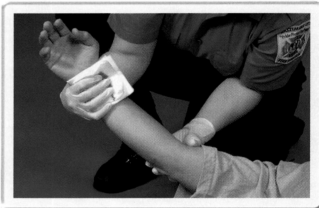

 Elevate extremity.

Elevate the extremity while maintaining direct pressure.
    Note: If the wound continues to bleed, continue to Step 4. If bleeding is controlled, proceed to Step 6.

Step 4 Apply an additional dressing to the wound without removing the first dressing.

If the wound continues to bleed, a bulk dressing may be needed. Leaving the first dressing in place, apply additional dressings to the wound. Continue to apply direct pressure with elevation.

   Note: If the wound continues to bleed, continue to Step 5. If bleeding is controlled, proceed to Step 6.

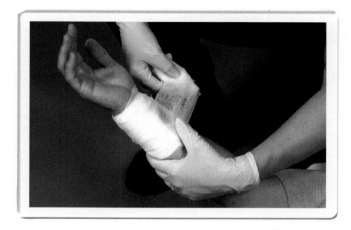

Step 5 Locate and apply pressure to appropriate arterial pressure point.

If bleeding is still not controlled, locate the artery above the wound. Apply pressure to the pressure point. If the initial pressure point fails to control bleeding, a more proximal artery should be tried.

   Recent studies have brought in to question the effectiveness of using pressure points in severe hemorrhage. It is acceptable, if allowed by protocol and local policy, to move directly to the use of a tourniquet without attempting pressure point control.

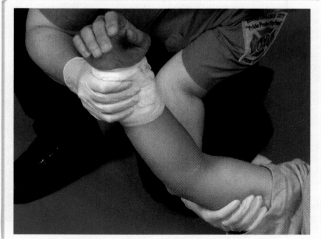

Step **5** continued

As a last resort to stop bleeding, a tourniquet may be applied. If a tourniquet is deemed necessary, it should be applied quickly and *not* released until after a physician has repaired the wound. Many rescuers use a blood pressure cuff as a tourniquet. This is acceptable as long as the cuff pressure can be maintained. A slow leak in cuff pressure can be severely damaging to the patient.

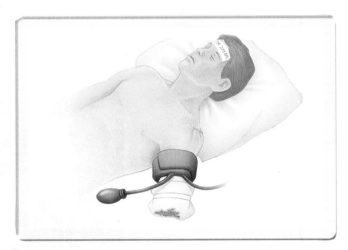

Step **6** ▶ **Bandage the wound.**

Once bleeding is controlled, cover the dressing completely with an appropriate bandaging technique.
    Note: Perform a patient assessment to evaluate the patient's condition. If the patient presents with signs and symptoms of hypovolemia, proceed to Step 7.

Step **7** ▶ **Properly position the patient.**

Place the patient supine and elevate the legs. In conscious patients, or patients who are breathing on their own, a modified Trendelenburg position is preferred over a true Trendelenburg position.

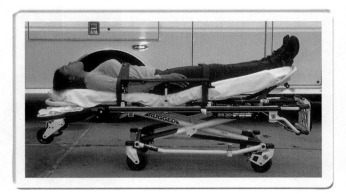

Step 8 **Apply high-concentration oxygen.**

Place the patient on high-flow, high-concentration oxygen via a nonrebreathing mask. Adjust oxygen therapy based on oxygen saturation as measured by pulse oximetry (S_pO_2) and end-tidal carbon dioxide.

▼

 Step 9 **Initiate steps to prevent heat loss from the patient.**

Place a blanket over the patient to keep the patient from losing body heat. Do not assume that outside temperatures are high enough that a blanket is not needed.

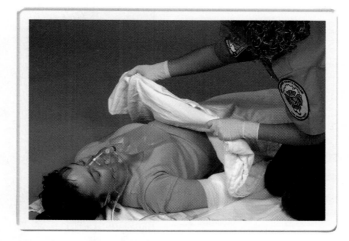

▼

 Step 10 **Begin immediate transportation.**

Hypovolemic shock is a serious medical condition. Immediate transportation to a trauma center is essential.

Bandaging Techniques for Specific Injuries

Performance Objective

The candidate should be able to perform the following bandaging techniques. Alterations to these techniques are permitted provided the objectives of the skill are met.

Equipment

The following equipment is required to perform this skill:
- Appropriate body substance isolation/personal protective equipment
- 4" × 4" gauze dressings
- 5" × 9" dressings
- 3" roller bandages
- 6" roller bandages
- Triangular bandages
- 1" tape (cloth or silk)

Equipment that may be helpful:
- Multitrauma dressings
- Elastic roller bandages
- Sterile saline (500 mL and 1,000 mL bottles)

Indications

- Specific to injury

Contraindications

- Specific to injury

Complications

- Excessive pressure can cause tourniquet effect with loss of distal circulation

Procedures

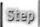 **Ensure body substance isolation before beginning procedures.**

Prior to beginning patient care, appropriate body substance isolation procedures should be employed.

▼

 Evaluate distal circulation (capillary refill or pulse), sensation, and motor function distal to injury as required (see Skill 61).

As appropriate and depending on the location of the injury, assess circulation, sensation, and motor function distal to the injury site.

▼

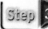 **Apply appropriate dressings and bandages specific to the injury.**

Using aseptic technique, apply sterile dressings and bandages to the injury. Procedures specific to common injuries are detailed in the following subsections.

Scalp Laceration (Without Skull Fracture)

Because of the injury location, no evaluation of distal circulation, sensation, or motor function is required.

Using aseptic technique, apply a sterile dressing to the wound. Apply several more pieces of dressing material on top of the dressing to add bulk.

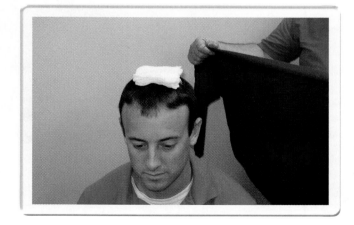

Step **3** continued

Apply direct pressure. The direct pressure must be continued until the bandage is applied and secured.

Make a 1″ fold along the base (long side) of a triangular bandage, and fold to the outside. Place the bandage over the top of the patient's head with the base positioned level with the eyebrows and the apex (point) behind the head.

Pull the two ends tightly around the back of the head, making sure the apex is underneath, and tie a half knot low on the back of the head.

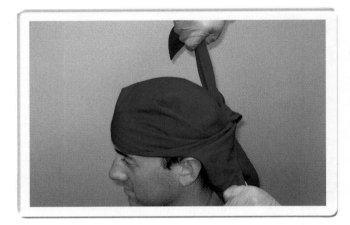

If the tails are long enough, return the two ends to the front of the head and tie a square knot. Tuck the ends to keep them out of the patient's eyes.

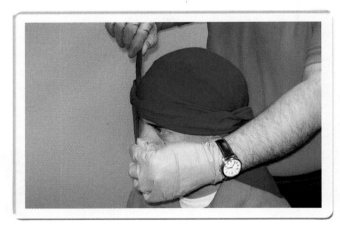

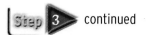 continued

Scalp Laceration (With Skull Fracture)

Because of the injury location, no evaluation of distal circulation, sensation, or motor function is required.

Using aseptic technique, apply a sterile dressing to the wound. Apply several more pieces of dressing material on top of the dressing to add bulk without placing direct pressure on the site. The added bulk must be sufficient to control hemorrhage without using direct pressure. It may be necessary to place large pieces of roller gauze bandage on the first dressing.

While holding the dressing materials in place, wrap a few turns of roller bandage around the head from forehead to back and anchor in place.

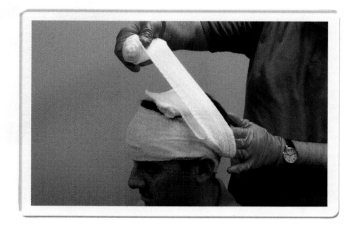

With recurrent turns, completely cover the top of the head and all dressing materials, including bulk.

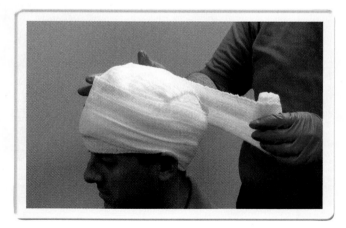

Secure in place using roller bandage applied around the forehead and back of head.

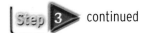

Step **3** ▶ continued

Eye Injury

Because of the injury location, no evaluation of distal circulation, sensation, or motor function is required.

All injuries that involve the globe of the eye should be covered with a moist, sterile dressing and bandaged without using pressure. Cups, pediatric oxygen masks, or commercially made eye shields should be used to avoid pressure of any kind.

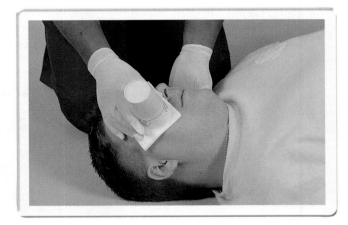

Both the injured and uninjured eye should be covered to avoid sympathetic movement of the injured eye as the uninjured eye tracks. Be sure not to bandage over the patient's nose or mouth.

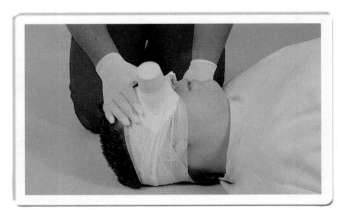

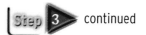

continued

Facial Cheek Laceration

Because of the injury location, no evaluation of distal circulation, sensation, or motor function is required.

Using aseptic technique, apply a sterile dressing over the cheek laceration. Have the patient open his or her mouth to check for a through-and-through laceration. If the laceration continues into the oral cavity, place a sterile dressing into the mouth, between the cheek and gum, leaving a corner of the dressing visible. This is important to prevent aspiration by the patient. Additional dressing materials may be applied to the external dressing to form a bulk dressing.

Holding the dressing in place, wrap a few turns of roller bandage around the forehead and back of head and anchor. On successive turns, bring the roller bandage over the dressing materials and pull tightly to achieve a pressure dressing.

Avoid covering the patient's mouth or nose. When bandages are properly applied, the patient should not have any bandaging materials below the eyebrow of the uninjured side. All dressing materials should be covered by the roller bandage.

Neck Laceration

Distal circulation should be assessed by checking the patient's level of consciousness and the carotid pulse above the injury site on the ipsilateral side.

Using aseptic technique, apply a sterile occlusive dressing (to prevent air embolism) to the laceration.

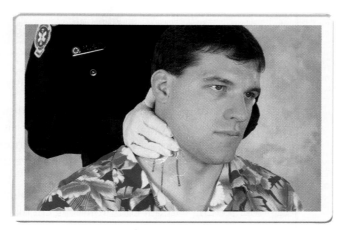

Secure with roller bandage wrapped around the injured side of the neck and the uninjured (opposite) armpit.

Reassess circulation and check that the airway has not been compromised.

Step **3** ▶ continued

Sucking Chest Wound

Distal circulation to sucking chest wounds should be assessed any time the wound is superior to the nipple line on the anterior chest. Circulation, sensation, and motor function should be assessed in the arm of the injured side; however, due to the seriousness of this condition, this assessment should be delayed until after the sucking chest wound has been treated.

Using aseptic technique, apply a sterile occlusive dressing to the laceration. Place a gauze dressing over the occlusive dressing and bandage in place on the superior, medial, and inferior sides. Leave the lateral side open to act as a flutter valve, allowing excess chest pressure to escape.

Watch your patient carefully. Should severe respiratory distress or other signs of a tension pneumothorax develop, remove the dressing and bandage to release the thoracic pressure. Once the tension pneumothorax has been reduced, replace the dressing and the three-sided bandage.

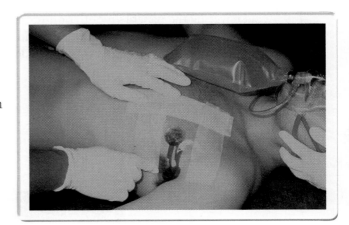

Joint Laceration

Assess circulation, sensation, and motor function distal to the injury site.

Using aseptic technique, apply a sterile dressing over the wound, covering the entire laceration. Place the extremity in a position of function (for instance, elbows should be flexed, placing the hand above the level of the elbow) and secure the dressing using a figure-of-8 (criss-cross) bandage with roller gauze.

Always wrap extremities from distal to proximal, using enough pressure to control bleeding without compromising circulation. All dressing material should be covered by the roller gauze.

Lacerations to upper extremities should be placed in a sling and secured with a swathe to avoid aggravation of the injury and for patient comfort (see Skill 66 for immobilization techniques). Reassess circulation, sensation, and motor function upon completion.

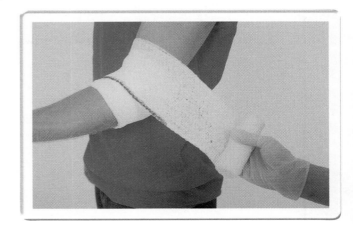

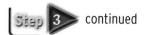 continued

Limb Laceration

Assess circulation, sensation, and motor function distal to the injury site.

Using aseptic technique, apply a sterile dressing over the wound, covering the entire laceration. Place the extremity in a position of function (for instance, elbows should be flexed, placing the hand above the level of the elbow) and secure the dressing using roller gauze.

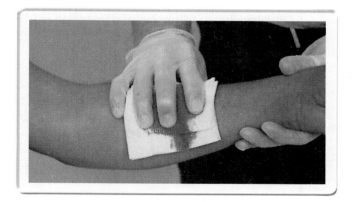

Always wrap extremities from distal to proximal, using enough pressure to control bleeding without compromising circulation. All dressing material should be covered by the roller gauze.

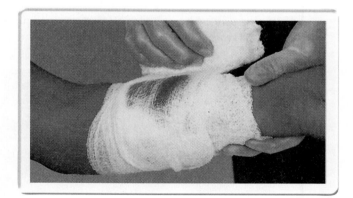

Lacerations to upper extremities should be placed in a sling and secured with a swathe to avoid aggravation of the injury and for patient comfort. Reassess circulation, sensation, and motor function upon completion.

Step 3 continued

Open (Compound) Fracture

The dressing and bandaging of the laceration associated with a compound fracture always takes precedence over the immobilization of the fracture.

Assess circulation, sensation, and motor function distal to the injury site.

Using aseptic technique, apply a dry, sterile dressing over the wound, covering the entire laceration and all exposed bone. Place additional dressing materials if necessary to form bulk. If bone ends are protruding from the wound, place roller bandage on the medial and lateral side of the wound, running parallel to the bone(s). Secure the dressing, bulk, and roller bandage in place using triangular bandages applied in the following manner.

Place the body of the triangular bandage over the dressing and bulk with the apex of the bandage distal to the injury. Carefully tuck the tails of the triangular bandage under the injured extremity. Pull the tails of the triangular bandage snug and tie proximal to the injury using a square knot. Wrap a second triangular bandage around the distal end of the first bandage to secure the apex of the bandage.

Reassess circulation, sensation, and motor function before proceeding with the immobilization of the fracture (see Skill 66 for immobilization techniques).

Impaled Object

Impaled objects should never be removed from the body unless they are to the facial cheek or the object interferes with the performance of cardiopulmonary resuscitation (CPR). Impaled objects in the facial cheek may be removed after inspection inside the mouth reveals that the penetrating end of the object has not penetrated other structures, and that it is a potential cause of airway obstruction. If an object must be removed to perform adequate CPR, pack the wound with gauze to tamponade the bleeding.

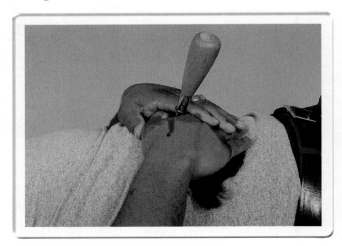

Distal circulation, sensation, and motor function should be assessed if the object is penetrating an extremity, shoulder, upper torso, groin, or hip.

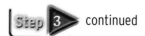 continued

Using aseptic technique, apply sterile dressings over the wound and around the impaled object. Stabilize the object by applying bulk dressings on all four sides.

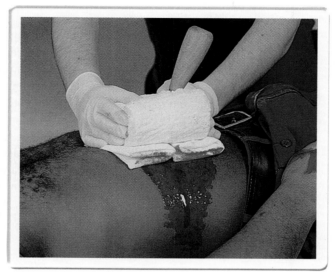

Bandage in place using sufficient pressure and bulk to control bleeding and stabilize the object without impeding circulation.

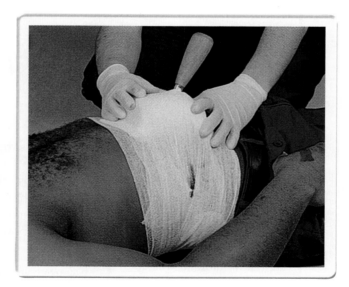

Reassess circulation, sensation, and motor function as appropriate.

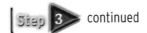

Step 3 continued

Amputations

Assessment of distal circulation, sensation, and motor function is impossible.

Using aseptic technique, apply a dry, sterile dressing to the stump of the extremity. Apply additional dressing materials as necessary to control hemorrhage. On rare instances, it may be necessary to apply a tourniquet above the injury to control bleeding. In most cases, however, direct pressure will be sufficient.

Anchor the roller bandage by wrapping a few turns around the extremity about 2 to 3 inches above the amputation. Using recurrent turns, completely cover the stump and all dressing materials. Secure by carefully tucking the end of the roller bandage.

Rinse the severed body part with sterile saline and blot dry with sterile dressing materials. Cover the severed end with dry, sterile dressings and wrap the entire part to keep it clean. Place the wrapped part in a plastic, watertight bag, and place on a bed of ice or in a container of ice water. Be sure to prevent the severed part from freezing. Transport the severed part with the patient to the hospital.

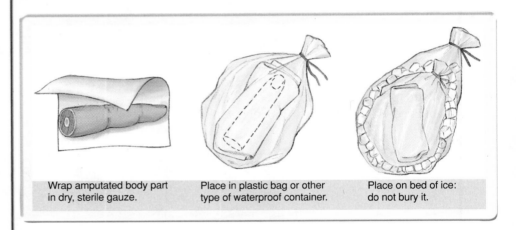

Wrap amputated body part in dry, sterile gauze.

Place in plastic bag or other type of waterproof container.

Place on bed of ice: do not bury it.

Burns

Smaller burns (less than 5% of the total body surface area) should be wrapped with dry dressings.

Cover all burned areas with sterile dressings using aseptic technique. Separate digits with gauze dressings unless fused together, and attempt to place them in a position of function. Gently wrap with loose, bulky roller bandage. Sling and swath upper extremity burns with the hand above the elbow.

Assess distal circulation often, if possible. Be prepared to loosen the bandage and reapply if circulation becomes compromised due to swelling.

If a burn involves a large percentage of the body, wrap the victim in a dry burn sheet. No additional bandaging is necessary for severe burns.

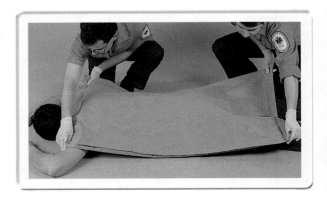

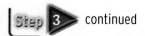
continued

Abdominal Organ Evisceration

Because of the injury location, no evaluation of distal circulation, sensation, or motor function is required.

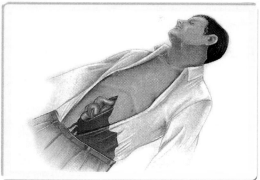

All protruding abdominal organs should be covered with a moist, sterile dressing using aseptic technique. Cover the moist dressing with an occlusive material (plastic package from multitrauma dressing, aluminum foil, etc.) to prevent wicking of contaminants. Do not attempt to replace the organs into the abdominal compartment.

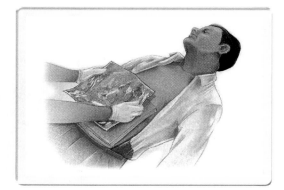

Secure the dressing in place using bandages or tape. Keep the eviscerated area and the patient warm.

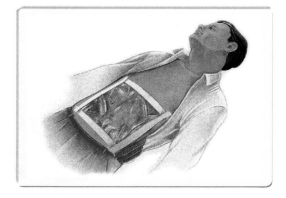

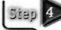 Reassess circulation, sensation, and motor function upon completion as required.

As appropriate and depending on the location of the injury, reassess circulation, sensation, and motor function as required upon completion.

64 Joint Injury

Performance Objective

Given a patient and a description of the patient's injuries, the candidate shall apply splinting techniques according to the principles of joint immobilization, in 10 minutes or less.

Equipment

The following equipment is required to perform this skill:
- Appropriate body substance isolation/personal protective equipment
- 3" roller bandages
- 6" roller bandages
- Triangular bandages
- 15" padded board splints
- 36" padded board splints
- 54" padded board splints

Equipment that may be helpful:
- Commercially made splinting kits
- Vacuum splint kits
- Ladder splints
- Long backboards
- Backboard straps

Indications

- Suspected fracture or dislocation of a joint

Contraindications

- None

Complications

- None

Procedures

 Step 1 Ensure body substance isolation before beginning procedures.

Prior to beginning patient care, appropriate body substance isolation procedures should be employed.

▼

 **Step 2** Direct application of manual stabilization of the injury.

Upon identifying a joint injury, ensure the joint is stabilized manually. A second rescuer should gently hold the injury while the first rescuer assesses the injury and prepares for the immobilization.

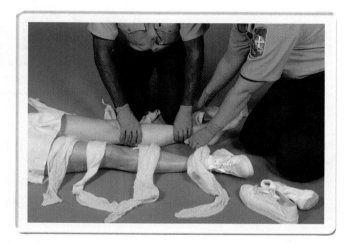

▼

 Step 3 Assess distal circulation, sensation, and motor function (see Skill 61).

A check of the distal circulation through capillary refill or pulse check must be performed when appropriate and possible. Assessment of sensation and motor function must be performed on all extremities.

Joint injuries found without a pulse, sensation, or motor function should not be manipulated without approval from medical control. Manipulation of joint injuries can create devastating neurovascular conditions.

▼

4 Select proper splinting material.

Based on the specific injury, gather and prepare the appropriate splinting materials. Be sure enough material is available to perform the entire procedure without stopping.

See Skill 66 for specific immobilization techniques for various types of injuries.

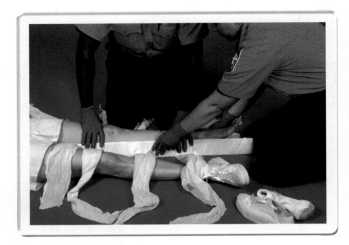

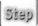 Secure and stabilize the bone above the injury site.

Apply and secure splinting material to the bone above the injury.

  Secure and stabilize the bone below the injury site.

Apply and secure splinting material to the bone below the injury.

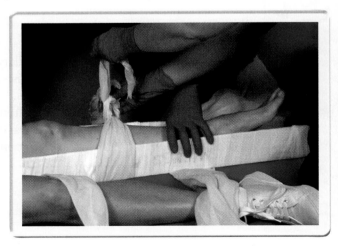

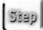 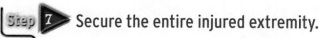
Step 7 Secure the entire injured extremity.

After completing the application of the initial splinting material, confirm that effective motion restriction has been achieved. Ensure that the injury does not bear distal weight.

▼

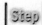
Step 8 Reassess distal circulation, sensation, and motor function.

A check of the distal circulation through capillary refill or pulse check must be performed when appropriate and possible. Assessment of sensation and motor function must be performed on all extremities.

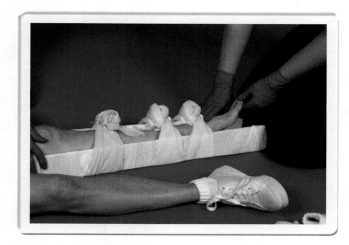

▼

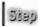
Step 9 Begin transport.

The patient should be readied for transportation to the emergency department. Simple joint injuries may be transported to non-trauma centers.

▼

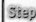
Step 10 Apply pain management.

Begin appropriate pain management. In many cases, ice or cold packs applied to the injury may be all that is available. In advanced life support systems, narcotic analgesics or inhaled anesthetics should be used.

Long Bone Injury

Performance Objective

Given a patient and a description of the patient's injuries, the candidate shall apply splinting techniques according to the principles of fracture immobilization, in 10 minutes or less.

Equipment

The following equipment is required to perform this skill:
- Appropriate body substance isolation/personal protective equipment
- 3" roller bandages
- 6" roller bandages
- Triangular bandages
- 15" padded board splints
- 36" padded board splints
- 54" padded board splints

Equipment that may be helpful:
- Commercially made splinting kits
- Vacuum splint kits
- Ladder splints
- Long backboards
- Backboard straps

Indications

- Suspected or confirmed fractures to long bones
- Muscular or soft-tissue injury to arms or legs

Contraindications

- None

Complications

- None

Procedures

Step 1 ▶ Ensure body substance isolation before beginning procedures.

Prior to beginning patient care, appropriate body substance isolation procedures should be employed.

▼

Step 2 ▶ Direct application of manual stabilization.

Upon identifying a long bone injury, ensure the joint is stabilized manually over open wounds with a dry, sterile dressing. A second rescuer should gently hold the injury while the first rescuer assesses the injury and prepares for the immobilization.

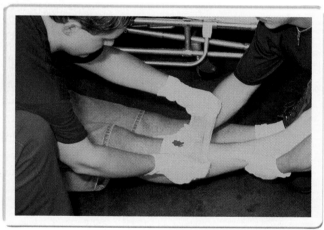

▼

Step 3 ▶ Assess distal circulation, sensation, and motor function (see Skill 61).

A check of the distal circulation through capillary refill or pulse check must be performed when appropriate and possible. Assessment of sensation and motor function must be performed on all extremities.

Angulated long bone injuries found without a pulse, sensation, or motor function should be slightly straightened with gentle traction in an attempt to return a blood flow into the extremity.

▼

Step **4** Select proper splinting material and measure splint.

Based on the specific injury, gather and prepare the appropriate splinting materials. Be sure enough material is available to perform the entire procedure without stopping.

Choose board splints or a commercially made device of appropriate size for the patient and the injury. Gently and without unnecessary movement, place the splint on the injured extremity.

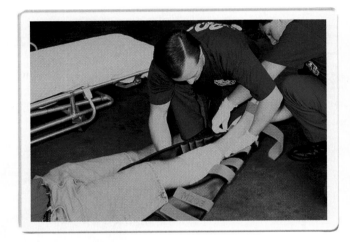

See Skill 66 for specific immobilization techniques for various types of injuries.

Step **5** Secure and stabilize the joint above the injury site.

Apply and secure splinting material to the joint above the injury.

Step **6** Secure and stabilize the joint below the injury site.

Apply and secure splinting material to the joint below the injury.

Step 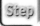 **7** Secure the entire injured extremity.

After completing the application of the initial splinting material, confirm that effective motion restriction has been achieved. Ensure that the injury does not bear distal weight.

Ensure position of function in hand or foot.

Before completion of the splinting process, ensure that the involved hand or foot is placed in proper position of function.

▼

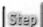 **Reassess distal circulation, sensation, and motor function.**

A check of the distal circulation through capillary refill or pulse check must be performed when appropriate and possible. Assessment of sensation and motor function must be performed on all extremities.

▼

Step 10 **Begin transport.**

The patient should be readied for transportation to the emergency department. Simple long bone injuries may be transported to non-trauma centers.

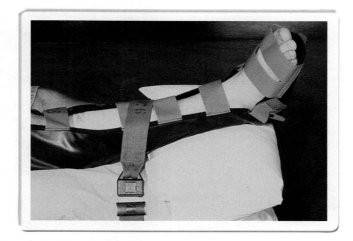

▼

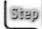 **Apply pain management.**

Begin appropriate pain management. In many cases, ice or cold packs applied to the injury may be all that is available. In advanced life support systems, narcotic analgesics or inhaled anesthetics should be used.

Performance Objective

The candidate should be able to perform the following immobilization techniques. Alterations to these techniques are permitted provided the objectives of the skill are met.

Equipment

The following equipment is required to perform this skill:
- Appropriate body substance isolation/personal protective equipment
- 3" roller bandages
- 6" roller bandages
- Triangular bandages
- 15" padded board splints
- 36" padded board splints
- 54" padded board splints

Equipment that may be helpful:
- Commercially made splinting kits
- Vacuum splint kits
- Ladder splints
- Long backboards
- Backboard straps (minimum of three)

Indications

- Specific to injury

Contraindications

- Specific to injury

Complications

- Specific to injury

Procedures

 Ensure body substance isolation before beginning procedures.

Prior to beginning patient care, appropriate body substance isolation procedures should be employed.

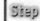 **Evaluate distal circulation, sensation, and motor function as required.**

As appropriate and depending on the location of the injury, assess circulation, sensation, and motor function distal to the injury site.

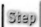 **Apply appropriate immobilization specific to the injury.**

Immobilize the injury. Procedures specific to common injuries are detailed in the following subsections.

Shoulder Injury

Assess circulation, sensation, and motor function distal to the injury.

Maintain the injury in the position found. Do not attempt to reposition the arm next to the body. Pillows or other forms of bulk may be needed to maintain the position of the arm. Apply a modified wrist sling around the opposite side of the neck.

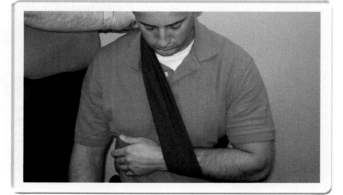

Secure with a minimum of two swathes. One of the two swathes should be positioned to prevent wrist drop.

Reassess circulation, sensation, and motor function.

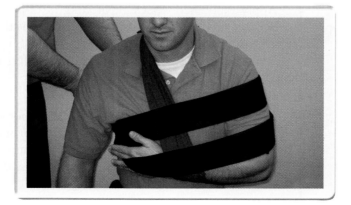

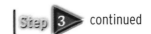

Step **3** ➤ continued

Scapula Fracture

Assess circulation, sensation, and motor function distal to the injury.

Maintain the injury in the position found. Do not attempt to reposition the arm next to the body. Apply a wrist sling around the neck.

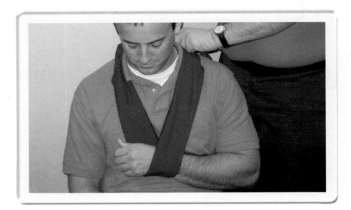

Secure with two swathes. One of the two swathes should be positioned to prevent wrist drop.

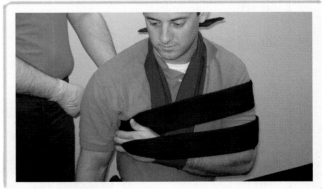

Reassess circulation, sensation, and motor function.

Clavicle Injury

Assess circulation, sensation, and motor function distal to the injury.

Apply a modified wrist sling around the opposite side of the neck.

Secure with two swathes. One of the two swathes should be positioned to prevent wrist drop (see the photos shown in the "Shoulder Injury" section).

Reassess circulation, sensation, and motor function.

Humerus Fracture

Assess circulation, sensation, and motor function distal to the injury.

Most fractured humeri are found with the arm next to the body. Generally a board splint is not needed to immobilize this injury.

However, if the arm is away from the body and cannot be gently brought into anatomic position without excessive pain to the patient, use a short arm board

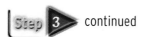

Step 3   continued

applied laterally. Apply a modified wrist sling around the opposite side of the neck. Secure with two swathes. One of the two swathes should be positioned to prevent wrist drop.

Reassess circulation, sensation, and motor function.

Elbow Injury: Joint Flexed, Arm Held Against Body

Assess circulation, sensation, and motor function distal to the injury.

Maintain the injury in the position found. No board splint is needed for this injury. Apply a wrist sling or modified wrist sling around the neck.

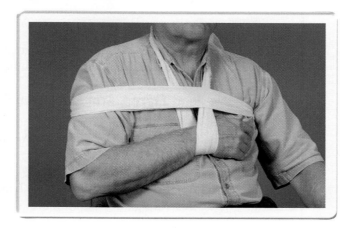

Secure with two swathes. One of the two swathes should be positioned to prevent wrist drop.

Reassess circulation, sensation, and motor function.

Elbow Injury: Joint Extended

Assess circulation, sensation, and motor function distal to the injury.

Maintain the injury in the position found. Apply a rigid splint from the upper arm to the fingertips. The board can be placed medial, lateral, or posterior depending on needs. Secure the splint with triangular bandages above and below the elbow, and above and below the wrist.

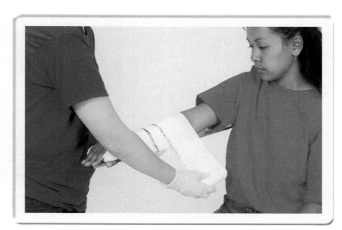

Step 3 continued

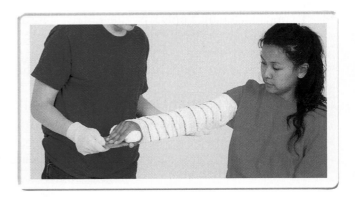

Elevate the injury with a pillow once the patient is supine.

Reassess circulation, sensation, and motor function.

Elbow Injury: Joint Flexed, Arm Away from Body

Assess circulation, sensation, and motor function distal to the injury.

Maintain the injury in the position found. Apply a rigid splint diagonal to the injury.

Secure the board to the humerus, below the elbow, and above and below the wrist. Either roller bandage or a triangular bandage may be used. Selection should be made depending on which can best secure the board with the least amount of movement. Roller bandage will work best most of the time. Keep the hand in a position of function if possible.

Move the arm into the body and apply a wrist sling around the neck. Secure with two swathes. One of the two swathes should be positioned to prevent wrist drop.

Reassess circulation, sensation, and motor function.

Radius or Ulna Fracture

Assess circulation, sensation, and motor function distal to the injury.

Position the arm with the elbow flexed, allowing the hand to rest higher than the elbow. Apply a rigid splint along the long axis of the arm from the elbow to the fingertips.

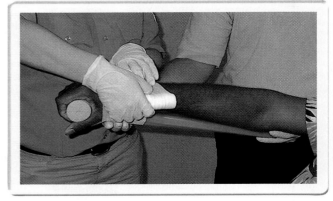

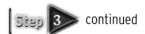

Step 3 continued

Keeping the hand in a position of function, secure the board above and below the injury and above and below the wrist using roller bandage or triangular bandages. Selection should be made depending on which can best secure the board with the least amount of movement. Roller bandage will work best most of the time.

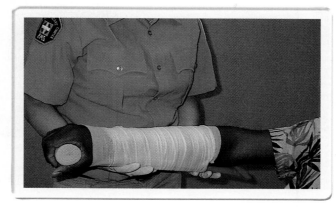

Move the arm into the body and apply a wrist sling around the neck. Secure with two swathes.

Reassess circulation, sensation, and motor function.

Wrist (Colles) Fracture

Assess circulation, sensation, and motor function distal to the injury.

Position the arm with the elbow flexed, allowing the hand to rest higher than the elbow.

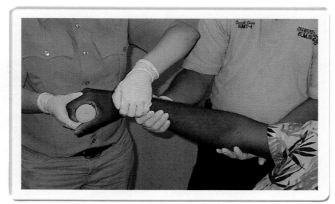

Apply a rigid splint along the long axis of the arm from the elbow to the fingers. Keeping the hand in a position of function, secure the board above and below the wrist using roller bandage.

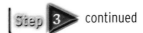

continued

Support all gaps using contour padding made from dressing material or roller bandage.

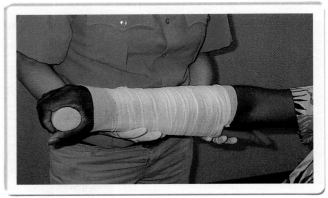

Move the arm into the body and apply a wrist sling around the neck. Secure with two swathes.

Reassess circulation, sensation, and motor function.

Femur Fracture: No Traction Splint Available or Compound Fracture

Assess circulation, sensation, and motor function distal to the injury.

Place a long board splint lateral to the leg, from the armpit past the ankle. A medium board splint should be applied medial to the leg from the groin past the ankle. Secure the boards above and below the knee, above and below the fracture site, and above and below the ankle. Position on a long backboard.

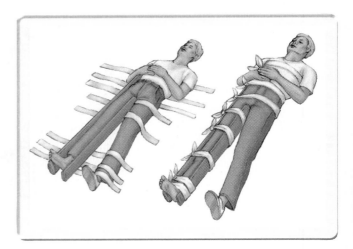

Reassess circulation, sensation, and motor function.

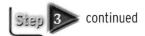

Step 3 continued

Femur Fracture: Proximal Injury

Assess circulation, sensation, and motor function distal to the injury.

The leg should be splinted in a 90/90 technique. Using pillows or other appropriate materials, position the injured thigh at a 90° angle to the torso.

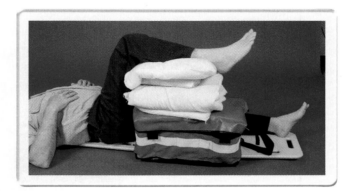

Secure the knee at a 90° angle to the thigh. Secure the entire leg to prevent movement during transport.

Reassess circulation, sensation, and motor function.

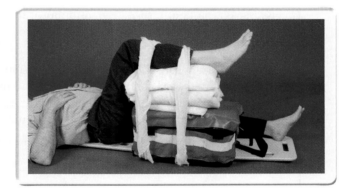

Hip or Pelvis Injury

Assess circulation, sensation, and motor function distal to the injury.

Place the patient on a long backboard. Stabilize the legs and hip in position found using pillows, blankets, or sheets. Secure with straps or triangular bandages.

Reassess circulation, sensation, and motor function.

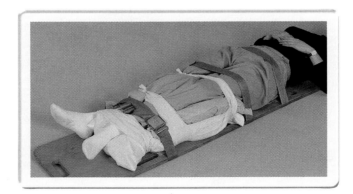

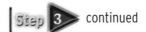

Step **3** continued

Knee Injury

Assess circulation, sensation, and motor function distal to the injury.

If the knee is flexed, splint the leg in the position found.

Place medium board splints on the lateral and medial sides of the leg. Secure using triangular bandages above and below the knee, and above and below the ankle.

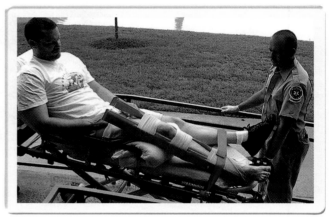

If the knee is straight, splint it straight.

Reassess circulation, sensation, and motor function.

Tibia or Fibula Fracture

Assess circulation, sensation, and motor function distal to the injury.

Place medium board splints on the lateral and medial sides of the leg. Secure using triangular bandages above and below the knee, and above and below the ankle.

Reassess circulation, sensation, and motor function.

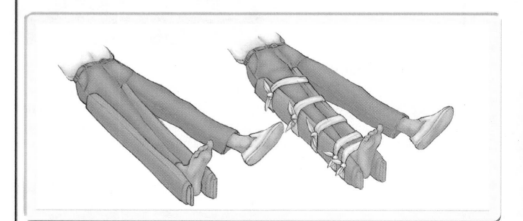

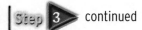 **3** ▶ continued

Ankle or Foot Injury

Assess circulation, sensation, and motor function distal to the injury.

Place medium board splints on the lateral and medial sides of the leg. Secure using triangular bandages above and below the ankle. A pillow may be used if it is long enough to immobilize the ankle completely.

Reassess circulation, sensation, and motor function.

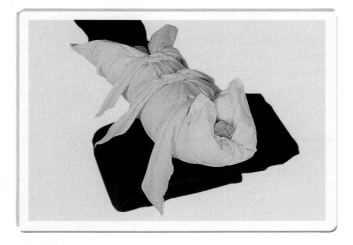

▼

 4 ▶ **Reassess circulation, sensation, and motor function upon completion as required.**

Reassess circulation, sensation, and motor function as required upon completion.

Spinal Motion Restriction—Seated

Performance Objective

Given a patient with a potential spinal injury, the candidate shall use the proper technique to immobilize the spine using short and long spinal immobilization devices, in 10 minutes or less.

Equipment

The following equipment is required to perform this skill:

- Appropriate body substance isolation/personal protective equipment
- Vest-style immobilization device, with
  - Neck pad
  - Chest and ischial straps
  - Head and chin straps
- Rigid extrication collars (various sizes or adjustable)
- Long backboard
- Backboard straps (minimum of three)
- Pillows

Equipment that may be helpful:

- Towels (for towel rolls and padding)
- Triangular bandages
- 3" roller bandages
- Web-type backboard straps

Indications

- Suspected or confirmed injury to the spine of a seated patient

Contraindications

- Multisystem trauma requiring rapid transport
- Environmental or situational hazards in which rapid removal is indicated

Complications

- Chest straps that are too tight may impede respiratory effort.

Procedures

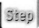 **Ensure body substance isolation before beginning procedures.**

Prior to beginning patient care, appropriate body substance isolation procedures should be employed.

 Direct assistant to place or maintain patient's head in the neutral, in-line position.

Have your partner take control of the seated patient's head and neck. This *must* be performed as soon as patient access is achieved. Ensure that the head and neck are maintained in the neutral position until they are *completely* stabilized with a rigid extrication collar and mechanical cervical motion restriction.

Tell the patient what is happening. Talking to the patient, conscious or not, and explaining what is happening will add to the success of the procedure.

 Assess distal circulation, sensation, and motor function in each extremity.

Check the distal circulation, sensation, and motor function in all four of the patient's extremities.

 **Apply an appropriately sized rigid extrication collar.**

Using an appropriate sizing method, choose the correct-sized rigid extrication collar for the patient. Explain to the patient the procedure for applying—and the need for—a rigid extrication collar. Apply the extrication collar without allowing flexion or extension of the patient's neck.

Manual immobilization must not be released to apply the extrication collar.

5 ▶ **Position the immobilization device behind the patient.**

Without compromising the integrity of the cervical spine, position the short device behind the patient. Begin by having your partner apply manual traction to the patient's head and neck while moving the patient's torso forward. All movement of the patient should be slow, steady, and coordinated. Usually a three count, given by the responder controlling the head, is used to ensure all responders work as a unit in the move.

Slide the immobilization device behind the patient and manipulate into position. While working the immobilization device behind the patient, be sure the device does not get caught on the patient's clothing or the car seat. Bring the side panels up into the axilla as high as possible without impeding circulation through the axillary artery.

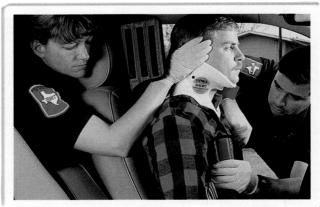

▼

 6 ▶ **Secure the device to the patient's torso.**

Instruct your partner to move the patient back into position against the back of the seat. Begin strapping the short device to the patient's chest. Attach all straps smoothly and snugly. Be sure to adjust each strap without twisting the device. The chest strap should be snug but should not compromise the patient's respiratory effort. Attach both ischial straps. These straps may be crossed or secured directly.

▼

Step **7** ▶ **Evaluate torso fixation.**

Before securing the head to the device, ensure the splint is firmly secured to the torso. The top strap should be securely tightened without impeding the patient's ventilatory effort. Adjust the device as necessary to ensure proper fit.

▼

Step 8 Evaluate and pad behind the patient's head as necessary.

It may be necessary to place a folded neck pillow behind the patient prior to achieving neutral alignment with the back of the board. Inspect the void between the patient and the device to determine the amount of padding required. When completed, the patient's face should be positioned looking directly forward, in a natural anatomic position. Be sure that the patient's neck is not flexed or hyper-extended.

Step 9 Secure the patient's head to the device.

Bring the head panels around both sides of the head and secure them in place with foam straps applied to the forehead. Chin straps may be needed as well. Neutral alignment of the patient's neck must be maintained by the partner throughout this step. Once this step is complete, tighten the chest strap. The head and neck must be in a neutral, in-line position when finished.

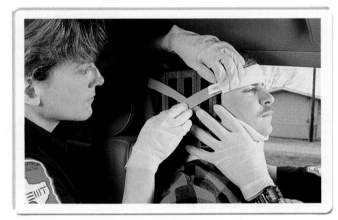

Step 10 Move the patient to a long backboard.

With the patient secured to the short device, move the patient to a long backboard.

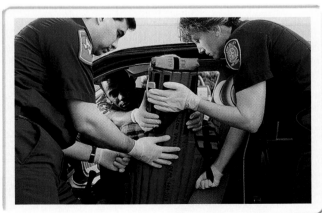

In the Field

Rapid Extrication

In situations in which the patient's condition or situation requires immediate removal from a vehicle, there is no time to apply a vest-style device. In these cases rapid extrication should be employed. This procedure begins identical to seated spinal motion restriction, but uses the rescuer's body as a support for the patient's torso as he or she is rotated to be laid onto a long backboard.

Follow these steps:
1. Support the cervical spine.
2. Apply a rigid extrication collar, sized appropriately for the patient.
3. Position the backboard on the cot or the seat next to the patient.
4. Carefully rotate the patient's upper and lower torso as a unit. Be sure the neck and legs follow appropriately.
5. Position the backboard under the patient's buttocks.
6. Lower the patient onto the backboard, maintaining neutral alignment of the spine.
7. Secure the patient to the backboard *before* removal from the vehicle and quickly assess pulse, sensation, and motor function in all four extremities.
8. Note in the patient care report the reason for the rapid extrication of the patient and the status of pulse, sensation, and motor function in all extremities before and after the move.

In the Field

Lifting and Carrying the Patient on a Long Backboard

It is always best to lift a backboard directly from the ground to the stretcher. When it is necessary to carry a patient on a backboard for any distance, the following techniques can be used.

- **Diamond carry.** This carry requires four rescuers. The two primary rescuers are positioned at the patient's head and feet, and use both hands to lift the patient. The remaining rescuers use one hand to carry the backboard from the center handholds. This carry is usually reserved for carrying the patient short distances.
- **One-handed carry.** This carry requires four or six rescuers. Each rescuer grasps a handhold at the chest or legs of the patient. If six rescuers are available, the additional two grab the center handholds. The patient is then lifted and carried to the desired location.

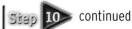 **10** continued

Place the end of the board under the patient's hip and rotate the patient *as a unit* in line with the long backboard. Carefully lower the patient onto the backboard.

Using longitudinal pulls, position the patient on the long backboard. Once the patient is properly positioned on the board, the ischial straps can be loosened. Strap and secure the patient to the long backboard. Remember that all patient movement must occur as a coordinated unit.

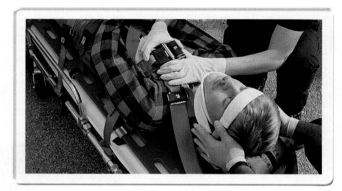

▼

 11 Reassess distal circulation, sensation, and motor function in each extremity.

Check the distal circulation, sensation, and motor function in all four of the patient's extremities.

Spinal Motion Restriction—Supine

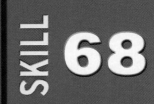

Performance Objective

Given a patient with a potential spinal injury, the candidate shall use the proper technique to immobilize the spine using short and long spinal immobilization devices, in 10 minutes or less.

Equipment

The following equipment is required to perform this skill:
- Appropriate body substance isolation/personal protective equipment
- Rigid extrication collars (various sizes or adjustable)
- Long backboard
- Backboard straps (minimum of three)
- Cervical immobilization device
- Pillows

Equipment that may be helpful:
- Towels (for towel rolls and padding)
- Web-type backboard straps
- Triangular bandages
- Adhesive tape

Indications

- Suspected or confirmed spinal injury

Contraindications

- None

Complications

- Decubitus ulcers
- Back pain

Procedures

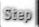 **Ensure body substance isolation before beginning procedures.**

Prior to beginning patient care, appropriate body substance isolation procedures should be employed.

 Direct assistant to place or maintain patient's head in the neutral, in-line position.

Have your partner take control of the patient's head and neck. This *must* be performed as soon as patient access is achieved. Ensure the head and neck are maintained in the neutral position until they are *completely* stabilized with a rigid extrication collar and mechanical cervical motion restriction.

    Tell the patient what is happening. Talking to the patient, conscious or not, and explaining what is happening will add to the success of the procedure.

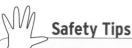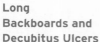

Safety Tips

Long Backboards and Decubitus Ulcers

Long backboards have been shown to greatly accelerate the incidence of decubitus ulcers in patients. Consider padding the entire length of the backboard, or using a scoop stretcher in lieu of a standard backboard. Scoop stretchers can be applied in an identical manner as described in this skill and simply broken apart upon arrival at the hospital.

 Assess distal circulation, sensation, and motor function in each extremity.

Check the distal circulation, sensation, and motor function in all four of the patient's extremities.

 Apply an appropriately sized rigid extrication collar.

Using an appropriate sizing method, choose the correct-sized rigid extrication collar for the patient. Explain to the patient the procedure for applying—and the need for—a rigid extrication collar. Apply the extrication collar without allowing flexion or extension of the patient's neck.

    Manual immobilization must not be released to apply the extrication collar.

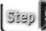

Step 5 Position the long backboard appropriately.

Position the long backboard beside the patient.

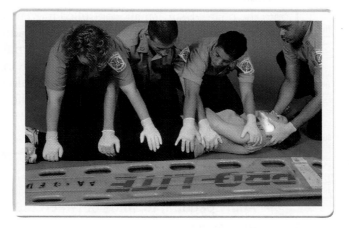

Step 6 Direct movement of the patient onto the long backboard without compromising the integrity of the spine.

With the aid of one or two *additional* rescuers, perform a log roll of the patient. The log roll should be performed by grasping the patient's torso and pelvis. With direction from the person stabilizing the head, roll the patient as a unit. A proper log roll should result in the entire spine being lifted without twisting or shifting.

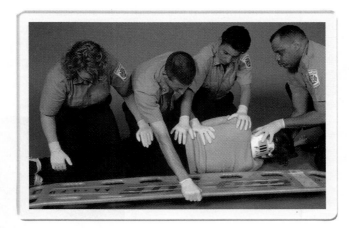

 In the Field

Rolling Patients
Log rolls and other procedures used to move a patient require a firm grasp of the patient, not the patient's clothing. Avoid attempting to move a patient by grabbing a collar, sleeve, or belt loop. Waistbands of pants are acceptable holding points only because they are usually sturdier than other pieces of clothing.

When controlling the head, a hold that incorporates the chest, neck, and head is much better than holding the head alone.

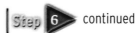 continued

Perform a quick and thorough examination of the patient's back and spine. Place the long backboard directly under the patient and roll the patient down onto the board. Using small, controlled movements, slide or lift the patient into proper position on the board. The patient should be positioned by sliding up or down along the long axis of the body, using a pulling motion. Pushing the torso up or over is never appropriate and may result in compression or separation of the spine. Each movement of the patient should be a coordinated event. In most cases the responder at the patient's head has the responsibility for signaling the other responders, usually with a three count, to ensure that all responders act as a unit.

 Apply padding to voids between the torso and the backboard as necessary.

Place padding in any voids found between the torso and the spine to reduce the possibility of spinal movement.

 Secure the patient's torso to the backboard.

Secure the patient to the board by placing a minimum of three straps. The first strap should be over the patient's chest, the second over the pelvis, and the third over the thighs. If the handholds and strapping holes on the backboard are not aligned to properly position the straps over the chest or abdomen, crossing the straps may be necessary. This is accomplished by running straps from a higher and a lower hole position on each side of the patient and crossing them as they are placed on the opposite side.

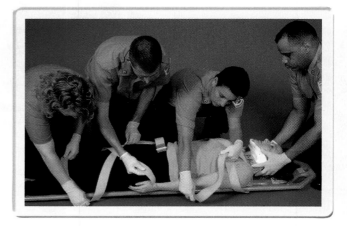

In the Field

Thinking Off the Board Long backboards have become the mainstay for trauma management. It has become customary for every trauma patient, with or without spinal injury, to be placed on a long backboard for transport. Although a safe move in many situations, this can be detrimental in others. One such case would be a patient with a diaphragmatic tear. These injuries can allow the abdominal organs to enter the thorax if the patient is laid down, causing difficulty breathing and agitation. In such cases the patient should be allowed to sit up as long as the blood pressure is not compromised. If spinal injury is suspected along with the torn diaphragm, support can be accomplished with a vest-type immobilization device. Always evaluate the need for a long backboard and spinal motion restriction before application. As with all aspects of medicine, these decisions should be based on the patient's best interest rather than reflex.

Step 9 Evaluate and pad behind the patient's head as necessary to maintain neutral, in-line position.

Evaluate the need for padding behind the head to ensure neutral position.

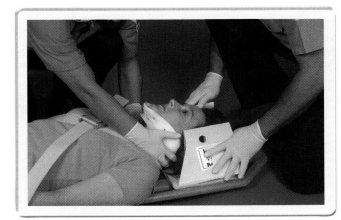

Most commercially made cervical immobilization devices (CIDs) have a small pad as a part of the device. *Do not* assume that the padding on the device is sufficient padding. When completed, the patient's face should be looking skyward in the supine position, parallel to the long backboard.

▼

 Step 10 Secure the patient's head to the long backboard.

Secure the patient's head to the long backboard using a cervical immobilization device, towel rolls, or other soft padding that restricts lateral movement. When complete, the head and neck must be in neutral, in-line position.

▼

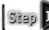 **Step 11** Secure the patient's legs to the backboard.

Place a pillow under the patient's knees to maintain a slightly bent position. This will place the back in the correct anatomic position. Ensure the patient's legs are secured to the long backboard by applying a fourth strap below the patient's knees.

▼

 Safety Tips

Helmet Removal
Helmets protect the patient from injury during an accident, but may pose obstacles to proper patient assessment and management if left in place. The decision to remove a helmet really is two-fold: Does the helmet disrupt cervical alignment, or can the airway be maintained? Before removing a helmet, evaluate the helmet and the situation.

- **Motorcycle helmets.** In most cases, motorcycle helmets should be removed prior to securing patients to long backboards. This will require two rescuers to work together. The first rescuer reaches into the helmet and supports the patient's head and neck. The second rescuer grasps the helmet by the chin straps and, pulling the straps out and up, gently removes the helmet.
- **Football helmets.** Football helmets are usually not removed in the prehospital setting. Since they are worn in conjunction with shoulder pads, cervical spine alignment is usually not compromised. By removing the face mask, easily accomplished with a tool called a Trainer's Angel, you can assess and maintain the airway. Removal of a football helmet without removal of the shoulder pads will require considerable padding to achieve cervical alignment and is usually not considered the standard of care.

Safety Tips

The Standing Patient With Spinal Injury

Occasionally, you will encounter a walking patient following an incident with a high index of suspicion for spinal injury. In such situations it is best to have the patient remain standing and perform spinal immobilization in the upright position.

 Step 12 Secure the patient's arms to the backboard.

Secure the patient's arms to the long backboard to prevent the arms from flailing when the board is lifted.

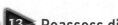

Step 13 Reassess distal circulation, sensation, and motor function in each extremity.

Check the distal circulation, sensation, and motor function in all four of the patient's extremities.

Traction Splinting—
Ratchet Device

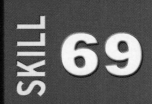

Performance Objective

Given a traction splint and a patient, the candidate(s) shall apply the traction splint to immobilize a closed fracture to the midshaft of the femur, in 10 minutes or less.

Equipment

The following equipment is required to perform this skill:

- Appropriate body substance isolation/personal protective equipment
- Ratchet-type traction splint, with:
  - Straps
  - Ankle hitch
  - Adjustable stand
- Long backboard
- Long backboard straps

Equipment that may be helpful:

- Triangular bandages
- Pillow

Indications

- Closed midshaft femur fracture

Contraindications

- Fractures of the proximal femur, hip, or knee
- Fractures of the lower leg on the same side

Complications

- None

Procedures

Ratchet-type traction splints require two people for proper application. Both partners have an equal responsibility to properly apply the device. Once the initial assessment has identified the fractured femur and the decision to apply a traction splint has been made, rescuers should work together using the following steps, with Rescuer One applying the splint and Rescuer Two pulling traction.

 Step 1 ▸ **Ensure body substance isolation before beginning procedures.**

Prior to beginning patient care, appropriate body substance isolation procedures should be employed.

▼

 Step 2 ▸

Rescuer One: Apply manual stabilization of the injured leg.

Upon recognition of a midshaft fracture to the femur, the first rescuer should stabilize the fracture by positioning his or her hands gently around the thigh. The objective is to reduce involuntary movement in the patient's leg muscles and to act as a shock absorber while the remainder of the leg is assessed.

Rescuer Two: Assemble and prepare splint.

Ensure the splint is adjusted to the proper size using the uninjured leg. The splint should be approximately 10 to 12 inches longer than the distance from the ischial tuberosity to the ankle. Prepare four straps and position them on the splint. It is best to position the straps toward the top of the splint and to pull the straps down into position as needed. Attempting to guess the proper position of the straps on the splint will usually lead to having to adjust straps up, working against the taper of the splint.

Release the traction ratchet and pull the strap out to its full length. Release and open the ischial strap.

▼

In the Field

What Is Traction?
Traction is the use of surrounding muscles to stabilize a fracture. Stretching the muscles supports the ends of the broken bone or separated joint. To achieve traction, only slight tension needs to be applied and maintained. The goal here is simply to pull on the muscles, not to realign the bone ends. Realignment or rearticulation is known as *reduction* and is performed only after further evaluation determines the correct course of action.

Step 3 **Rescuer One: Stabilize lower leg.**

Support the lower leg while the ankle hitch is applied.

Pressure should be enough that movement at the ankle does not reach the femur, but not so much that the lower leg is injured.

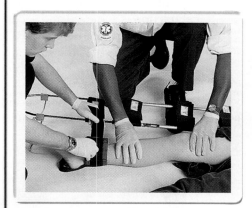

Rescuer Two: Assess distal circulation, sensation, and motor function. Apply ankle hitch.

If not already performed, carefully remove the patient's shoe.

Check the distal circulation through pulse check or capillary refill. Also assess the distal sensation and motor function.

With proper padding applied circumferentially around the ankle, apply an ankle hitch to the patient. The ankle hitch must be applied in a position to pull traction along the long axis of the bones of the lower leg. Minimal manipulation should be used to prevent additional injury to the fracture and surrounding soft tissue.

▼

Step 4 **Rescuer One: Position hands to lift thigh.**

Move hands up the leg and position under the thigh, one hand on each side of the fracture site.

Rescuer Two: Position hands to pull traction.

Support the limb as you position your hands to pull traction.

▼

Step 5 ▶ Rescuer One: Lift thigh.

Give your partner the direction to lift the patient's leg and pull traction while you lift the thigh.

Maintaining proper body position will reduce the risk of back injury to the responder.

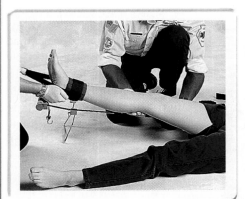

Rescuer Two: Lift leg and pull traction.

Working with your partner, gently lift the leg, pulling traction as you elevate. Sufficient elevation should be achieved to allow your partner to apply the splint under the leg. Once elevation and traction are achieved, the leg *must* remain in this position until mechanical traction is achieved and secured. Mechanical traction is secured after your partner secures the strap around the patient's ankle to the traction splint.

Maintaining proper body position will reduce the risk of back injury to the responder.

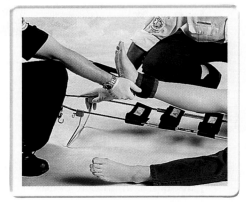

Step 6 **Rescuer One: Apply splint.**

Position the ischial pad under the patient's thigh and firmly against the ischium.

Apply padding across the inguinal region from both sides of the frame. Fasten the ischial strap tight enough to hold the splint, but not enough to impede circulation. Ensure the patient's genitalia are not trapped by the strap. Connect the ankle hitch to the frame and take up slack.

Using a mechanical ratchet or a windlass, tighten the connection of the ankle hitch. Once manual traction has been equaled, no further traction should be pulled (only 10% of the patient's weight is needed). If a windlass was used, secure the windlass to the frame to prevent traction from being lost.

Rescuer Two: Maintain control and elevation of the leg.

As mechanical traction is obtained, maintain elevation of the leg.

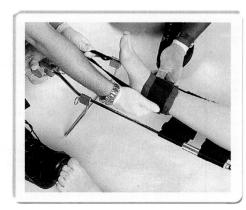

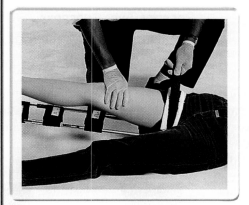

Step 7 **Rescuer One: Secure ankle hitch.**

Apply the splint strap just above the ankle. Mechanical traction is now complete.

Step 8 **Rescuer One: Apply remaining straps and lower the stand.**

Start by placing a strap below the ischial strap and continue down the leg, placing one strap above the fracture site, one strap below the fracture site, and the final straps below the knee. If cravats are being used, they should be tight enough to lift the leg into alignment with the ankle hitch. Cravats should be positioned to avoid placement directly over or around the fracture itself. However, Velcro straps can be placed over the fracture site if necessary. Knots should be tied to the splint and not over the patient's leg.

Lower the traction splint stand.

Rescuer Two: Lower splint and reassess patient.

Gently lower the splint to rest on the stand, and maintain control to prevent excessive movement.

Step 9  **Rescuer One: Reevaluate the proximal and distal securing devices.**

Inspect the splint to ensure the device is working properly. Check the ischial strap (proximal securing device) to ensure it remains secure. The ankle hitch (distal securing device) should be checked to ensure that it remains snug and pulls straight along the long axis of the leg and does not pull from or on the foot.

Rescuer Two: Reassess distal circulation, sensation, and motor function.

Check the distal circulation through pulse check or capillary refill. Also assess the distal sensation and motor function.

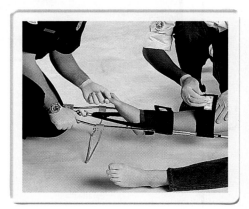

Step 10 Secure the torso and splint to the long backboard to immobilize the hip.

Once the traction splint has been applied, the patient should be moved onto a long backboard and secured so that the end of the traction splint is supported. Ensure that the stand remains on the long backboard so that the splint remains elevated.

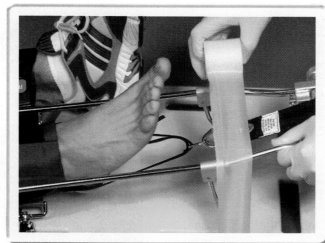

Traction Splinting—Sager-Type Device

Performance Objective

Given a traction splint and a patient, the candidate shall apply the traction splint to immobilize a closed fracture to the midshaft of the femur, in 10 minutes or less.

Equipment

The following equipment is required to perform this skill:
- Appropriate body substance isolation/personal protective equipment
- Sager-type traction splint, with
  - Straps
  - Ankle hitch
- Long backboard
- Long backboard straps

Equipment that may be helpful:
- Triangular bandages
- Pillow

Indications

- Closed midshaft femur fracture

Contraindications

- Fractures of the proximal femur, hip, or knee
- Fractures of the lower leg on the same side

Complications

- None

Procedures

Step 1  Ensure body substance isolation before beginning procedures.

Prior to beginning patient care, appropriate body substance isolation procedures should be employed.

▼

Step 2  Direct application of manual stabilization of the injured leg.

Upon recognition of a midshaft fracture to the femur, direct another rescuer to stabilize the fracture site.

The fracture site should be stabilized by positioning your hands gently around the thigh. The objective is to reduce involuntary movement in the patient's leg muscles and to act as a shock absorber while the remainder of the leg is assessed. During the application of the ankle hitch, move your hands down to hold the lower leg. Pressure should be enough that movement at the ankle does not reach the femur, but not so much that the lower leg is injured.

▼

Step 3  Assess distal circulation, sensation, and motor function.

Check the distal circulation through pulse check or capillary refill. Also assess the distal sensation and motor function.

▼

Step 4  Position the splint.

Position the splint between the patient's legs, resting the ischial perineal cushion (the saddle) against the ischial tuberosity, with the shortest end of the articulating base toward the ground. In the case of a unilateral fracture, the splint should be placed in the perineum on the side of the injury. In bilateral fractures, excluding pelvic trauma, the splint should be placed on the side with the greatest degree of injury.

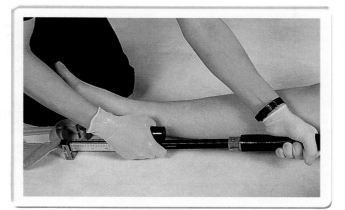

▼

Step 5 ▶ **Apply the thigh strap and adjust the splint.**

Apply the thigh strap around the upper thigh of the fractured limb. Push the ischial perineal cushion gently down while at the same time pulling the thigh strap laterally against the ischial tuberosity. Tighten the thigh strap snugly. Lift the spring clip to extend the inner shaft of the splint until the crossbar rests adjacent to the patient's heels.

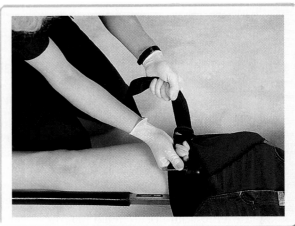

Step 6 ▶ **Apply the ankle harness.**

Position the ankle harness beneath the heel(s) and just above the ankle(s).

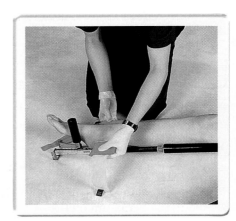

Fold down the number of comfort cushions needed to engage all of the ankle above the medial and lateral malleoli. Using the attached hook and loop straps, wrap the ankle harness around the ankle to secure snugly. Pull control tabs to engage the ankle harness tightly against the crossbar.

Step 7 ▶ **Apply quantifiable dynamic traction.**

Grasp the padded shaft of the splint with one hand and the traction handle with the other. Gently, extend the inner shaft of the splint until the desired amount of traction is recorded on the traction scale.

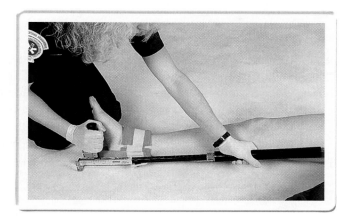

It is suggested to use 10% of the patient's body weight per fractured femur, up to 7 kg (15 lb) per leg (this would be a maximum of 14 kg [30 lb] for bilateral fractures).

▼

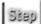 **Step 8** ▶ **Position and secure the support straps. (Velcro straps may be applied directly over the fracture site.)**

At the hollow of the knees, gently slide the large elastic leg cravat through and upward to the thigh. Repeat this process with the remaining cravats to minimize lower and midlimb movement.

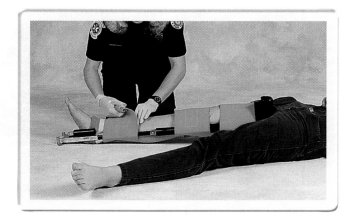

▼

Adjust straps and secure the feet.

Adjust the thigh strap at the upper thigh, making sure it is snug and secure. Ensure that all elastic leg cravats are secure. Apply the figure-of-eight strap around the feet to prevent rotation of the leg(s).

 Reevaluate the proximal and distal securing devices.

Inspect the splint to ensure the device is working properly. Check the ischial strap (proximal securing device) to ensure it remains secure. The ankle hitch (distal securing device) should be checked to ensure that it remains snug and pulls straight along the long axis of the leg and does not pull from the foot.

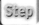 **Reassess distal circulation, sensation, and motor function.**

Check the distal circulation through pulse check or capillary refill. Also assess the distal sensation and motor function.

 Secure the torso and splint to the long backboard to immobilize the hip.

Once the traction splint has been applied, the patient should be moved onto a long backboard and secured so that the end of the traction splint is supported.

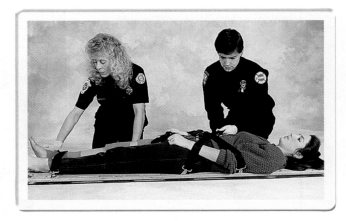

Pneumatic Antishock Garment

Performance Objective

Given a patient, the candidate shall demonstrate the proper application of the pneumatic antishock garment (PASG) using the criteria herein described, in 5 minutes or less.

Equipment

The following equipment is required to perform this skill:
- Appropriate body substance isolation/personal protective equipment
- Pneumatic antishock garment
- Long backboard
- Long backboard straps

Indications

- Hemorrhagic shock
- Pelvic fracture
- Lower-body air splint

Contraindications

- Pulmonary edema
- Patients too large or too small for the device
  - Do not place children in a single leg of an adult device.
  - Use devices specifically designed for pediatric patients only if they fit the child. Increased abdominal pressure can cause severe respiratory compromise.

Complications

- Pulmonary edema
- Accelerated blood loss

Procedures

Step **Ensure body substance isolation before beginning procedures.**

Prior to beginning patient care, appropriate body substance isolation procedures should be employed.

Step **Assess distal circulation, sensation, and motor function.**

Check the distal circulation through pulse check or capillary refill. Also assess the distal sensation and motor function.

In the Field

Use of Pneumatic Antishock Garments

There is little evidence to support the use of pneumatic antishock garments. If used at all, they should be used cautiously and limited to pelvic fractures or as a lower-body air splint.

Step **Prepare patient for application of the PASG.**

Remove the patient's pants and underwear. Ensure that all sharp objects have been removed from the inflation area. This will prevent the garment from becoming damaged and unable to accomplish its purpose.

The PASG should be applied with the patient on a long backboard. Some systems will place the PASG on the board before the patient, then position it on the patient after the log roll.

Step  **Position and align garment.**

Place the PASG under the patient's legs and carefully work it under the patient's hip.

Remember: This patient may have a lower spine injury. Caution should be used to prevent additional injury.

Position the top of the garment below the patient's lower rib margin. The midsection should be carefully aligned along the spine.

Note: Clothes should be removed before applying the PASG in the field.

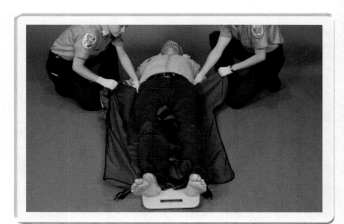

Step 5 ▶ Secure leg sections.

Snugly wrap the leg sections around the patient's legs. Because of the design of the garment, it will be easiest to wrap the left leg first and then the right. However, wrapping the right leg first will accomplish the same objective.

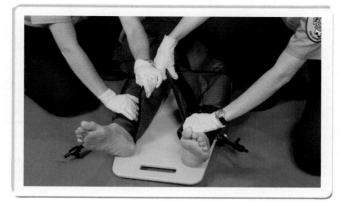

Step 6 ▶ Secure abdominal section.

Snugly apply the abdominal section. If the patient's abdomen is too large for the abdominal section to fit (from pregnancy, obesity, or just largeness), inflation of the garment is contraindicated in most situations.

Step 7 ▶ Inflate garment.

Close the valve to the abdominal section and ensure that the valves to both leg sections are open.

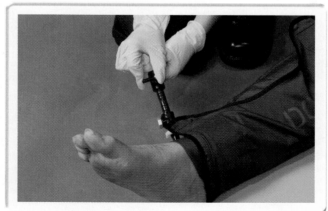

Using the foot pump, inflate both leg sections. Close the leg valves. Open the abdominal section valve and inflate. Close the abdominal valve. If desired, all three compartments can be inflated at one time. Stop inflating when the Velcro starts to crackle off the pop-off valve or the pop-off valve opens.

8 **Set valves to prevent loss of air from garment.**

Recheck the valves for all sections of the PASG, making sure they are closed.

▼

 9 **Transport patient.**

Use of a PASG on a patient requires transportation to a trauma center. Transport should begin without delay.

Performance Objective

Given a patient who meets the criteria for decompression of a tension pneumothorax and all of the appropriate equipment, the candidate shall demonstrate the procedures to safely perform needle decompression, in 3 minutes or less.

Equipment

The following equipment is required to perform this skill:
- Appropriate body substance isolation/personal protection equipment
- Prepackaged pneumothorax decompression kit (highly recommended), containing:
  - 16-gauge catheter or larger (some are wire-wrapped catheters that prevent collapse)
  - Scalpel
  - One-way valve
  - Connecting tubing with three-way valve
  - Seal or petroleum dressing
- Stethoscope
- Tape
- Cleaning solution
  - Chlorhexidine preps
  - Povidone-iodine preps
  - Alcohol preps

Equipment that may be helpful:
- Multiple pneumothorax sets

Indications

- Tension pneumothorax, with rapid development into critical respiratory distress or cardiac arrest, from thoracic trauma

Contraindications

- None

Complications

No complications *if performed correctly*. However, the following may occur if performed improperly:
- Inadvertent puncture of costal vessels and nerves
- Subcutaneous emphysema
- Puncture/laceration of pulmonary tissue:
  - Leading to hemothorax
  - Leading to worsening pneumothorax

Procedures

Step **Ensure body substance isolation before beginning procedures.**

Prior to beginning patient care, appropriate body substance isolation procedures should be employed.

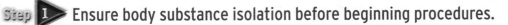

▼

Step  **Maintain sterility and safety throughout procedure.**

Ensure that all sterile equipment and the aseptic field are not contaminated. Maintain safety with needles, and use body substance isolation appropriately.

▼

In the Field
Signs of Tension Pneumothorax

Shock (a late sign), decreased breath sounds, and hyperresonance to percussion on the same side of the chest indicate a tension pneumothorax until proven otherwise.

Step  **Assess breath sounds, jugular vein distension, and tracheal shift.**

Verify the presence of a tension pneumothorax by assessing the patient's breath sounds, jugular vein distension, and degree of tracheal shift. Remember that jugular vein distension is a late sign and that a tracheal shift may not appear above the sternal notch. Confirmation should be made based on the patient's worsening dyspnea, decreased breath sounds, mechanism of injury, and hyperresonant chest. In cases of cardiac arrest from trauma, only a mechanism of injury to the chest and pulseless electrical activity may indicate the presence of a tension pneumothorax.

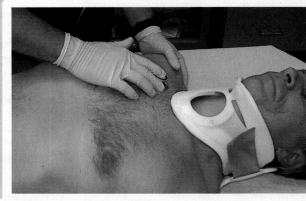

▼

Step 4 ▶ **Assemble equipment.**

Gather the necessary equipment to perform the needle decompression. Pre-packaged needle decompression kits are best, especially kits that contain wire-wrapped catheters. If a prepackaged set is not available, the equipment must be gathered from standard equipment. This will include at least one 2″, 14-gauge or larger catheter. A pneumothorax that results from a large tear will require several catheters to completely relieve the excess pressure. Chlorhexidine or povidone-iodine swabs and alcohol swabs will be needed to cleanse the puncture site, and some form of one-way valve will be needed for each inserted catheter.

Commercially made one-way valves are available and should be inserted with the wedge of the valve pointed away from the patient. If a one-way valve must be created, the finger of a rubber glove taped to the end of the catheter works very well if performed properly. Tape a longer finger to the end of the catheter and make a small slit down the center of the glove finger's tip to create the valve.

 Step 5 ▶ **Locate and prep puncture site.**

Local protocols will dictate exact locations for needle placement for decompression. In most cases it will involve an anterior approach along the midclavicular line in the second, third, or fourth intercostal space. In general, as long as the needle is placed superior and lateral to the nipple line, the puncture will be in an appropriate place. Some systems use the midaxillary approach. For very large-breasted women or for obese people, this may be the most appropriate option. However, in most cases the use of the midaxillary approach is reserved for the placement of chest tubes used to remove hemothoraces. In the presence of a hemothorax, the midaxillary approach can cause the needle to fill with blood, clot, and worsen the pneumothorax.

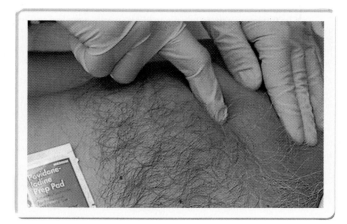

Cleanse injection site to kill microbial agents on the patient's skin. Using povidone-iodine or chlorhexidine, scrub in a circular motion, starting from the inside and wiping out. Alcohol may be used after povidone-iodine to

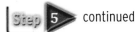 continued

provide better visualization. Chlorhexidine is clear, so secondary wiping is not necessary. If the patient is allergic to iodine or shellfish, do not use povidone-iodine. Chlorhexidine should not be used on neonates. Alcohol is acceptable as a last resort when allergies or other situations in which povidone-iodine or chlorhexidine are contraindicated. The routine use of alcohol is below the standard of care.

▼

 Insert needle.

Push the IV catheter through the intercostal space by running the needle over the top of the rib. Be sure not to go under the rib. Passing the needle under the rib greatly increases your chances of puncturing a costal artery, vein, or nerve. A considerable amount of force may be necessary.

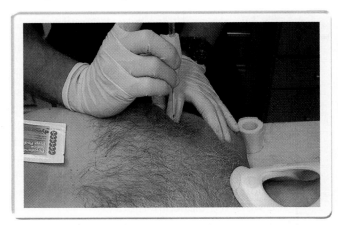

▼

Remove stylet and secure catheter.

When the catheter has entered the pleural space, remove the needle stylet from the catheter. Listen for air exchange, and be careful for the expulsion of small drops of blood as air escapes. Dispose of the needle in a puncture-resistant sharps container. Secure the catheter in place.

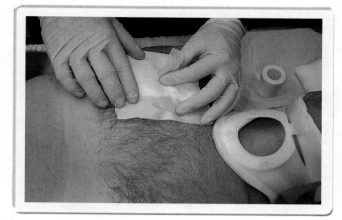

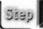 **Attach one-way valve.**

If required in the system, attach the one-way valve to the end of the IV catheter. Make sure the valve allows air out and prevents air from entering the chest.

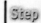 **Reassess patient.**

Reassess the patient's breath sounds, respiratory effort, and circulation. Be prepared to insert additional catheters or to perform other procedures as necessary.

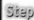 **Consider rapid transport.**

Because a tension pneumothorax is a critical condition, consider the effectiveness of the needle decompression and the need for rapid transport.

 Properly dispose of contaminated equipment.

Dispose of needles and all sharp instruments with blood or bodily fluid contamination in puncture-resistant sharps containers. Other materials that have been contaminated by blood or body fluids should be disposed of in biohazard bags. Waste materials that are not contaminated by blood or body fluids can be disposed of in normal trash receptacles.

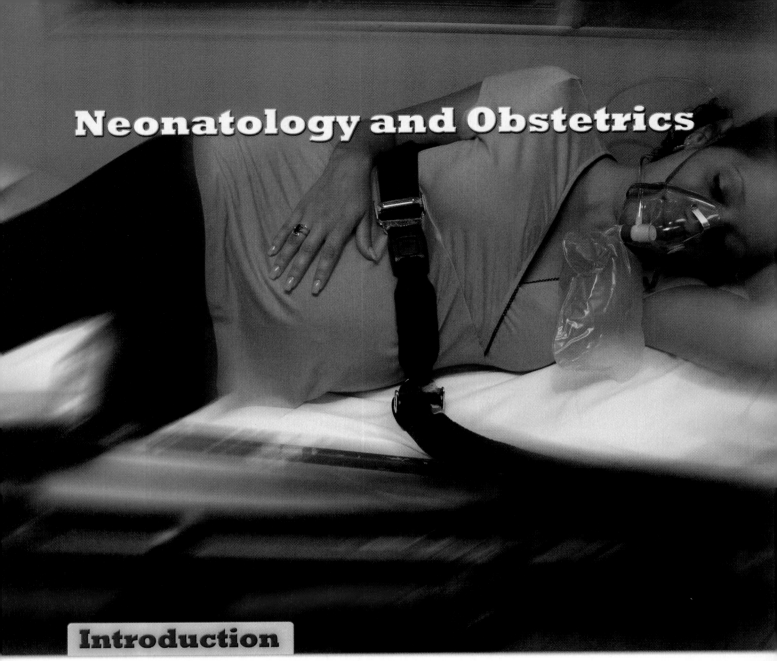

Neonatology and Obstetrics

Introduction

Although childbirth is a natural process that will occur with or without you, it is important to maintain the knowledge and skills to manage childbirth, potential complications of delivery, and the postdelivery care of the newborn. A patient could require your assistance at any given time.

The skills in this section demonstrate the proper assessment, preparation, and procedures for natural childbirth as well as the management of a breech delivery and a prolapsed cord.

Performance Objective

Given a pregnant patient with a term pregnancy and all necessary equipment, the candidate shall demonstrate the proper assessment, preparation, and procedures for the delivery of an infant, within 10 minutes or less.

Equipment

The following equipment is required to perform this skill:

- Appropriate body substance isolation/personal protective equipment
- Obstetrical kit, to include:
  - Bulb syringe
  - Umbilical clamps or ties (three)
  - Scalpel or umbilical shears
  - Sterile gloves
  - Drapes
  - Abdominal pads
  - 5″ × 9″ absorbent pads (chucks)
  - Foil blanket
  - 4″ × 4″ gauze pads
  - Plastic bag (for placenta), with tie

Equipment that may be helpful:

- Clean sheets
- Multitrauma dressings
- Receiving blanket
- Infant knit cap

Indications

- Natural childbirth when delivery is imminent
  - Delivery is imminent when the baby's head is visible in the birth canal (also known as crowning).

Contraindications

- Complications of delivery
- Single footling breech
- Limb presentation
- Prolapsed cord

Complications

Maternal
- Perineal tear
- Uterine rupture
- Postpartum hemorrhage

Neonatal
- Breech birth
- Nuchal cord
- Prolapsed cord

Procedures

Step 1 Ensure body substance isolation before beginning procedures.

Prior to beginning patient care, appropriate body substance isolation procedures should be employed.

▼

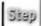**Step 2** Prepare equipment and position mother.

Open the obstetrical kit and check to make sure all the necessary equipment is present. This kit should contain draping for the mother, a scalpel, at least three umbilical cord ties or clamps, sterile gloves, a foil blanket, a bulb syringe, a plastic bag for the placenta, several 4″ × 4″ gauze pads, and some 5″ × 9″ absorbent pads (chucks).

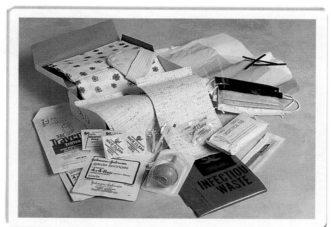

Prepare for the delivery by opening a 4″ × 4″ gauze pad and unwrapping it to 8″ × 8″. Push the tip of the bulb syringe through the gauze pad and tie the four corners around the top. This will give you a better grip on the wet rubber syringe when it is time to use it.

Position the mother near the end of a bed if possible. Have her lie supine with her knees bent and feet spread apart. Administer oxygen by nasal cannula or nonrebreathing mask. If time permits, an IV should be started with normal saline or lactated Ringer's.

▼

In the Field

Childbirth and Emergency Childbirth

Childbirth is a natural event that is not by nature an emergency. For millions of years, mammals, including humans, have been having babies with little need for medical attention.

In some cases, however, childbirth can pose a serious danger to the mother, the baby, or both. A detailed history should reveal known complications. In these cases, emergency transport should be performed in order to reduce the risks of field delivery. Attempting to physically delay delivery can be very dangerous and should never be attempted without a physician's order.

3 > **Position barrier devices and draping.**

All personnel who will be in the immediate area of the delivery should follow full body substance isolation precautions. Gloves, goggles, and masks should be donned as soon as possible and before any contact with the perineum or baby.

If time permits, place the drapes over the mother's legs and abdomen. The chuck should be placed under the buttocks.

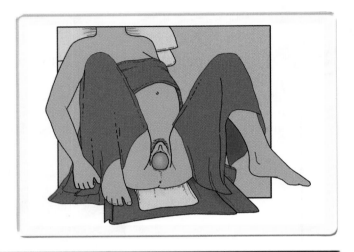

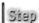 **Coach mother and communicate with team members.**

Until the baby's head is visible in the vaginal opening, transport should be continued. No effort to get the mother to push should be made.

As the head begins to appear in the vaginal opening, inform the mother that the baby is coming. Have her push with the contractions, and stop and breathe deeply after each push. It is a good idea to utilize the training of the mother's delivery coach if that coach is present.

Open communications should be given so that the mother and all team members know the progress of the delivery and can anticipate what steps will need to be performed next.

Step 5 Guide head and prevent explosive delivery.

As the head delivers, apply gentle pressure to the perineum and presenting part to prevent an explosive delivery.

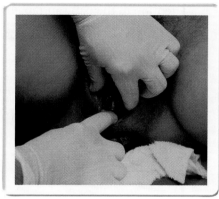

If the amniotic sac has not ruptured it may be necessary to break the membrane with your finger. Keep the baby's head up to prevent contact with any vaginal discharge, urine, or fecal material that may be present.

If the umbilical cord is around the baby's neck, act quickly to remove it. Attempt to reposition it by lifting it over the baby's head. If you are unable to do this, quickly apply two umbilical cord clamps and cut the cord. Continue with normal delivery.

Step 6 Suction baby's mouth and nose.

Once the baby's head is completely delivered, have the mother stop pushing and rest for a short time. Have her breathe easily, or pant if necessary. Suction the baby's mouth and nose with a bulb syringe and check for the presence of meconium. Since babies are obligate nose breathers, the mouth should always be cleaned first to prevent aspiration of mucus in the oropharynx.

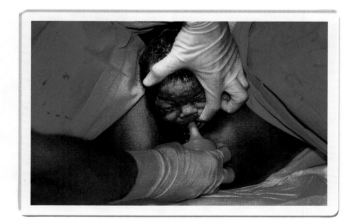

Step **7** ▶ **Continue with delivery.**

Continue with the delivery by having the mother continue to push with each contraction. This final step should be very quick. You will need to pay close attention to the baby and maintain a firm grasp. Record the time of birth.

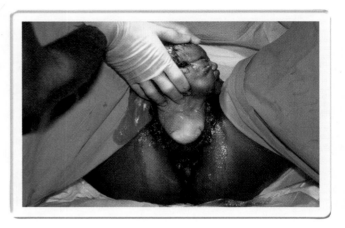

▼

Step **8** ▶ **Suction baby's mouth and nose.**

Lay the baby down and quickly suction the mouth and nose again.

▼

Step **9** ▶ **Cut and clamp cord.**

Apply two umbilical cord clamps or ties approximately 8″ to 10″ from the baby, 2″ to 3″ apart. Cut between the clamps. A slight amount of bleeding is expected initially. However, if the bleeding continues, especially from the baby's end, a second cord clamp or tie should be applied near the first. It is a good habit to apply a tie below the clamp on the baby's cord as an added safety measure.

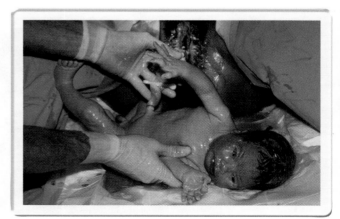

▼

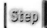 Step **10** ▶ **Dry the baby.**

Dry the baby of amniotic fluid without removing the vernix and wrap him or her in a blanket. The blanket should be positioned to cover the top of the baby's head to prevent heat loss. Placing the baby on her or his side with the head slightly lower than the rest of the body will facilitate drainage and ease breathing.

▼

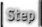 Step **11** ▶ **Stimulate breathing.**

In most cases, the delivery and drying process will be enough to stimulate breathing. If breathing does not start soon after birth, stimulate respiratory effort by rubbing the baby's back or by flicking or tapping the soles of the feet. Further, more aggressive stimulation is not necessary. If this action does not stimulate breathing, more advanced supportive care is required (see the box entitled *Neonatal Resuscitation*).

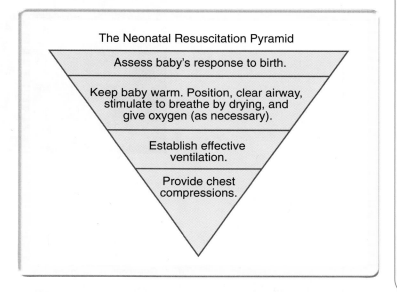

The Neonatal Resuscitation Pyramid

- Assess baby's response to birth.
- Keep baby warm. Position, clear airway, stimulate to breathe by drying, and give oxygen (as necessary).
- Establish effective ventilation.
- Provide chest compressions.

▼

 In the Field

Neonatal Resuscitation
After delivery of a baby, it is important to perform an adequate assessment to determine if he or she is doing well. A simple APGAR usually is not sufficient to determine the need for resuscitation. The American Heart Association and the American Academy of Pediatrics have come together to create the neonatal resuscitation pyramid. This pyramid guides the process of resuscitation of a struggling newborn. Although not all newborns will need the full gamut of resuscitation efforts, all newborns need the procedures specified in the top level of the pyramid.

Step **12** **Evaluate baby and mother, and deliver placenta.**

The baby should be evaluated using the APGAR score (see the table entitled *The APGAR Score*). A measurement should be taken after 1 minute and again 5 minutes later.

Once the baby is delivered and cared for, evaluate the mother. Evaluate the perineum for tears and vaginal bleeding. Perineal tears should be dressed while waiting for placental delivery. Bleeding from the vaginal opening could be coming from the vaginal wall or from the uterus. Uterine bleeding can be controlled by fundal massage or having the baby nurse.

The placenta should deliver in 5 to 15 minutes, but transport should not be delayed while waiting for it.

Keep the placenta as clean as possible and place it in a plastic bag. The placenta should be delivered to the hospital with the mother and baby.

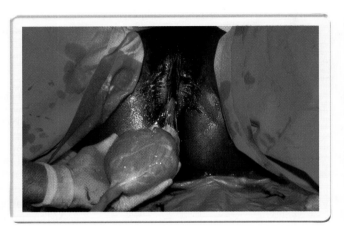

The APGAR Score		
Condition	Description	Score
Appearance–skin color	Completely pink Body pink, extremities blue Centrally blue, pale	2 1 0
Pulse rate	>100 <100 Absent	2 1 0
Grimace–irritability	Cries Grimaces No response	2 1 0
Activity–muscle tone	Active motion Some flexion of extremities Limp	2 1 0
Respiratory–effort	Strong cry Slow and irregular Absent	2 1 0

Step 13 Properly dispose of contaminated equipment.

Dispose of any sharp instruments with blood or body fluid contamination in puncture-resistant sharps containers. Other material that has been contaminated by blood or body fluids should be disposed of in biohazard bags. Waste materials that are not contaminated by blood or body fluids can be disposed of in normal trash receptacles.

▼

Step 14 Document.

Document the delivery of the baby on the mother's patient report. However, the baby should have a separate patient report that represents the assessment and any procedures performed during the care of the newborn.

Breech Delivery

Performance Objective

Given a pregnant patient with breech presentation, the candidate shall demonstrate the assessment and procedures for a breech delivery, within 10 minutes or less.

Equipment

The following equipment is required to perform this skill:
- Appropriate body substance isolation/personal protective equipment
- Obstetrical kit, to include
  - Bulb syringe
  - Umbilical clamps or ties (three)
  - Scalpel or umbilical shears
  - Sterile gloves
  - Drapes
  - Abdominal pads
  - 5" × 9" absorbent pads (chucks)
  - Foil blanket
  - 4" × 4" gauze pads
  - Plastic bag (for placenta), with tie

Equipment that may be helpful:
- Clean sheets
- Multitrauma dressings
- Receiving blanket
- Infant knit cap

Indications

- Breech presentation that fails to continue delivery once the legs and body have delivered

Contraindications

- None in emergency situations

Complications

- None in emergency situations

Procedures

 Ensure body substance isolation before beginning procedures.

Prior to beginning patient care, appropriate body substance isolation procedures should be employed.

▼

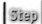 **Prepare equipment and position mother.**

Open the obstetrical kit and check to make sure all the necessary equipment is present. This kit should contain draping for the mother, a scalpel, at least three umbilical cord ties or clamps, sterile gloves, a foil blanket, a bulb syringe, a plastic bag for the placenta, several 4″ × 4″ gauze pads, and some 5″ × 9″ absorbent pads (chucks).

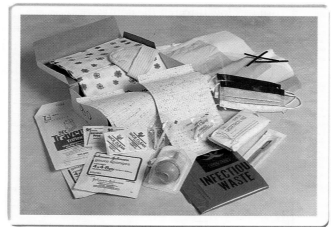

Prepare for the delivery by opening a 4″ × 4″ gauze pad and unwrapping it to 8″ × 8″. Push the tip of the bulb syringe through the gauze pad and tie the four corners around the top. This will give you a better grip on the wet rubber syringe when it is time to use it.

Position the mother near the end of a bed if possible. Have her lie supine with her knees bent and feet spread apart. Administer oxygen by nasal cannula or nonrebreathing mask.

▼

Step 3 ▶ Position barrier devices and draping.

Field delivery of a breech birth is not desirable because the possibility of complications is extremely high. Cesarean delivery is preferred if delivery can be delayed until arrival at the hospital.

All personnel who will be in the immediate area of the delivery should follow full body substance isolation precautions. Gloves, goggles, and masks should be donned as soon as possible and before any contact with the perineum or baby.

If time permits, place the drapes over the mother's legs and abdomen. The chuck should be placed under the buttocks.

▼

Step 4 ▶ Coach mother and communicate with team members.

Until the presenting part is visible in the vaginal opening, transport should be continued. Make every effort to discourage the mother to push by having her pant or blow through the contractions.

As the feet or buttocks appear in the vaginal opening, inform the mother that the baby is coming, and that the presentation is breech.

Do not encourage pushing until the option of delaying delivery no longer exists. At that point, have the mother push with the contractions, and stop and breathe deeply after each push. It is a good idea to utilize the training of the mother's delivery coach if that coach is present.

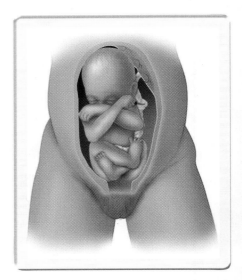

Open communications should be given so that the mother and all team members know the progress of the delivery and can anticipate what steps will need to be performed next.

▼

Step 5 ▷ Guide baby and prevent explosive delivery.

As the feet and body deliver, gently control the mother's pushing force with gentle pressure to the perineum and presenting part to prevent an explosive delivery.

If the amniotic sac has not ruptured it may be necessary to break the membrane with your finger. Keep the baby up to prevent contact with vaginal discharge, urine, or fecal material that may be present.

If the umbilical cord is around the baby's neck, attempt to reposition it by lifting it over the body. If you are unable to do this, evaluate the blood flow through the cord and the tightness around the neck. Cutting the cord may remove the most reliable oxygen supply the baby has.

▼

Step 6 ▷ Consider need for immediate transport.

Since the head will require more time to deliver than the body, consider whether immediate transport should begin. If the head does not deliver in the next 3 to 5 minutes, transport will be the only acceptable option. Continue to Step 8.

▼

Step 7 ▷ Gently guide head.

If the head delivers, continue with care of the baby and mother as in a normal cephalic delivery (see Skill 73).

▼

Step 8 ▷ Create airway.

If after 3 to 5 minutes the head has not delivered, an airway into the vagina must be made. With a fresh sterile glove, place two fingers, palm toward the baby, into the mother's vagina to the level of the baby's nose. Spread the fingers apart to form a V. If possible, pull the vaginal wall away from the baby's face. You may have to hold this position throughout transport and into the delivery room.

▼

Step 9 ▷ Assess further needs.

Assess further needs for the baby and the mother. In most cases, rapid transport and notification of the breech presentation to the receiving facility are all that is required.

Prolapsed Cord

Performance Objective

Given a pregnant patient with cord presentation, the candidate shall demonstrate the assessment and procedures for a prolapsed cord, within 10 minutes or less.

Equipment

The following equipment is required to perform this skill:
- Appropriate body substance isolation/personal protective equipment
- Obstetrical kit, to include
  • Bulb syringe
  • Umbilical clamps or ties (three)
  • Scalpel or umbilical shears
  • Sterile gloves
  • Drapes
  • Abdominal pads
  • 5" × 9" absorbent pads (chucks)
  • Foil blanket
  • 4" × 4" gauze pads
  • Plastic bag (for placenta), with tie

Equipment that may be helpful:
- Clean sheets
- Multitrauma dressings
- Receiving blanket
- Infant knit cap

Indications

- Presentation of the umbilical cord prior to the delivery of the baby

Contraindications

- None in emergency situations

Complications

- None in emergency situations

Procedures

 Step 1 Ensure body substance isolation before beginning procedures.

Prior to beginning patient care, appropriate body substance isolation procedures should be employed. All personnel who will be in the immediate area of the delivery should follow full body substance isolation precautions. Gloves, goggles, and masks should be donned as soon as possible and before any contact with the perineum or umbilical cord.

▼

 Step 2 Assess presenting part.

Assess the presenting part to determine the amount of umbilical cord present. Gently assess the cord and determine the presence of a pulse. Prepare for immediate transport.

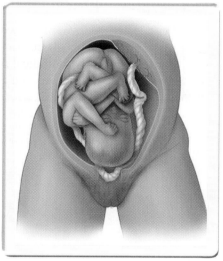

▼

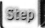 **Position mother and apply oxygen.**

Position the mother in a high Trendelenburg position (supine with lower extremities elevated approximately 12″) or a knee-chest position (see note below), and coach the mother not to push. Elevation of the inferior uterus is essential to shift the weight of an engaging fetus off the cervix. Administer 100% supplemental oxygen via nonrebreating mask.

Note: Use of the knee-chest position in the back of a moving ambulance can be extremely hazardous. The high Trendelenburg position is preferred while in transport.

With a prolapsed cord, the mother must be in the knee-chest position in order to perform Step 4. It will be important for the vehicle operator to understand the precarious position of the patient.

▼

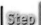 **Place gloved hand into vaginal opening and push baby's head back into uterus.**

With a sterile glove, place two fingers, palm toward baby, into the vaginal opening. Push the baby's head back into the uterus and remove pressure from the cord. Reassess the umbilical pulse. Cover any exposed cord with moistened dressings. It will be necessary to hold this position throughout transport.

Neonatal Resuscitation

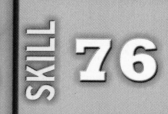

Performance Objective

Given a neonate patient in distress following delivery, the candidate shall demonstrate the proper sequence and techniques following pediatric advanced life support neonatal resuscitation outlines, in 10 minutes or less.

Equipment

The following equipment is required to perform this skill:

- Appropriate body substance isolation/personal protection equipment
- Neonatal or infant bag-valve device with various sized masks
- Oxygen cylinder, regulator, and key
- End-tidal carbon dioxide meter
- Intubation equipment appropriate for patient
- IV access equipment appropriate for patient
- Neonatal medications as needed for patient
- Suction equipment with adjustable manometer
- Pulse oximeter with neonatal sensor

Indications

- Newborn patients not responding to the normal stimuli to breathe or otherwise exhibiting signs of distress
- Cardiac arrest in newborns

Contraindications

- None

Complications

- None if properly applied

Procedures

 Step 1 ▶ Ensure body substance isolation before beginning procedures.

Prior to beginning patient care, appropriate body substance isolation procedures should be employed.

▼

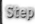 **Step 2 ▶ Assess history.**

Prior to the birth of the newborn, perform a history and assessment to determine the likelihood that the newborn will need resuscitation. Preterm delivery is the most common risk factor; however, lack of prenatal care or other characteristics that may be known by the mother should also be considered.

Identify the need for resuscitation by assessing four simple characteristics:

1. Was the newborn at or after a full term of gestation?
2. Is the amniotic fluid clear, with no signs of meconium or infection?
3. Is the newborn breathing or crying?
4. Does the newborn appear to have good muscle tone?

If the answer to all four of these questions is yes, there is no need for resuscitation. Move to the basic care of the newborn, which should include providing warmth, clearing the airway, drying, and assessing the infant's tissue color.

If the answer to any of the preceding questions is no, proceed through the following steps.

▼

 Step 3 ▶ Dry, warm, position, suction, and stimulate the newborn and assess further needs.

Upon delivery, wrap the newborn in a blanket and cut the cord. Quickly dry the newborn of the amniotic fluid and position with the head down. Suction the mouth and nose (if meconium aspiration has occurred, follow the procedure for removal before proceeding). Stimulate the newborn's respirations by gently rubbing the back or flicking the feet with your finger. Assess the need for further interventions by performing an assessment of the newborn.

▼

Administer oxygen.

Oxygen is needed when the newborn fails to breathe adequately or central cyanosis is present. One hundred percent oxygen should be administered by the blow-by technique or a simple neonatal face mask held against the face.

 Establish effective ventilation.

If the newborn is apneic or has gasping respirations, the newborn's heart rate is less than 100 beats/min, or central cyanosis persists despite oxygen administration, positive pressure ventilation is indicated.

Ventilations should be performed at a rate of 40 to 60 breaths/min and should be of adequate depth to obtain chest rise. Because neonatal lungs are tight initially, the first few ventilations may require more force then subsequent ventilation. Many infant bag-mask devices have pop-off valves to prevent overpressurization of an infant's lungs. If a pop-off valve exists on the bag-mask device, hold it closed during the initial ventilations. Initial lung compliance in newborns will require higher pressures than will be allowed with a pop-off valve.

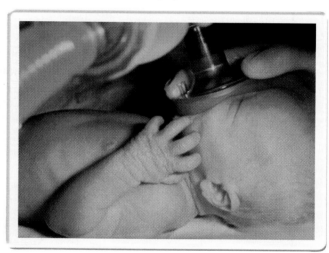

Step 6 **Consider intubation.**

Intubation should be considered when long-term ventilations are expected. The newborn should be intubated using a straight blade only, size 0 or 1. The size of the endotracheal tube can be determined by comparing the tube to the size of the newborn's little finger. In general, a newborn who weighs:

- Less then 1 kg (2 lb) will require a 2.5 endotracheal tube
- Between 1 and 2 kg (2–4 lb) will require a 3.0 endotracheal tube
- Between 2 and 3 kg (4–6 lb) will require a 3.5 endotracheal tube
- Over 3 kg (6 lb) will require a 4.0 endotracheal tube

The tube should be inserted until the black line rests at the level of the vocal cords.

The placement of an 8F to 10F orogastric tube is recommended if ventilations will be performed for an extended period of time.

In the Field

Indications for Endotracheal Intubation of a Newborn

- Inability to ventilate effectively by bag-mask device
- Necessity to perform tracheal suctioning, especially if meconium is present and infant is depressed at birth
- Necessity for prolonged ventilation

Step 7 **Assess need for chest compressions.**

Closed chest compressions are indicated any time the newborn's heart rate is less than 60 beats/min and not rapidly increasing with ventilations. Compressions should be performed at a rate of 120 per minute with the sternum depressed ½" to ¾" each time, using a 3:1 ratio of compressions to ventilations.

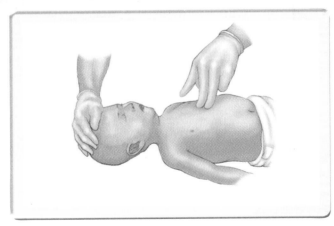

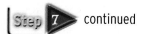

continued

The standard infant CPR finger placement is acceptable, or the chest can be compressed by placing both thumbs on the newborn's sternum and wrapping the fingers around the chest.

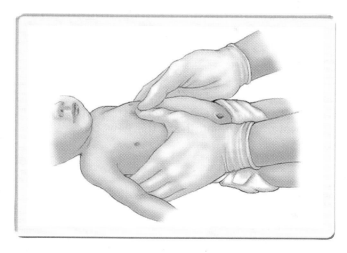

Step 8 ▶ Establish vascular access and consider medications.

Vascular access is usually best achieved through the umbilical route in neonates. Scalp and leg veins are also acceptable. Medications should be initiated as needed following pediatric advanced life support recommendations for dosing and intervals.

Meconium Aspiration

Performance Objective

Given a neonatal patient born with meconium present in the amniotic fluid and all necessary equipment, the candidate shall demonstrate the correct technique for the removal of meconium from the newborn's airway, in 3 minutes or less.

Equipment

The following equipment is required to perform this skill:
- Appropriate body substance isolation/personal protection equipment
- Obstetrical kit
- Laryngoscope handle and blades (straight only)
- Endotracheal tubes, uncuffed (2.5 to 4.0)
- Malleable intubation stylet (appropriate size for endotracheal tube)
- Water-soluble lubricant
- Towel or other padding
- Suction device and tubing
- Bag-mask device
- Oxygen cylinder, regulator, and key

Equipment that may be helpful:
- Meconium aspirator

Indications

- Meconium aspiration is a serious condition that must be corrected to prevent neonatal mortality. Thick meconium aspiration must be cleared using the procedure described. Thin meconium, evidenced by a thin green coloration to the amniotic fluid, can be cleared using simple mouth and nose suctioning with a bulb syringe.

Contraindications

- Thin or light meconium aspiration

Complications

- Bradycardia

Procedures

 Step 1 **Ensure body substance isolation before beginning procedures.**

Prior to beginning patient care, appropriate body substance isolation procedures should be employed.

▼

 Step 2 **Determine/recognize possibility of meconium aspiration.**

Recognize the presence of meconium in the amniotic fluid. This is done through direct evaluation of the amniotic fluid (noting a pea green color rather than a clear fluid with white flakes), examination of the newborn's skin (stained with meconium), history from the mother or witness about the color of the fluid, or visual inspection of the nasal aspirant.

▼

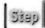 **Step 3** **Prepare equipment.**

Gather the necessary equipment by opening and preparing the obstetrical kit. Locate the drapes and place them over the mother if time permits. A 4″ × 4″ gauze sponge should be tied around the bulb syringe to make it easier to grasp.

In addition, you will need a suction unit set up with nothing attached to the working end of the suction connective tubing. A laryngoscope with a No. 1 Miller blade and a set of small endotracheal tubes (2.5 to 4.0) are also required. A meconium aspirator, a small plastic device that fits over the end of the endotracheal tube and connects to the suction tubing, is helpful but not required.

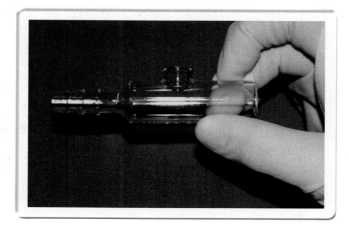

Because there is a possibility that the newborn may require supportive action, ready an infant bag-mask device and have oxygen ready.

▼

Step **4** Suction mouth/nose with bulb syringe upon delivery of head.

Upon delivery of the newborn's head, have the mother relax long enough for suctioning of the mouth and nose to occur. Using a bulb syringe, suction as much fluid as possible from the mouth and nose.

▼

Step **5** Continue delivery.

Continue with the delivery of the newborn. Have the mother begin pushing again until the newborn has completed delivery. Because meconium aspiration can be an extreme emergency, clamp and cut the umbilical cord very quickly. Position the newborn and prepare to intubate. Minimal stimulation should be applied to prevent initiation of spontaneous ventilations.

▼

Step **6** Intubate.

Follow the procedures for infant intubation. Place an uncuffed endotracheal tube into the newborn's trachea. When the tube has been placed, do not begin ventilations.

▼

Step **7** Apply suction and remove.

Attach suction connective tubing directly to the endotracheal tube adapter and remove the endotracheal tube with the suction running. If a meconium aspirator is available, place the aspirator between the endotracheal tube and the suction catheter and apply suction by covering the hole just like a suction wand.

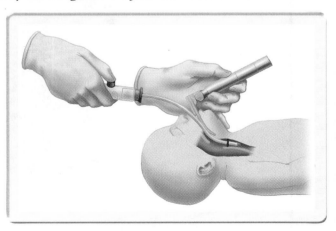

▼

Repeat Step 4 until airway is clear.

Evaluate the meconium removed. If the meconium is thick and abundant, repeat the intubation and suction sequence. If possible, a new, sterile endotracheal tube should be used after each intubation. Continue to reassess and suction until the airway is clear. Two to three times should be enough.

Remember that meconium is very thick and cannot come up a suction catheter applied inside the infant's endotracheal tube. Adding fluid down the endotracheal tube may not be of sufficient quantity to loosen the meconium. Simple intubation and direct suction is the preferred method of clearing meconium aspiration.

▼

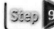 **Stimulate breathing.**

Quickly dry the newborn of amniotic fluid and wrap in a blanket. This activity should be enough to stimulate respiration. If, however, the newborn does not begin adequate ventilations, stimulate the breathing by tapping or flicking the soles of the feet or by rubbing his or her back.

▼

 Assess the newborn.

Assess the newborn's respirations and heart rate to determine other actions required. An APGAR score should be taken at 1 minute and again at 5 minutes, but it is not the most efficient means of determining neonatal distress.

The APGAR Score

Condition	Description	Score
Appearance–skin color	Completely pink	2
	Body pink, extremities blue	1
	Centrally blue, pale	0
Pulse rate	> 100	2
	< 100	1
	Absent	0
Grimace–irritability	Cries	2
	Grimaces	1
	No response	0
Activity–muscle tone	Active motion	2
	Some flexion of extremities	1
	Limp	0
Respiratory–effort	Strong cry	2
	Slow and irregular	1
	Absent	0

Follow standard pediatric advanced life support neonatal resuscitation standards to determine the necessary interventions.

Umbilical Vein Catheterization

Performance Objective

Given a neonate with a healthy umbilical cord and appropriate equipment, the candidate shall properly place an IV catheter into the umbilical vein, in 3 minutes or less.

Equipment

The following equipment is required to perform this skill:
- Appropriate body substance isolation/personal protection equipment
- Sharps container
- IV pole
- Selection of IV solutions (normal saline, lactated Ringer's)
- Administration sets: Macro/micro/extension tubing
- Selection of IV catheters (20, 22 gauge)
- 3-mL syringe
- Tape or commercially made IV securing system
- 4" × 4" gauze pads
- Umbilical cord tape
- Scalpel
- Cleaning solution
  - Povidone-iodine preps
  - Alcohol preps
- Bulky dressing

Equipment that may be helpful:
- Towels

Indications

- Any neonate in the first few hours of life who is in need of IV access

Contraindications

- Birth defects of the umbilical cord (such as omphalocele)

Complications

- Placement of the catheter into the portal vein can cause liver injury (hepatic hemorrhage) and does not allow medications to mix with blood before reaching the liver

Procedures

 Step 1 Ensure body substance isolation before beginning procedures.

Prior to beginning patient care, appropriate body substance isolation procedures should be employed.

▼

 Step 2 Assemble equipment.

Gather the necessary equipment for starting an IV line, including fluid, administration set (preferably a volutrol), tape, sterile 4″ × 4″ gauze, povidone-iodine swabs, and alcohol swabs. A 20- or 22-gauge, 1″ or 1.5″ catheter should be prepared by removing the needle stylet and attaching a 3-mL syringe filled with normal saline. Carefully flush 1 to 2 mL of saline through the end of the catheter.

▼

 Step 3 Prep the site.

Prepare the umbilical cord by cleaning with povidone-iodine swabs from the navel to the cord clamp. Light rubbing is all that is necessary. Chlorhexidine is contraindicated in neonates.

▼

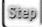 **Step 4 Cut the cord.**

With a sterile scalpel, cut the umbilical cord 0.5″ to 1″ from the skin attachment of the navel. Slight bleeding is normal and expected.

▼

Step 5 ▷ Place catheter.

Holding the cord snugly to minimize bleeding, place the catheter (attached to a syringe) into the umbilical vein with a slight twisting motion.

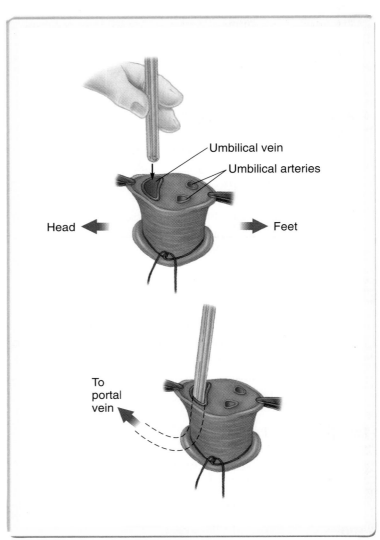

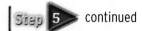Step 5 ▶ continued

Pull back on the syringe plunger as you insert the catheter into the vein. The catheter should be inserted only until blood return appears in the syringe.

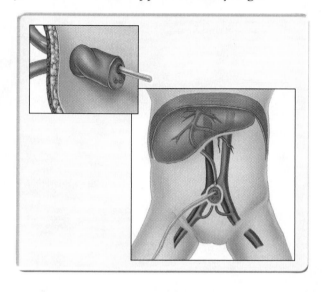

▼

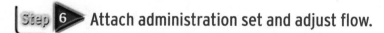Step 6 ▶ **Attach administration set and adjust flow.**

Attach the administration set to the catheter and adjust to the ordered rate or very slow to keep open (TKO). A quick flush with 5 mL of normal saline may be performed before securing the catheter.

▼

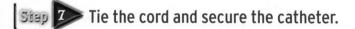Step 7 ▶ **Tie the cord and secure the catheter.**

Tie the cord with a loop of umbilical cord tape. *Do not* use a cord clamp because it will occlude the catheter. Be sure the cord tape is tight enough to prevent bleeding but not too tight to occlude the IV flow.

Tape the catheter to the umbilical cord.

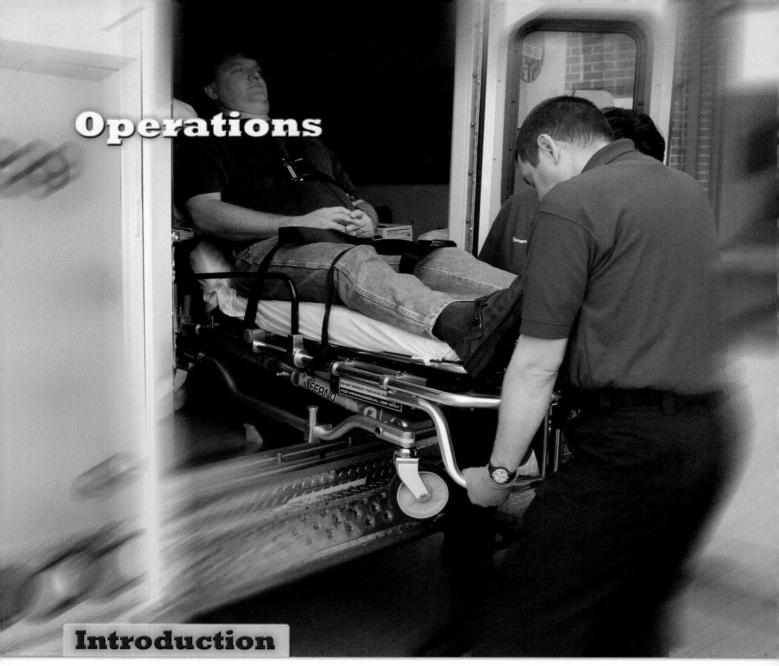

Operations

Introduction

Operational skills are performed on almost every call and many of the skills are more for the benefit of the responder than the patient. The number one responsibility of the responder is personal safety. In fact, in order of importance, the responder comes first, bystanders and family second, and the patient third. If a responder gets injured, it takes away from the number of responders available to care for the patient; if bystanders or the patient's family get injured, it takes additional responders away from the patient.

The patient's best interests are served when responders take care of themselves and family first. The skills in this section demonstrate how to perform operational skills while keeping responders, bystanders, and patients safe.

Cot Operation

Performance Objective

Given a cot and a patient, the candidates will be able to secure the patient comfortably to the cot, raise the cot to a transport position, move the cot to the ambulance, raise the cot to the loading position, and load and un-load the cot, in 10 minutes or less.

Equipment

The following equipment is required to perform this skill:
- Appropriate body substance isolation/personal protective equipment
- Multilevel ambulance cot

Indications

- Transport of a patient on a cot

Contraindications

- Patients above the maximum weight rating of the cot

Complications

- Back injury to the operator

Procedures

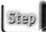 **Step 1** **Ensure body substance isolation before beginning procedures.**

Prior to beginning patient care, appropriate body substance isolation procedures should be employed.

▼

 Step 2 **Secure patient.**

With the patient positioned on the cot, gently raise the head of the cot to a position of comfort not to exceed 45°. Place straps on the patient's chest and thighs and secure.

▼

 Step 3 **Raise cot for transport.**

Lifting from the head and foot of the patient, raise the cot to position three, four, or five.

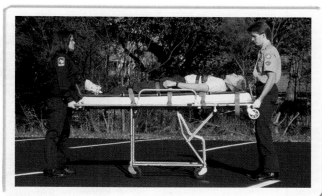

Safety Tips

Raising Cots
Raising the cot to a higher position is not recommended for routine transport of patients. These higher positions are not stable should sudden shifting of the patient occur.

▼

 Step 4 **Move the patient on the cot.**

With one person at the foot and another at the head, move the patient with the cot to the desired location. It is usually best to move the patient feet first, and on inclines and stairs always keep the patient's head up and feet down.

▼

Step 5 Raise cot to loading position and load cot.

Lifting from the head and foot of the patient, raise the cot to the appropriate loading position.

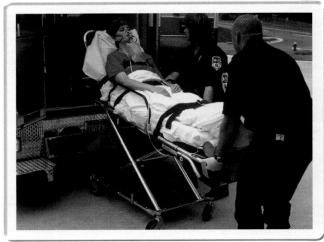

Place the back wheels onto the rear platform of the ambulance. While the person at the patient's foot lifts the cot and releases the locking mechanism, the second person lifts the undercarriage.

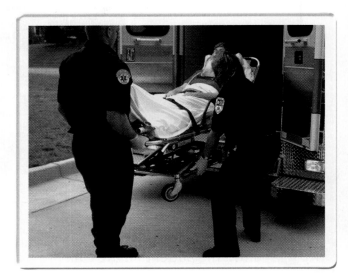

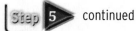 continued

Roll cot into the ambulance and lock it in place.

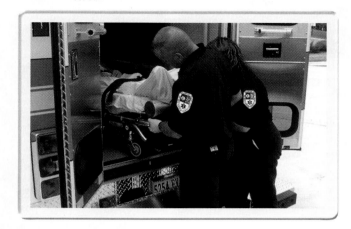

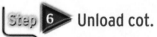 Step 6 **Unload cot.**

Release the locking mechanism for the cot. With one person positioned at the patient's feet, begin unloading the cot by lifting and rolling the cot. The second person should guide the undercarriage to the ground and ensure the wheels have locked before completely removing the cot from the ambulance.

Performance Objective

Given a patient in a variety of positions on the ground, chair, or bed, the candidates shall demonstrate safe lifting techniques, in 1 minute or less.

Equipment

The following equipment is required to perform this skill:
- Appropriate body substance isolation/personal protective equipment
- Multilevel ambulance cot
- Standard bed sheet

Indications

- Movement of a patient

Contraindications

- None

Complications

- Improper lifting can result in injury to rescuers or the patient.

Procedures

Standard Lift

This technique is used to lift a cot, backboard, scoop stretcher, or other heavy loads.

 Ensure body substance isolation before beginning procedures.

Prior to beginning patient care, appropriate body substance isolation procedures should be employed.

▼

 Squat using proper body mechanics.

With your feet spread comfortably, about shoulder width apart, squat into position by bending the knees. Keep your back straight.

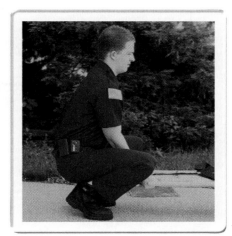

▼

 Grasp the object to be lifted.

Grasp the cot or other object to be lifted with your palms facing out. Keep your arms close to the center of your body.

▼

Step **4**   **Perform lift.**

Lift the cot or other object by straightening the knees. The back should remain straight, and your arms should remain close to your body.

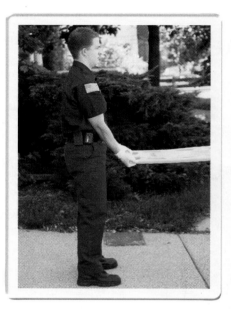

Step **5**   **Lower patient.**

To lower the patient, reverse the steps.

Two-Person Extremity Lift Technique

This technique is used to lift a non-trauma patient from the ground to the cot.

 Ensure body substance isolation before beginning procedures.

Prior to beginning patient care, appropriate body substance isolation procedures should be employed.

▼

 Rescuer One: Raise patient's upper body.

Rescuer Two: Prepare to lift the lower body.

Kneeling behind the patient, grasp the patient's wrists. Hold the arms into the chest. Pull the patient into a seated position.

Place your hands under the patient's knees.

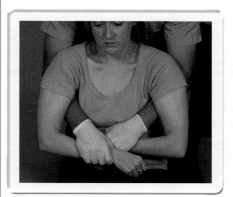

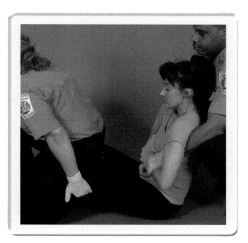

▼

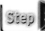

Step **3** ▶ **Both Rescuers: Lift the patient.**

Working together and using the standard lifting technique, lift the patient.

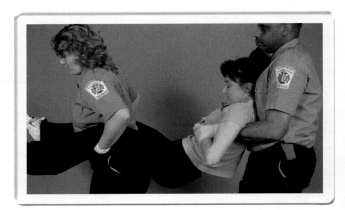

▼

Step **4** ▶ **Position the patient.**

Carefully lower the patient onto the cot. Position as appropriate and secure.

Bed-to-Cot Transfer: Sheet Technique

This technique is used to move a non-trauma patient from a bed to the cot using the sheet technique. The procedure requires a minimum of two people. With larger patients, as many as six people may be required.

 Step 1 ▶ **Ensure body substance isolation before beginning procedures.**

Prior to beginning patient care, appropriate body substance isolation procedures should be employed.

▼

 Step 2 ▶ **Log roll the patient.**

Log roll the patient to the side of the bed.

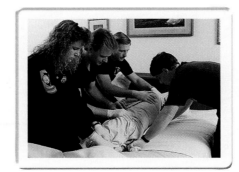

▼

 Step 3 ▶ **Prepare the sheet.**

Using a standard bed sheet or a draw sheet, roll the edges to make a handle.

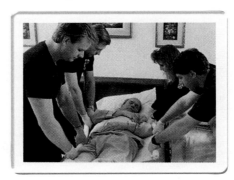

▼

4 **Position patient.**

Lifting as a team, move the patient to the edge of the bed. Ensure the patient does not roll out of the bed before the transfer is complete.

▼

 5 **Move and position the patient.**

As before and working as a team, lift the patient carefully onto the cot. Position patient as appropriate and secure.

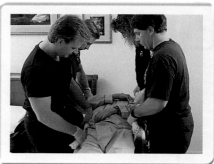

Bed-to-Cot Transfer: Direct Lift Technique

This procedure is used to move a non-trauma patient from a bed to the cot using the direct lift technique. This requires a minimum of two people. With larger patients, three people may be required.

 Ensure body substance isolation before beginning procedures.

Prior to beginning patient care, appropriate body substance isolation procedures should be employed.

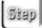 **Position the cot.**

Set up for this transfer by placing the head of the cot at the patient's feet, or the foot of the cot at the patient's head. This will allow you to lift the patient, rotate 90°, and place the patient.

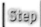 **Prepare patient for move.**

Working as a team, place your arms under the patient. Be sure to support the head and shoulders, the midback, the hips, and the lower legs.

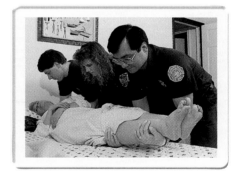

4 Lift patient.

Working as a team, lift the patient by rolling him or her into your chest and then standing upright.

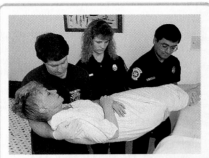

 5 Move and position patient.

Move the patient to the cot and lower patient carefully. Position as appropriate and secure.

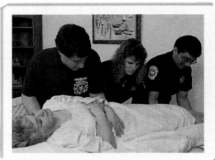

Infection Control Techniques

81

Performance Objective

Given standard patient contact situations, the candidate will demonstrate appropriate body substance isolation, disposal of contaminated sharps, and disposal of contaminated equipment and materials, in 1 minute or less.

Equipment

The following equipment is required to perform this skill:
- Appropriate body substance isolation/personal protective equipment
- Wraparound-style eye protection, designed to prevent splash behind the lenses
- Surgical mask
- HEPA filter mask
- Disposable gown
- Puncture-resistant sharps container
- Biohazard disposal box, with red bags

Indications

- Known cases of infectious patients
- Preparation for care of patients where infectious risk is unknown
- Clean-up following patient care

Contraindications

- None

Complications

- None

Procedures

Disposing of Contaminated Sharps

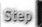 **Ensure body substance isolation before beginning procedures.**

Prior to beginning patient care, appropriate body substance isolation procedures should be employed.

▼

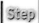 **Place sharps in puncture-resistant container.**

As soon as possible following use, contaminated sharps should be put into a specifically designed, puncture-resistant container. Never shove a needle into the container. Do not recap the needle before placing it into the container.

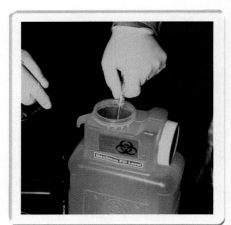

▼

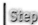 **Seal and dispose of puncture-resistant container.**

When the sharps container is two thirds to three fourths full, secure the cover. Place in a biohazard disposal box.

Disposing of Contaminated Equipment and Materials

 Ensure body substance isolation before beginning procedures.

Prior to beginning patient care, appropriate body substance isolation procedures should be employed.

▼

 Place contaminated disposable equipment and materials in biohazard bag.

Place disposable equipment and materials in a specifically designed biohazard disposal bag.

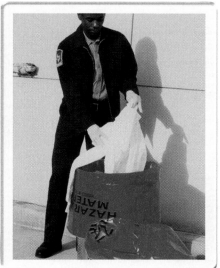

▼

 Dispose of biohazard bag.

Place the full biohazard disposal bag into a biohazard disposal box.

▼

 Seal the biohazard box.

Seal the biohazard box *before* it becomes completely full.

Crime Scene Operations

Performance Objective

Given a patient found in an active crime scene, the candidate will demonstrate proper patient and evidence management in cooperation with law enforcement, in 2 minutes or less.

Equipment

The following equipment is required to perform this skill:
- Appropriate body substance isolation/personal protective equipment
- Paper bags

Indications

- Operations in an active crime scene

Contraindications

- None

Complications

- None when properly applied

Procedures

Working in the Crime Scene

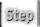 **Ensure body substance isolation before beginning procedures.**

Prior to beginning patient care, appropriate body substance isolation procedures should be employed.

▼

 Minimize contact with the scene.

Everything surrounding the patient contains potential evidence. Touch or move only those items that are absolutely necessary. It is best to eliminate unnecessary equipment and personnel by placing them outside the actual crime scene. Even the cot can be placed outside the immediate area in most cases.

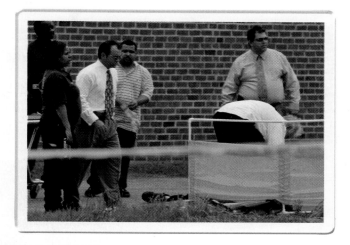

▼

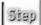 **Minimize contamination.**

Be careful not to contaminate the scene with "ambulance droppings." As the time and the situation permits, place wrappings and packaging in appropriate containers. This should be performed as equipment and supplies are opened and before the packaging materials reach the ground. Any wrappings that reach the ground should be left to avoid gathering or destroying evidence that may exist underneath. Be careful about where you position equipment bags, monitors, and cots.

▼

Step   **Document.**

After finishing patient care, document for law enforcement personnel everything in the crime scene that was moved or touched in the care of the patient. A sketch of the scene may be helpful. This should be performed on a report separate from the patient care record. It is helpful for the police investigation for you to give your name and contact information. This will allow them to contact you if any questions arise concerning the operation in the crime scene.

Preserving Evidence

Step   **Ensure body substance isolation before beginning procedures.**

Prior to beginning patient care, appropriate body substance isolation procedures should be employed.

▼

Step  **Cut necessary clothing from the patient.**

Remove clothing by cutting carefully. Do not use stab holes, gunshot holes, or rips caused by assault as starting points for cutting. Do not shake the clothing in order to preserve trace evidence.

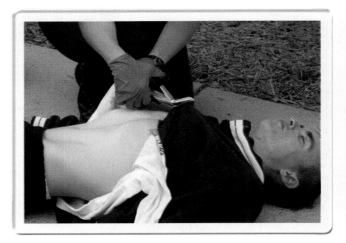

▼

Step 3 ▶ Collect patient's clothing.

Place any clothing removed from the patient into individual paper bags. Placing pieces of clothing in the same bag or clothing in plastic bags will cause evidence to blend or sweat.

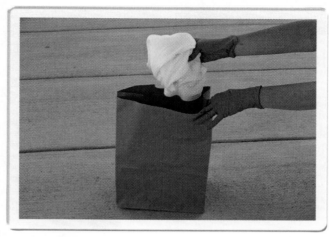

▼

Step 4 ▶ Protect the patient's hands.

Place paper bags over the patient's hands to protect evidence.

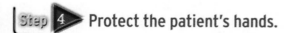

▼

Step 5 ▶ Use caution bandaging wounds.

Use caution cleaning up any wounds present on the patient. Bandaging and dressing should be limited to wounds that absolutely require bleeding control.

Performance Objective

Given a violent patient in danger of harming himself or herself or others, and working with other rescuers, the candidate(s) shall demonstrate the proper procedure for subduing and restraining the patient, in 2 minutes or less.

Equipment

The following equipment is required to perform this skill:
- Appropriate body substance isolation/personal protective equipment
- Multilevel ambulance cot
- Commercially made restraints for wrists and ankles
- Backboard straps

Indications

- Violent patients who must be restrained for their own safety or the safety of others

Contraindications

- Personnel who are not trained or prepared to physically restrain the patient
- Patients with weapons

Complications

- Injury to rescuers
- Injury to the patient
- Cardiac arrest from excited delirium or other metabolic states associated with stimulant intoxication (in-custody death syndrome)

Procedures

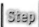 **Ensure body substance isolation before beginning procedures.**

Prior to beginning patient care, appropriate body substance isolation procedures should be employed.

▼

  Request police and remove others from danger.

As soon as the danger has been identified, call for police assistance. Remove unnecessary personnel from the scene and maintain a safe distance.

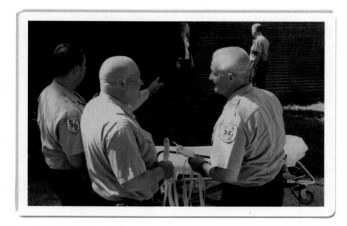

▼

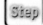 **Attempt to calm the patient verbally.**

Using a calm voice, talk to the patient and attempt to calm him or her. To avoid confusion, only one responder should communicate with the patient. Avoid threatening, derogatory, or demanding tones as you attempt to gain the patient's cooperation. You should start by asking questions to determine the cause of the bizarre and dangerous behavior. As you ask questions, avoid questions starting with "why." Why questions force patients to justify their actions. Our intent is not for the patients to *justify* what they are doing but instead to *identify* what they are doing. Be prepared to spend time talking to your patient. As long as the patient keeps talking and is not posing an immediate threat to himself, herself, or others, time is on your side.

▼

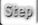 **Advise patient of need for restraint and continue to give opportunity to comply.**

If negotiation and conversation fail, it is necessary to give the patient specific instructions as to how to behave. These instructions should be specific, with a reasonable time frame in which to comply. Included in these instructions should be a warning that further actions will result in the need to be physically restrained.

▼

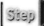 **Formulate plan and make assignments.**

While the person who is performing the negotiations talks to the patient, other members of the patient care team should formulate plans for restraining the patient. These plans should include who will be responsible for controlling which body part. It is best for three to four people to attempt the restraint. Fewer people are often insufficient, and more people often get in the way. As you plan your actions, assign people to the following sites:

- One person should approach from behind to control the patient's legs.
- One person should be assigned to each arm and be prepared to approach from the sides.
- One person should approach from behind to grab the patient's head.
- Any additional personnel should be held in reserve to assist as needed.
- If chemical assistance will be given, the medication should be prepared and the syringe hidden from the patient. The injection site should be predetermined.

 In the Field

Chemical Assistance to Restraint

If allowed by protocol, sedative or antipsychotic medications may be used to reduce the patient's desire and ability to resist. These medications should be given as soon as possible after the patient is physically controlled and can be given directly through the patient's clothing if necessary. Patients should be assessed quickly to ensure ventilation and circulation after the patient becomes calm or sleepy.

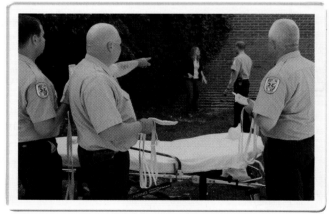

▼

Step 6 Surround patient and give last opportunity to comply.

Get into the proper position to subdue the patient. The person who is doing the negotiation should continue to talk to the patient and attempt to get the patient to comply.

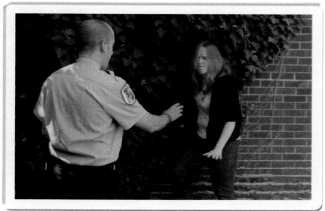

 In the Field

Management of Subdued Patient With Excited Delirium

- Support ventilations
- Maintain patient in supine or recovery position
- Begin fluid administration
- Normal saline, to keep open (TKO)
- Administer benzodiaze-pines
- Consider sodium bicarbonate

 Step 7 Grab and control the patient.

Immediately after the patient has failed to comply when given her or his final opportunity, move forward and gain control. Remember the following rules as you approach and grab the patient:

- Act fast and act together to control the patient. Do not give the patient an opportunity to develop her or his own counterplan.
- Restrain each arm by grabbing the patient by the upper arm while controlling the lower arms. Grabbing the wrists gives the patient room to wiggle free.
- Restrain the legs by grabbing the lower thighs together and pulling backward. Approaching from behind reduces the chances of being kicked. If the patient attempts to kick backward, the rescuers who are controlling the arms can use his or her altered balance to put the patient on the ground.
- Restrain the head to control the general movement of the body. Be careful not to get any part of your body in a position to be bitten. Also use caution not to strangle the patient by grabbing around the neck.

In the Field

Tasers

Police are now utilizing Tasers and other electrical stun devices as a means of controlling uncooperative and noncompliant suspects. These devices are in and of themselves nonlethal. However, there have been numerous cases where patients have died shortly after the use of a Taser. In nearly all cases, these deaths have resulted not from the Taser but from the use of stimulants that the patient had used before being tased. To ensure proper assessment and care of those who have been tased, it is important for police agencies and EMS to establish strict policies concerning the assessment of every patient.

The Taser probes are small darts about the size of a 25-gauge needle. They can be easily removed by simply pulling straight back quickly. These are considered to be contaminated sharps and should be handled appropriately. Probes should not be removed in the field if they are located in the eye, hands, female breast, or genitalia.

It is possible for EMS personnel to touch a patient while they are being tased without any detriment to themselves, as long as they do not place any part of their body between the probes. This is important to know in cases where a tased patient may require multiple exposures before being physically restrained.

Documentation should include the condition of the patient before and after the Taser has been used and the location of the probes.

 Step 8 ▶ **Place the patient on the cot.**

There may be a brief period during which the patient is lying on the ground either prone or supine. This position should be extremely brief to prevent issues with positional asphyxia.

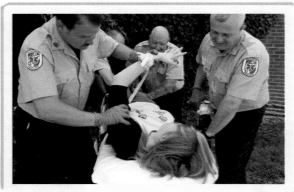

When the patient is controlled, move the patient onto the cot.

Working in unison, put the patient on the cot as soon as possible. Avoid the use of handcuffs before the patient is placed on the cot. Because the patient will need to have his or her hands secured with a wider and padded restraint, handcuffs will create more problems than they will solve.

▼

 Step 9 ▶ **Secure the patient to the cot.**

Apply straps to the patient's chest, hips, and thighs. Wrist restraints should be applied and tied to the sides of the cot. Ankle restraints may be applied if needed. Commercially made restraints are best because they are wide and padded. If unavailable, triangular bandages or fluffy roller gauze can be made into a restraint as well. Be sure the restraints do not cut off the patient's distal circulation. If the patient begins spitting, place a barrier over his or her mouth.

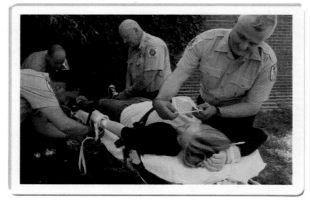

▼

10 **Assess and manage the patient.**

When the patient is secured to the cot, perform the necessary physical examination. This may be as simple as identifying that the patient continues to breathe and is conscious. Any further assessment may simply raise the patient's aggressiveness and force him or her to fight the restraint.

Patients who lose consciousness during restraint need immediate assistance. Ensure that the patient is breathing adequately. Assess the patient's temperature, and manage hyperthermia accordingly. Patients who have been taking stimulants may benefit from benzodiazepines even if they do not seem agitated at the time.

Credits

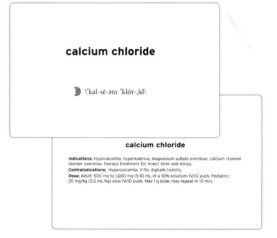

adenosine (Adenocard)

))) \ə -'den-ə-,sēn\

Indications: Conversion of paroxysmal supraventricular tachycardia (PSVT) to sinus rhythm; may convert re-entry supraventricular tachycardia (SVT) due to Wolff-Parkinson-White (WPW) syndrome.
Contraindications: Second- or third-degree heart block or sick sinus syndrome, A-fib/flutter, V-tach, hypersensitivity to adenosine, poison-induced tachycardia.
Dose: Adult: 6 mg over 1-3 sec, followed by 20 mL saline flush; if no response after 1-2 min, repeat with 12 mg over 1-3 sec (to maximum dose of 30 mg). Pediatric: 0.1-0.2 mg/kg rapid IV; maximum single dose 12 mg.

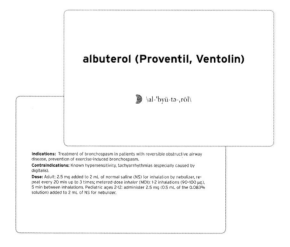

calcium chloride

))) \'kal-sē-əm 'klôr-,īd\

calcium chloride

Indications: Hypocalcemia, hyperkalemia, magnesium sulfate overdose, calcium channel blocker overdose, therapy treatment for insect bites and stings.
Contraindications: Hypercalcemia, V-fib, digitalis toxicity.
Dose: Adult: 500 mg to 1,000 mg (5-10 mL of a 10% solution) IV/IO push. Pediatric: 20 mg/kg (0.2 mL/kg) slow IV/IO push. Max 1 g dose; may repeat in 10 min.

albuterol (Proventil, Ventolin)

))) \al-'byü-tə-,rōl\

Indications: Treatment of bronchospasm in patients with reversible obstructive airway disease, prevention of exercise-induced bronchospasm.
Contraindications: Known hypersensitivity, tachyarrhythmias (especially caused by digitalis).
Dose: Adult: 2.5 mg added to 2 mL of normal saline (NS) for inhalation by nebulizer, repeat every 20 min up to 3 times; metered-dose inhaler (MDI): 1-2 inhalations (90-100 µg), 5 min between inhalations. Pediatric ages 2-12: administer 2.5 mg (0.5 mL, of the 0.083% solution) added to 2 mL of NS for nebulizer.

PharmaFlash Cards

American Academy of Orthopaedic Surgeons
Bob Elling
Kirsten Elling

ISBN-13: 978-0-7637-6913-0
Flashcards • 80 Cards • © 2009

The Perfect Study Aid!

These handy pharmacology flashcards will help you learn critical information about each medication you will use in the field. They are also an ideal tool for you to refresh your knowledge of critical medications.

The name of the drug is printed on the front of each card, along with a pronunciation key. The back of the card lists indications, contraindications, and adult and pediatric doses.

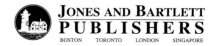

Case Studies for the Paramedic Series

Each text in the *Case Studies for the Paramedic Series* contains 20 case studies representing a variety of emergencies that you may encounter in the field. Superb supplements to classroom and textbook learning, these case studies allow you to practice applying knowledge to cases before actually going on an emergency call.

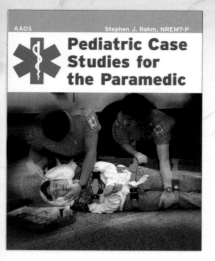

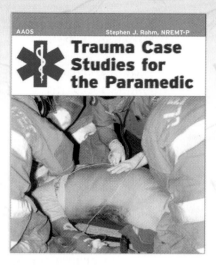

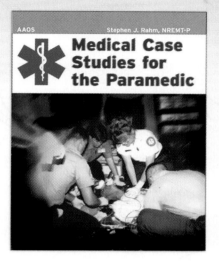

Pediatric Case Studies for the Paramedic

American Academy of
Orthopaedic Surgeons
Stephen J. Rahm

ISBN-13: 978-0-7637-2582-2
Paperback • 212 Pages
© 2006

Trauma Case Studies for the Paramedic

American Academy of
Orthopaedic Surgeons
Stephen J. Rahm

ISBN-13: 978-0-7637-2583-9
Paperback • 200 Pages
© 2005

Medical Case Studies for the Paramedic

American Academy of
Orthopaedic Surgeons
Stephen J. Rahm

ISBN-13: 978-0-7637-2581-5
Paperback • 196 Pages
© 2004

*"I really enjoyed the **Medical Case Studies for the Paramedic** book. I used it as the final practical exam for my students and was really impressed by the narratives, assessments, and especially liked the case study and answer questions. I will be adding it to my suggested reading list of helpful books for my next class."*

–Toni Roberson
Alamance Community College
Graham, North Carolina

Place your risk-free order today!

A Dynamic Test Preparation Tool

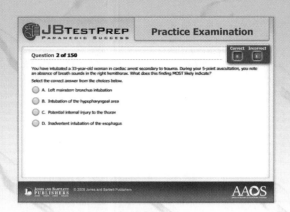

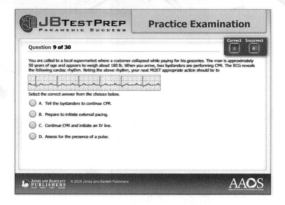

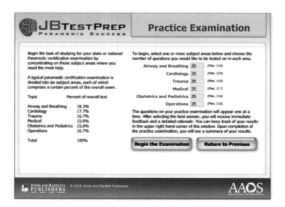

JBTest Prep: Paramedic

American Academy of Orthopaedic Surgeons
Stephen J. Rahm

ISBN-13: 978-0-7637-5784-7
Online • © 2010

Begin the task of studying for your state or national Paramedic certification examination by concentrating on those subject areas where you need the most help.

This dynamic program is designed to prepare you to sit for your state or national Paramedic certification examination by including the same type of questions you are likely to encounter in a similar electronic environment.

JBTest Prep: Paramedic provides a series of self-study modules, offering practice examinations and simulated certification examinations using case-based questions and detailed rationales to help you hone your knowledge of the subject matter.

By the time you are done, you will feel confident and prepared to complete the final step in the certification process—passing the examination!

Take an interactive tour through *JBTest Prep* online at
http://www.jblearning.com/testingServices.cfm

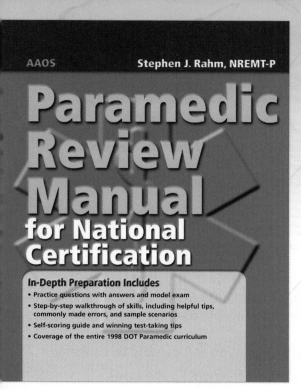

Paramedic Review Manual for National Certification

American Academy of Orthopaedic Surgeons
Stephen J. Rahm

ISBN-13: 978-0-7637-5518-8
Paperback • 156 Pages • © 2004

Prepare for state and national exams with this essential resource!

The *Paramedic Review Manual for National Certification* is designed to prepare you to sit for the national certification exam by including the same type of skill-based and multiple-choice questions that are likely to appear on the exam. The review manual will evaluate your mastery of the material presented in your paramedic training program. You will be able to complete practice quizzes and identify any weak areas, allowing for adjustment in your pre-exam studies. Copies of the performance skill sheets, requirements for successful completion of each skill, and common errors made during the performance of each skill are also included.

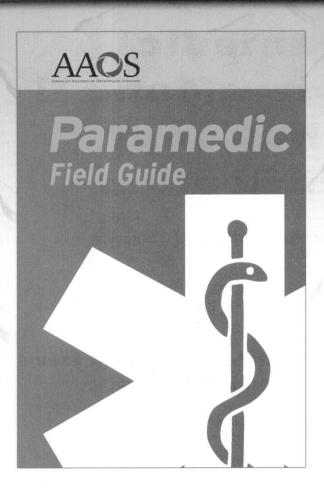

Paramedic Field Guide

American Academy of Orthopaedic Surgeons
Bob Elling
Marilynn Jackson
Lee Jackson

ISBN-13: 978-0-7637-5122-7
Spiral • 352 Pages • © 2008

This full-color, spiral-bound field guide contains a wealth of information that you will need at your fingertips..

Using this field guide, you will be able to confirm:

- Appropriate pediatric ET tube sizes
- Emergency measures in the event of an infectious exposure
- Signs and symptoms of acute illnesses
- Conditions that warrant supplemental oxygen administration
- Fracture classifications based on displacement
- Much more!

Take your paramedic training into the field with the most comprehensive field guide available!

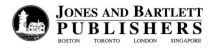

JONES AND BARTLETT PUBLISHERS
BOSTON   TORONTO   LONDON   SINGAPORE